Echinoderms Metabolites: Structure, Functions and Biomedical Perspectives II

Echinoderms Metabolites: Structure, Functions and Biomedical Perspectives II

Editors

Vladimir I. Kalinin
Alexandra S. Silchenko

MDPI • Basel • Beijing • Wuhan • Barcelona • Belgrade • Manchester • Tokyo • Cluj • Tianjin

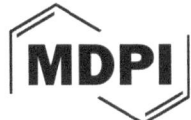

Editors
Vladimir I. Kalinin
G.B. Elyakov Pacific Institute of Bioorganic
Chemistry of the Far East Branch of the
Russian Academy of Sciences
Russia

Alexandra S. Silchenko
G.B. Elyakov Pacific Institute of Bioorganic
Chemistry of the Far East Branch of the
Russian Academy of Sciences
Russia

Editorial Office
MDPI
St. Alban-Anlage 66
4052 Basel, Switzerland

This is a reprint of articles from the Special Issue published online in the open access journal *Marine Drugs* (ISSN 1660-3397) (available at: https://www.mdpi.com/journal/marinedrugs/special_issues/Echinoderms_Metabolites_II).

For citation purposes, cite each article independently as indicated on the article page online and as indicated below:

LastName, A.A.; LastName, B.B.; LastName, C.C. Article Title. *Journal Name* **Year**, *Volume Number*, Page Range.

ISBN 978-3-0365-5129-6 (Hbk)
ISBN 978-3-0365-5130-2 (PDF)

© 2022 by the authors. Articles in this book are Open Access and distributed under the Creative Commons Attribution (CC BY) license, which allows users to download, copy and build upon published articles, as long as the author and publisher are properly credited, which ensures maximum dissemination and a wider impact of our publications.

The book as a whole is distributed by MDPI under the terms and conditions of the Creative Commons license CC BY-NC-ND.

Contents

About the Editors vii

Vladimir I. Kalinin and Alexandra S. Silchenko
Echinoderms Metabolites: Structure, Functions and Biomedical Perspectives II
Reprinted from: *Mar. Drugs* **2022**, *20*, 492, doi:10.3390/md20080492 1

Reem Abuzaytoun, Suzanne M. Budge, Wei Xia and Shawna MacKinnon
Unusual Ether Lipids and Branched Chain Fatty Acids in Sea Cucumber (*Cucumaria frondosa*) Viscera and Their Seasonal Variation
Reprinted from: *Mar. Drugs* **2022**, *20*, 435, doi:10.3390/md20070435 7

Nadezhda E. Ustyuzhanina, Maria I. Bilan, Andrey S. Dmitrenok, Eugenia A. Tsvetkova, Sofya P. Nikogosova, Cao Thi Thuy Hang, Pham Duc Thinh, Dinh Thanh Trung, Tran Thi Thanh Van, Alexander S. Shashkov, Anatolii I. Usov and Nikolay E. Nifantiev
Fucose-Rich Sulfated Polysaccharides from Two Vietnamese Sea Cucumbers *Bohadschia argus* and *Holothuria (Theelothuria) spinifera*: Structures and Anticoagulant Activity
Reprinted from: *Mar. Drugs* **2022**, *20*, 380, doi:10.3390/md20060380 19

Alla A. Kicha, Anatoly I. Kalinovsky, Timofey V. Malyarenko, Olesya S. Malyarenko, Svetlana P. Ermakova, Roman S. Popov, Valentin A. Stonik and Natalia V. Ivanchina
Disulfated Ophiuroid Type Steroids from the Far Eastern Starfish *Pteraster marsippus* and Their Cytotoxic Activity on the Models of 2D and 3D Cultures
Reprinted from: *Mar. Drugs* **2022**, *20*, 164, doi:10.3390/md20030164 33

Alexandra S. Silchenko, Anatoly I. Kalinovsky, Sergey A. Avilov, Pelageya V. Andrijaschenko, Roman S. Popov, Ekaterina A. Chingizova, Vladimir I. Kalinin and Pavel S. Dmitrenok
Triterpene Glycosides from the Far Eastern Sea Cucumber *Psolus chitonoides*: Chemical Structures and Cytotoxicities of Chitonoidosides E_1, F, G, and H
Reprinted from: *Mar. Drugs* **2021**, *19*, 696, doi:10.3390/md19120696 51

Elena A. Zelepuga, Alexandra S. Silchenko, Sergey A. Avilov and Vladimir I. Kalinin
Structure-Activity Relationships of Holothuroid's Triterpene Glycosides and Some In Silico Insights Obtained by Molecular Dynamics Study on the Mechanisms of Their Membranolytic Action
Reprinted from: *Mar. Drugs* **2021**, *19*, 604, doi:10.3390/md19110604 69

Alexandra S. Silchenko, Anatoly I. Kalinovsky, Sergey A. Avilov, Pelageya V. Andrijaschenko, Roman S. Popov, Pavel S. Dmitrenok, Ekaterina A. Chingizova and Vladimir I. Kalinin
Triterpene Glycosides from the Far Eastern Sea Cucumber *Thyonidium* (=*Duasmodactyla*) *kurilensis* (Levin): The Structures, Cytotoxicities, and Biogenesis of Kurilosides A_3, D_1, G, H, I, I_1, J, K, and K_1
Reprinted from: *Mar. Drugs* **2021**, *19*, 187, doi:10.3390/md19040187 91

Roman S. Popov, Natalia V. Ivanchina and Pavel S. Dmitrenok
Application of MS-Based Metabolomic Approaches in Analysis of Starfish and Sea Cucumber Bioactive Compounds
Reprinted from: *Mar. Drugs* **2022**, *20*, 320, doi:10.3390/md20050320 117

Timofey V. Malyarenko, Alla A. Kicha, Valentin A. Stonik and Natalia V. Ivanchina
Sphingolipids of Asteroidea and Holothuroidea: Structures and Biological Activities
Reprinted from: *Mar. Drugs* **2021**, *19*, 330, doi:10.3390/md19060330 151

About the Editors

Vladimir I. Kalinin

Vladimir I. Kalinin has a PhD in Chemistry and Dr. Sc. in Biology (biochemistry). In 1979 he began work in the G.B. Elyakov Pacific Institute of Bioorganic Chemistry of the Far Eastern Branch of the Russian Academy of Sciences (Vladivostok, Russia), where he has been leading scientist since 1998. His scientific interests are: structure, biological activities, taxonomical distribution, chemotaxonomy significance and the evolution of sea cucumber triterpene glycosides. Kalinin is the author and co-author of more than 80 book chapters and scientific articles, etc., in international scientific journals referred by SCOPUS and WOS, such as *Marine Drugs, Molecules, Tetrahedron, Journal of Natural Products* (Lloydia), *Natural Product Research, Natural Product Communications, Carbohydrate Research, Journal of Theoretical Biology, Toxicon, Biological Systematics and Ecology*, etc. He is Associate Editor of *Natural Product Communications*, a member of the *Marine Drugs* Editorial Board, and Guest Editor of the *Marine Drugs* Special Issues titled "Marine Glycoconjugates, Trends and Perspectives", "Echinoderms metabolites: structure, function and biomedical perspectives" and "Echinoderms metabolites: structure, function and biomedical perspectives II". He was also a participant of expeditions on r/v "Professor Bogorov" and "Akademik Oparin" in the Indian and Pacific Oceans.

Alexandra S. Silchenko

Alexandra S. Silchenko graduated from Far Eastern State University, the Department of General Biology, Ecology and Soil Science (Vladivostok) in 2000. In the same year she began work in the G.B. Elyakov Pacific Institute of Bioorganic Chemistry of the Far Eastern Branch of the Russian Academy of Sciences, where has been a senior scientist since 2016. Silchenko received her PhD in Chemistry in 2006 and her Dr. Sc. in Chemistry in 2020. In 2007, she was awarded the G.B. Elyakov award of FEB RAS for her series of publications on triterpene glycosides from sea cucumbers. Her scientific interests are: the isolation of natural products, structure elucidation, biological activities, taxonomical distribution, chemotaxonomy and the biosynthesis of sea cucumber triterpene glycosides. Silchenko is the author and co-author of more than 80 scientific articles and book chapters in international scientific journals indexed by SCOPUS and WOS, such as *Marine Drugs, Molecules, Tetrahedron, Journal of Natural Products* (Lloydia), *Natural Product Research, Natural Product Communications, Carbohydrate Research, Biological Systematics and Ecology*, etc. She is a reviewer in *Natural Product Communications* and *Marine Drugs* and Guest Editor of the MDPI Special Issue: "Echinoderms Metabolites: Structure, Functions and Biomedical Perspectives II".

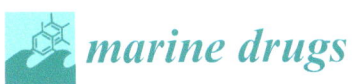

Editorial

Echinoderms Metabolites: Structure, Functions and Biomedical Perspectives II

Vladimir I. Kalinin * and Alexandra S. Silchenko *

G.B. Elyakov Pacific Institute of Bioorganic Chemistry, Far Eastern Branch of the Russian Academy of Sciences, Pr. 100-letya Vladivostoka 159, 690022 Vladivostok, Russia
* Correspondence: kalininv@piboc.dvo.ru (V.I.K.); silchenko_als@piboc.dvo.ru (A.S.S.);
  Tel.: +7-914-705-08-45 (V.I.K.)

Citation: Kalinin, V.I.; Silchenko, A.S. Echinoderms Metabolites: Structure, Functions and Biomedical Perspectives II. *Mar. Drugs* **2022**, *20*, 492. https://doi.org/10.3390/md20080492

Received: 21 July 2022
Accepted: 28 July 2022
Published: 29 July 2022

Publisher's Note: MDPI stays neutral with regard to jurisdictional claims in published maps and institutional affiliations.

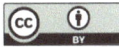

Copyright: © 2022 by the authors. Licensee MDPI, Basel, Switzerland. This article is an open access article distributed under the terms and conditions of the Creative Commons Attribution (CC BY) license (https://creativecommons.org/licenses/by/4.0/).

Echinoderms belong to the phylum Echinodermata (from the Ancient Greek words "echinos" (hedgehog) and "derma" (skin)). They possess radial symmetry, and have a unique water vascular (ambulacral) system. The phylum includes the classes Ophiuroidea (brittle stars), Asteroidea (starfish), Crinoidea (sea lilies or feather stars), Echinoidea (sea urchins) and Holothuroidea (sea cucumbers). All of them have a calcareous skeleton, which is reduced to ossicles in the sea cucumbers. Echinoderms inhabit all ocean depths and include more than 7000 living species. Echinoderms are a unique source of different metabolites that have a wide spectrum of biological activities. The representatives of Echinodermata have evolutionary acquired the exceptional mechanism of decreasing the level of free 5,6-unsaturated sterols in their cell membranes by sulfation of food sterols. Moreover, the starfish and holothurians are able to transform these 5,6-unsaturated sterols to stanols or 7,8-unsaturated sterols. This ability has arisen in parallel to the capacity of the representatives of these classes to synthesize and keep their own 5,6-sterol-dependent membranolytic toxins. Such toxins include triterpene oligoglycosides for the sea cucumbers and steroid oligoglycosides for the starfish. These metabolites have protective and ecological significance for the producers. Starfish and brittle stars biosynthesize numerous polyhydroxysteroids and their derivatives as food emulgators, which give them unique food plasticity. The echinoderms contain naphthoquinone pigments and carotenoids. The naphthoquinone derivatives are specifically characteristic of the sea urchins. The lipids of echinoderms are also uncommon, including cerebrosides and gangliosides characteristic of other Deuterostomia, namely, Chordata and Hemichordata. Echinoderms also contain lectins, glycan-specific glycoproteins that have immunity functions for the producers, glycosaminoglycans and fucoidans. Hence, plenty of unusual biologically active metabolites originated from the echinoderms [1].

This Special Issue begins from the articles dedicated to the sea cucumber triterpene glycosides. The first one by Silchenko et al. concerns the isolation, structural elucidation, cytotoxic activities and biogenesis of nine new non-holostane (having no lactone) triterpene glycosides from the Far Eastern sea cucumber *Thyonidium* (=*Duasmodactyla*) *kurilensis* (Levin), namely, kurilosides A_3, D_1, G, H, I, I_1, J, K and K_1. In addition to the native compounds, two desulfated derivatives, DS-kurilosides L and M, with interesting structural features were obtained from inseparable glycoside fraction. DS-kuriloside L has a trisaccharide branched chain, and DS-kuriloside M is characterized by a new hexa-*nor*-lanostane aglycone with a 7(8)-double bond instead of the 9(11)-double bond that is inherent for all other glycosidic aglycones from this sea cucumber. Their structures were elucidated by 2D NMR and HR-ESI-MS procedures. Five new carbohydrate chains and two new aglycones (having a 16β,20(S)-dihydroxy fragment and a 16β-acetoxy,20(S)-hydroxy fragment) were discovered in these glycosides. The analysis of the structural features of the aglycones and the carbohydrate chains of all the glycosides of *T. kurilensis* allows the creation of the schemes of their biosynthetic network. The cytotoxic activities of these compounds against mouse neuroblastoma Neuro-2a and normal epithelial JB-6 cells, as well as hemolysis against mouse erythrocytes, were investigated. The glycosides that have free hydroxyl groups in the aglycones were not active, whereas the other ones have moderate activities [2].

The second article by Silchenko et al. concerns chemical structures and cytotoxicity of triterpene glycosides from the Far Eastern sea cucumber *Psolus chitonoides*. The authors isolated four new triterpene disulfated glycosides: chitonoidosides E_1, F, G and H. Two of them (chitonoidosides E_1 and G) are hexaosides, differing from each other by the terminal (sixth) sugar residue, one is a pentaoside (chitonoidoside H) and one is a tetraoside (chitonoidoside F). The structures were elucidated using 2D NMR and HR-ESI-MS procedures. The most interesting structural feature of chitonoidoside G is the aglycone of a recently discovered new type, with an 18(20)-ether bond instead of a corresponding lactone. Rarely found terminal 3-O-methylxylose residue was a part of the carbohydrate chain of chitonoidoside E_1. The sulfate group in the uncommon position 4 of terminal 3-O-methylglucose is a distinctive feature of chitonoidosides F and H. The hemolytic activities of all the studied glycosides, including previously isolated chitonoidoside E against human erythrocytes and cytotoxicity against several human cancer cell lines, such as adenocarcinoma HeLa, colorectal adenocarcinoma DLD-1 and monocytes THP-1, were also studied [3].

The third article by Zelepuga et al. concerning sea cucumber metabolites describes the structure–activity relationships (SARs) for a broad series of sea cucumber glycosides in relation to different tumor cell lines and erythrocytes. The results showed a very complicated character of the SARs for this class of compounds depending both on the structures of aglycones and carbohydrate chains and their combinations, including positions and number of sulfate groups. The most interesting part of the article is devoted to in silico modulation of the interaction of several glycosides from *Eupentacta fraudatrix* with model erythrocyte membranes by simulations of full-atom molecular dynamics (MD). The modeling revealed that the glycosides bound to the membrane through hydrophobic interactions and hydrogen bonds. The mode of such interactions may be very different and depends on the aglycone structure, especially the side chain structural peculiarities. Different mechanisms of glycoside/membrane interactions were found. The first one was realized through the pore formation (by cucumariosides A_1 and A_8), which was preceded by the bonding of the glycosides with the membrane cholesterol, sphingomyelin and phospholipids. The carbohydrate chain serves as an anchor bonding to the polar heads of phospholipids. Later-occurring noncovalent intermolecular interactions inside multimolecular membrane complexes and their stoichiometry differed for these glycosides because they were mainly dependent from the aglycone structures. Cucumarioside A_1 had holostane aglycone with a 24(25)-unsaturated side chain penetrated to the outer membrane leaflet, which caused the formation of a "pore-like" assemblage. Cucumarioside A_8 has hydroxy-groups at C-18 and C-20 instead of 18(20)-lactone, which promoted the initial stage of its integration to the membrane that was followed by the deepening of the aglycone to the outer membrane leaflet, causing the subsequent rearranging of the inner leaflet. Noticeably, powerful interactions between glycoside molecules inside the pore-like complex and phospholipids were observed for cucumarioside A_8. The second mechanism was realized by cucumarioside A_2 having a 24-OAc group through the formation of phospholipid and cholesterol clusters in the outer and inner membrane leaflets, correspondingly. The glycoside/phospholipid interactions were also more preferable than the glycoside/cholesterol interactions. However, the glycoside interaction agglomerated the cholesterol molecules from the inner membrane leaflet. The modulation of the interaction of cucumarioside A_7, having the 24-hydroxyl group, with the model membrane revealed only weak bonding with phospholipid polar heads and the full absence of glycoside/cholesterol interactions. All the results correlated well with the experimental in vitro hemolytic activity of these substances. The obtained data open wide the possibility for understanding plenty of the experimental information concerning the membranolytic activities of the sea cucumber glycosides [4].

The next article by Kicha et al. concerns the isolation and structural elucidation of four new and one known steroid disulfates, including (20R)-7-oxo-24-methylcholesta-5,24(28)-diene-3β,21-di-O-sodium sulfate, (20R)-7-oxo-24-methyl-5α-cholest-24(28)-ene-3β,21-di-O-sodium sulfate, (20R)-24-methyl-7β-hydroxy-5α-cholest-24(28)-ene-3β,21-di-O-sodium sulfate, (20S)-cholesta-5,24-diene-3β,22-di-O-sodium sulfate, and (20R)-24-methylcholesta-5,24(28)-diene-3β,21-di-O-sodium sulfate from the starfish *Pteraster marsippus* [5]. The 2D NMR and HR-ESI-MS procedures were used for the structural elucidations. It is known that characteristics of the secondary metabolites of ophiuroids are mainly steroidal disulfated diols, triols, and rarely, tetraols that differ from other sulfated compounds of echinoderms in the positions of sulfoxy groups at 3α- and 21 in 5β-, Δ^5-, and very rarely, 5α-cholestane cores. The common sulfated compounds from starfish have hydroxyl or sulfoxy groups occupying five or more positions [6]. It is of interest that similar ophiuroid-type polyxydroxysteroids, containing sulfoxy groups at 3α- (or 3β-) and 21 positions in 5α- or Δ^5-cholestane nuclei were found in some species belonging to the family Pterasteridae (Velatida, Asteroidea), whereas the polyhydroxylated steroids and asterosaponins, common in other starfish, were absent in the starfish of this family. The currently obtained results correlate well with this trend. The cytotoxicities of a series of the isolated compounds were studied on models of 2D and 3D colonies of cancer cells, but the activities were weak or moderate [5].

The article by Malyarenko et al. is a review concerning the structure and biological activities of sphingolipids from starfish and sea cucumbers, namely, ceramides, cerebrosides and gangliosides. The gangliosides are the most complex sphingolipids characteristic of vertebrates, but have been found in the echinoderms also, which reflects a common origin of the Deuterostomia. The review comprehensively summarizes the data on sphingolipids of the sea cucumbers and starfish, which are the most studied among all the echinoderms, from the past twenty years. The structures, properties and peculiarities of biogenesis of ceramides, cerebrosides and gangliosides are discussed. The review makes obvious a great structural diversity and the presence of some unique structural features in these classes of starfish and sea cucumber lipids. It was shown that starfish and sea cucumber cerebrosides are perspective candidates for practical application in the human diet and in the composition of food supplements. Noticeably, the authors use in a non-traditional sense the term "molecular species" as an inseparable fraction of a certain class of lipids (really a sub-class) instead of the more common understanding of the term as a synonym for an individual substance characterized by a specific composition and the allocation of fatty acids in sphingolipids or the length of aliphatic chains in a sphingosine base. As a result, the phrases similar to, "Generally, about one hundred individual cerebrosides and their molecular species have been isolated from these animals", are very characteristic of the review [7].

The article by Canadian researchers concerns characterization of unusual ether lipids and branched fatty acids from the viscera of commercially harvested North Atlantic sea cucumber *Cucumaria frondosa* and its seasonal variation [8]. The purpose of this investigation is to expand the nutraceutical use of the lipids from the viscera of this sea cucumber, but not the proteins, and different biologically active substances from the body walls and muscular bands only. The authors found that the highest total lipid content is in the winter season and diacylglycerols are predominant components. The triacylglycerols dominate in the summer season. The branched 12-methyltetradecanoic acid is a major component in diacylglycerols, and as a result, its total content seems to be maximal in the winter period also. The authors concluded that these observations should be taken into account during the harvesting of the sea cucumber. The authors used HPLC for the isolation of different classes of lipids and applied NMR spectroscopy for their characterization. They carried out the hydrolysis followed by derivatization of fatty acids and their analysis used traditional capillary GLC/MS. Such methodology seems to be quite adequate for the goals of the investigation.

The next review by Popov et al. concerns the application of MS-based metabolomics in the analysis of starfish and sea cucumber bioactive compounds [9]. It considers the use of metabolomic approaches for the study of polar steroids, triterpene glycosides and polar lipids. The authors note that elucidating the structure of starfish and sea cucumber metabolites is a very difficult task, comprising the isolation of individual compounds and followed by the application of modern MS and NMR techniques. They stressed that the use of an MS-based metabolomic method provides a possibility to study very complicated mixtures of echinoderm metabolites without the isolation of individual compounds. The authors describe the most characteristic features of MS-based approaches including sample preparation and MS analysis steps. Concluding the results of the MS-based metabolomic studies of secondary metabolites of starfish and sea cucumbers, the authors showed that the method makes it easy to carry out the detection and identification of polar steroids, triterpene glycosides and lipids in the organism-producer and to propose their preliminary structures. It allows the search for new biologically active molecules effectively and allows the authors to conclude their taxonomic distribution, biogenesis, and even biological functions. The MS-based metabolomic approach can be used successfully for comparing metabolomic profiles of different echinoderm species and populations for ecological, dietary, biosynthesis and chemotaxonomic studies [9]. It is necessary to note that the effectiveness of the discussed approach is highly dependent on the availability of the database containing the established structures of related compounds. Since the unambiguous identification and characterization of the compounds is a challenge for metabolomic research, it can be effectively applied only in combination with the isolation of individual substances and the elucidation of their structures.

The article by Ustyuzhanina et al. concerns the structural characteristics and blood anticoagulated activity of a series of fucose-rich sulfated polysaccharides from two Indo-West Pacific sea cucumbers *Bohadschia argus* and *Holothuria spinifera* collected from Vietnamese shallow waters [10], including fucosylated chondroitin sulfates FCS-BA and FCS-HS, along with fucan sulfates FS-BA-AT and FS-HS-AT. Extensive NMR analysis was used for the structural characterization of the polysaccharides. The authors showed that the fucosylated chondroitin sulfates contain a chondroitin core $[\rightarrow 3)$-β-D-GalNAc-$(1\rightarrow 4)$-β-D-GlcA-$(1\rightarrow]n$ bearing sulfated fucosyl branches at O-3 of every GlcA residue. These fucosyl residues were different in the pattern of sulfation. It was found that fucan sulfate FS-BA-AT is a regular linear polymer of 4-linked α-L-fucopyranose 3-sulfate. Because of the considerable sulfate content, FS-BA-AT is not active as an anticoagulant. The structure of fucan sulfate FS-HS-AT is a mixture of chains identical to FS-BA-AT and the other chains are built up of randomly sulfated alternating 4- and 3-linked residues of α-L-fucopyranose [10].

Thus, the articles published in the Special Issue largely reflect the structural diversity of echinoderm metabolites including triterpene glycosides and fucosylated chondroitin sulfates, as well as branched fatty acids, di- and triacylglycerols and other lipid classes from the sea cucumbers, polyhydroxysteroids from starfish and different classes of sphingolipids from sea cucumbers and starfish. Finally, the MS-based metabolomic approach, which is very helpful for the estimation of such diversity, is discussed. The materials from the Special Issue also illustrate the biomedical potential of the presented metabolites as cytotoxins and anticoagulants. The in silico approach broadens the possibilities to investigate the mechanisms of the action of membranolytic compounds.

Author Contributions: Conceptualization, V.I.K. and A.S.S.; writing—original draft preparation, V.I.K.; writing—review and editing, V.I.K. and A.S.S. All authors have read and agreed to the published version of the manuscript.

Funding: This research received no external funding.

Conflicts of Interest: The authors declare no conflict of interest.

References

1. Kalinin, V.I. Echinoderms metabolites: Structure, function, biomedical perspectives. *Mar. Drugs* **2021**, *19*, 125. [CrossRef] [PubMed]
2. Silchenko, A.S.; Kalinovsky, A.I.; Avilov, S.A.; Andrijaschenko, P.V.; Popov, R.S.; Dmitrenok, P.S.; Chingizova, E.A.; Kalinin, V.I. Triterpene glycosides from the far eastern sea cucumber *Thyonidium* (=*Duasmodactyla*) *kurilensis* (Levin): The structures, cytotoxicities, and biogenesis of kurilosides A_3, D_1, G, H, I, I_1, J, K, and K_1. *Mar. Drugs* **2021**, *19*, 187. [CrossRef] [PubMed]
3. Silchenko, A.S.; Kalinovsky, A.I.; Avilov, S.A.; Andrijaschenko, P.V.; Popov, R.S.; Chingizova, E.A.; Kalinin, V.I.; Dmitrenok, P.S. Triterpene glycosides from the Far Eastern sea cucumber *Psolus chitonoides*: Chemical structures and cytotoxicities of chitonoidosides E_1, F, G, and H. *Mar. Drugs* **2021**, *19*, 696. [CrossRef] [PubMed]
4. Zelepuga, E.A.; Silchenko, A.S.; Avilov, S.A.; Kalinin, V.I. Structure-activity relationships of holothuroid's triterpene glycosides and some in silico insights obtained by molecular dynamics study on the mechanisms of their membranolytic action. *Mar. Drugs* **2021**, *19*, 604. [CrossRef] [PubMed]
5. Kicha, A.A.; Kalinovsky, A.I.; Malyarenko, T.V.; Malyarenko, O.S.; Ermakova, S.P.; Popov, R.S.; Stonik, V.A.; Ivanchina, N.V. Disulfated ophiuroid type steroids from the Far Eastern starfish *Pteraster marsippus* and their cytotoxic activity on the models of 2D and 3D cultures. *Mar. Drugs* **2022**, *20*, 164. [CrossRef] [PubMed]
6. Levina, E.V.; Andriyaschenko, P.V.; Kalinovsky, A.I.; Stonik, V.A. New ophiuroid-type steroids from the starfish *Pteraster tesselatus*. *J. Nat. Prod.* **1998**, *61*, 1423–1426. [CrossRef] [PubMed]
7. Malyarenko, T.V.; Kicha, A.A.; Stonik, V.A.; Ivanchina, N.V. Sphingolipids of Asteroidea and Holothuroidea: Structures and biological activities. *Mar. Drugs* **2021**, *19*, 330. [CrossRef] [PubMed]
8. Abuzaytoun, R.; Budge, S.M.; Xia, W.; MacKinnon, S. Unusual ether lipids and branched chain fatty acids in sea cucumber (*Cucumaria frondosa*) viscera and their seasonal variation. *Mar. Drugs* **2022**, *20*, 435. [CrossRef] [PubMed]
9. Popov, R.S.; Ivanchina, N.V.; Dmitrenok, P.S. Application of MS-based metabolomic approaches in analysis of starfish and sea cucumber bioactive compounds. *Mar. Drugs* **2022**, *20*, 320. [CrossRef] [PubMed]
10. Ustyuzhanina, N.E.; Bilan, M.I.; Dmitrenok, A.S.; Tsvetkova, E.A.; Nikogosova, S.P.; Hang, C.T.T.; Thinh, P.D.; Trung, D.T.; Van, T.T.T.; Shashkov, A.S.; et al. Fucose-rich sulfated polysaccharides from two Vietnamese sea cucumbers *Bohadschia argus* and *Holothuria* (*Theelothuria*) *spinifera*: Structures and anticoagulant activity. *Mar. Drugs* **2022**, *20*, 380. [CrossRef] [PubMed]

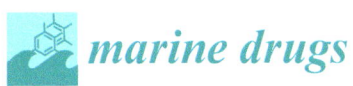

Article

Unusual Ether Lipids and Branched Chain Fatty Acids in Sea Cucumber (*Cucumaria frondosa*) Viscera and Their Seasonal Variation

Reem Abuzaytoun [1,*], Suzanne M. Budge [2], Wei Xia [3] and Shawna MacKinnon [4]

1. Department of Chemistry and Physics, Mount Saint Vincent University, Halifax, NS B3M 2J6, Canada
2. Department of Process Engineering and Applied Science, Dalhousie University, Halifax, NS B3H 4R2, Canada; suzanne.budge@dal.ca
3. Mara Renewables Corporation, Dartmouth, NS B2Y 4T6, Canada; wxia@maracorp.ca
4. Agriculture and Agri-Food Canada, Kentville, NS B4N 1J5, Canada; shawna.mackinnon2@agr.gc.ca
* Correspondence: reem.abuzaytoun@msvu.ca; Tel.: +1-902-441-2650

Abstract: The sea cucumber, *Cucumaria frondosa*, is harvested primarily for its muscular bands and body wall. Development of a nutraceutical product based on lipid recovered from its viscera would give commercial value to the entire organism; however, such development requires knowledge of the lipid and fatty acid (FA) profiles of the viscera. Here, we describe the lipid and FA composition of viscera recovered from *C. frondosa* harvested in coastal waters in the northwest Atlantic, taking into account variation due to harvest season. We found highest lipid content at ~29% in winter, with diacylglyceryl ethers (DAGE) comprising ~55% of the total lipid mass and triacylglycerols (TAG), phospholipids (PL) and monoacylglycerol ethers (MAGE) at 5–25% each. The branched chain FA, 12-methyltetradecanoic acid (12-MTA), represented 42% of total FA mass in DAGE. In summer, lipid content was lower at 24% and TAG was the dominate lipid, with proportions more than double that found in winter (45% vs. 20%); DAGE in summer dropped to ~30% of total lipids. In TAG, 12-MTA was much lower than found in DAGE in winter, at only 10% but eicosapentaenoic acid (EPA) content was ~20%, which brought the total EPA% to 28% of total FA—the highest among all three seasons. There was little effect of season on MAGE or PL proportions. These data can help harvesters maximize catch efforts in terms of lipid yield and profile.

Keywords: diacylglycerol ether; 1-*O*-alkylglyceryl ether; nutraceutical oils; bêche-de-mer

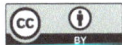

Citation: Abuzaytoun, R.; Budge, S.M.; Xia, W.; MacKinnon, S. Unusual Ether Lipids and Branched Chain Fatty Acids in Sea Cucumber (*Cucumaria frondosa*) Viscera and Their Seasonal Variation. *Mar. Drugs* 2022, 20, 435. https://doi.org/10.3390/md20070435

Academic Editors: Vladimir I. Kalinin and Alexanra S. Silchenko

Received: 31 May 2022
Accepted: 27 June 2022
Published: 29 June 2022

Publisher's Note: MDPI stays neutral with regard to jurisdictional claims in published maps and institutional affiliations.

Copyright: © 2022 by the authors. Licensee MDPI, Basel, Switzerland. This article is an open access article distributed under the terms and conditions of the Creative Commons Attribution (CC BY) license (https://creativecommons.org/licenses/by/4.0/).

1. Introduction

The sea cucumber, *Cucumaria frondosa*, is widely distributed in the cold waters off the coast of the United States and Canada. Along Nova Scotia and New Brunswick, Canada, *C. frondosa* is harvested as a by-catch [1] and, presently, only the muscular bands and body wall have commercial value; the viscera, representing 50% of the sea cucumber biomass, is discarded [2]. In 2018 the sea cucumber fisheries in Newfoundland reported landings of 5500 tons that were estimated to have a $6,000,000 value to the fishery [3]. The lipid extracted from the viscera has recently been identified as a potential source of marine lipids for nutraceutical applications [4]. However, little is known about the lipid and fatty acid (FA) composition of sea cucumber viscera.

Freeze-dried powders of *C. frondosa* harvested off the coast of Newfoundland [4] were reported to contain up to nine lipid classes including hydrocarbons, steryl esters, ethyl ketones, triacylglycerols (TAG), free fatty acids (FFA), alcohols, sterols, and phospholipids (PL). However, other studies of related species in the Holothurian class of sea cucumber, including *C. japonica*, *C. okhotensis*, *C. fraudatrix* and *Stichopus japonicas*, have identified ether lipids, specifically 1-*O*-alkylglyceryl ethers [5,6]. Diacylglyceryl ethers (DAGE) and monoacylglyceryl ethers (MAGE) have been reported in several marine animals, such as in the livers of dogfish and shark [7] and deep-sea squids (*Berryteuthis magister*) [8]. In the last two decades, ether lipids have attracted the interest of researchers due to their health promoting effects in humans, specifically for their potential in cancer therapy but also because they have been used to improve the bioavailability of other lipid molecules such as butyric acid or omega-3 FA [9–12].

A branched chain FA, 12-methyltetradecanoic acid (12-MTA), has also been reported in *C. frondosa*. For instance, in fresh and rehydrated powders of *C. frondosa* consisting of body walls and internal organs, 12-MTA was present at 4–9% of total FA mass [13]. However, neither Vaidya and Cheema [2] nor Mamelona et al. [4] identified this FA in their evaluation of *C. frondosa*. All three studies did quantify eicosapentaenoic acid (EPA) at proportions ranging from 17 to 52%, with the wide variation due to the type of sample evaluated; the lowest EPA proportion was found in the sample consisting of only viscera. As an omega-3 FA, EPA is well-known for its role in prevention of cardiovascular disease [14], while 12-MTA has been shown to have anti-inflammatory, anti-cancer and wound healing activity [15]. Thus, *C. frondosa* viscera lipids may contain a number of important bioactive components.

Our main objective was to characterize the lipid content and composition of *C. frondosa*. Since most marine animals show seasonal variation in those parameters due to both environmental factors and reproduction cycles [16], we also aimed to determine the differences in major lipid classes and FA profiles. Specifically, we describe here the variation in lipid classes and their lipid-specific FA proportions across three harvesting seasons in a single year with a goal of providing critical information in the development and marketing of sea cucumber viscera and lipids derived from it.

2. Results

The total lipid content of the viscera ranged from ~21–29% dwb (dry weight basis) with the winter harvest showing significantly higher levels (ANOVA; $p < 0.05$) than that observed for spring and summer (Table 1). Moisture content was lowest in winter at ~75%. Spring and summer samples were equivalent in terms of lipid and moisture content. EPA was the major PUFA and ranged from ~25–28%, with highest proportions in summer. In total lipids, PUFA varied between 27–30% of total FA mass with highest levels observed in the summer harvest (Table 1). The FA 12-MTA varied in a similar fashion with almost twice the proportion in winter. Total branched chain FA showed greater variation, with levels from 18–31% and largest amounts in winter.

Table 1. Seasonal variation in total lipid and moisture content of viscera of *C. frondosa* ($n = 3$; mean ± (SD)). Total lipid and moisture are expressed relative to total mass. Fatty acid (FA) content is mass % of total FA in the lipid extract. Values in the same row with different letters are significantly different ($p < 0.05$).

Component	Winter		Spring		Summer	
Total lipid (wwb *)	7.36	(0.21) [a]	4.93	(0.34) [b]	5.30	(0.29) [b]
Total lipid (dwb *)	28.87	(1.92) [a]	20.81	(1.22) [b]	23.83	(1.46) [b]
Moisture content (%)	74.47	(1.09) [b]	76.29	(0.08) [a]	77.75	(0.37) [a]
Total EPA (%)	24.74	(0.68) [b]	25.38	(0.18) [b]	28.23	(0.40) [a]
Total PUFA (%)	27.31	(0.62) [c]	28.03	(0.27) [b]	29.72	(0.42) [a]
12-MTA (%)	21.27	(0.77) [a]	19.17	(0.93) [b]	11.79	(0.78) [c]
Total Branched FA (%)	31.13	(0.75) [a]	27.84	(0.94) [b]	18.21	(0.87) [c]

* wwb = wet weight basis; dwb = dry weight basis.

HPLC analysis indicated that viscera lipids consisted predominantly of TAG and DAGE, with their identities confirmed through elution of authentic standards (Supplementary Figure S1). Undifferentiated PL were prominent peaks and eluted with the most polar mobile phase. Minor peaks coincided with retention times of FFA, DAG and MAG standards. TLC analysis largely confirmed the identities of peaks a, b, c and f in the HPLC chromatogram

(Supplementary Figure S1), with the presence of four TLC bands corresponding to TAG, DAGE, FFA, and PL. MAG eluted with PL in the TLC analysis. A fifth band, eluting between FFA and PL, could not be conclusively identified as its R_f did not match that of any available lipid standards. Based on the presence of DAGE, it was assumed to be MAGE. This also suggested that the 'DAG peak' (peak d in Supplementary Figure S1) identified by HPLC was in fact MAGE; however, without a MAGE standard, the identity could not be confirmed, and, thus, NMR and GC-MS analysis were pursued.

The main lipid class in viscera of sea cucumber harvested in the winter and spring was DAGE which represented ~55% and ~40% of total recovered lipids, respectively (Figure 1), while TAG was the main lipid class found in the summer and represented ~45% of total recovered lipids. For both DAGE and TAG, lipid contents varied by season (ANOVA; Tukey's test; $p < 0.05$). There was significantly more MAGE in the spring season than the other two (ANOVA; Tukey's test; $p < 0.05$); PL concentrations were lowest in summer.

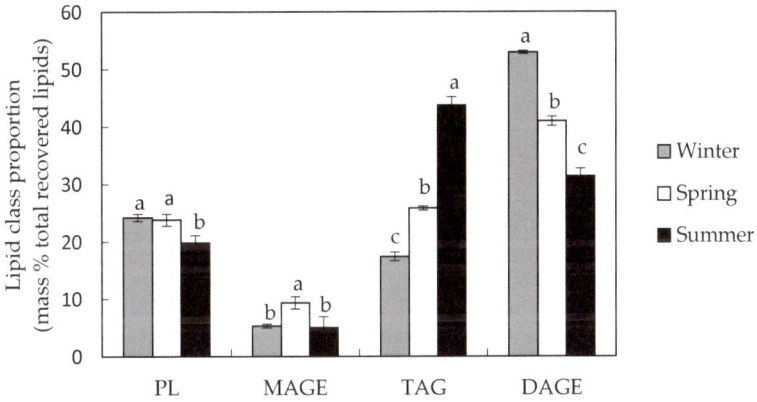

Figure 1. The approximate mass percentage of each lipid class in *C. frondosa* viscera extract relative to total lipids recovered from TLC plates (mean ± SD, n = 3). Values with different letters within a lipid class are significantly different (ANOVA; $p < 0.05$). The percentage of FFA was below detection limits. The PL proportion included a small contribution from MAG.

NMR analysis of the tentatively identified MAGE band contained peaks between 70–75 ppm in ^{13}C NMR spectra (Supplementary Figure S2a) and at ~3.5 ppm in the ^{1}H NMR (Supplementary Figure S2b) spectra which supported the presence of compounds containing ether bonds [17]. The identity of the MAGE bands was further confirmed using GC-MS analysis of the saponified and acetylated MAGE and DAGE bands and the DAGE standard. Analysis by EI of both of the saponified, acetylated bands yielded TIC with peaks that had similar spectra to the saponified and acetylated 1-O-hexadecyl-2,3-hexadecanoyl glycerol standard, indicating that ether structures were likely present. The saponified, acetylated DAGE standard analyzed by CI contained a single component with base peak at m/z 341, representing a $[M - 59]^+$ fragment. Based on this fragment, masses and tentative identities were assigned to the other peaks in the two bands. The major alkyl structures were 16:0 and 18:0, with 18:0 dominating in MAGE and roughly equivalent amounts of both in DAGE (Figure 2). Proportions of all other alkyl groups were similar in the two lipids. Seasonality was not evaluated in DAGE and MAGE.

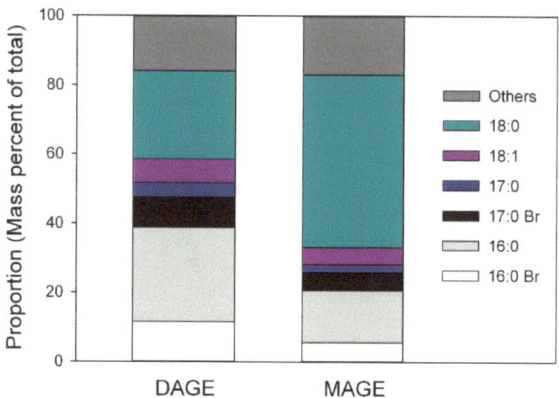

Figure 2. Approximate proportions of major alkyl structures in DAGE and MAGE in viscera lipids of *C. frondosa*.

FA composition varied by lipid class and season. The major FA identified in DAGE was 12-MTA, with highest proportions in winter/spring at 41–42% (Table 2). Other prominent branched chain FA included 4,8,12-Me-13:0, 8,12-Me-14:0, and 12-Me-15:0, with levels varying from 2–8% and generally following the same pattern as 12-MTA with lowest amounts in summer. Monounsaturated 16:1n-7 was present in second greatest amounts at ~20% with slightly lower levels in summer. The only prominent polyunsaturated FA was EPA with highest levels of ~9% in summer. In contrast, EPA was the major FA in MAGE in winter/spring at ~62% while 12-MTA was present at only ~5% in all seasons. In total, branched chain FA were present at 8–12% of total FA. In both lipid classes, EPA, branched chain FA, and 16:1n-7 accounted for ~78–85% of the total FA identified, showing very little diversity in structure in the ether lipids.

Table 2. Proportions of FA (mass% total FA identified) in ether lipids isolated from *C. frondosa* viscera ($n = 3$; mean ± (SD)). Values with different letters (e.g., [a–c] for MAGE; [e–g] for DAGE) within a FA and lipid class are significantly different (ANOVA, Tukey's test; $p < 0.05$).

	MAGE						DAGE					
	Winter		Spring		Summer		Winter		Spring		Summer	
4,8,12-Me-13:0	0.42	(0.00) [b]	0.38	(0.02) [c]	0.57	(0.05) [a]	3.65	(0.05) [e]	3.32	(0.19) [f]	2.51	(0.34) [g]
Me-14:0(a) *	0.10	(0.00) [a]	0.09	(0.00) [a]	0.11	(0.01) [a]	0.85	(0.03) [e]	0.84	(0.04) [e]	0.80	(0.01) [f]
Me-14:0(b) *	0.17	(0.03) [b]	0.17	(0.02) [b]	0.39	(0.04) [a]	0.75	(0.01) [e]	0.75	(0.02) [e]	0.74	(0.04) [e]
Me-14:0(c) *	0.08	(0.00) [b]	0.06	(0.00) [c]	0.11	(0.00) [a]	0.67	(0.03) [e]	0.57	(0.02) [f]	0.45	(0.04) [g]
12-MTA	4.81	(0.19) [a]	4.95	(0.28) [a]	5.79	(0.32) [a]	42.21	(0.61) [e]	41.09	(0.81) [e]	37.12	(0.01) [f]
8,12-Me-14:0	0.44	(0.03) [a]	0.30	(0.03) [b]	0.52	(0.02) [a]	3.33	(0.45) [e]	2.14	(0.29) [f]	2.74	(0.14) [g]
12-Me-15:0	2.09	(0.38) [b]	2.31	(0.24) [b]	3.98	(0.20) [a]	7.06	(0.22) [e]	6.84	(0.48) [e]	5.19	(0.02) [f]
8,12-Me-15:0	0.13	(0.04) [ab]	0.11	(0.01) [b]	0.19	(0.04) [a]	0.48	(0.01) [e]	0.44	(0.07) [e]	0.31	(0.01) [f]
ai-17:0	0.11	(0.01) [ab]	0.09	(0.01) [b]	0.13	(0.00) [a]	0.56	(0.02) [f]	0.57	(0.03) [f]	0.77	(0.02) [e]
14:0	0.16	(0.01) [b]	0.17	(0.02) [b]	0.56	(0.05) [a]	0.53	(0.03) [f]	0.61	(0.01) [f]	1.40	(0.16) [e]
15:0	0.03	(0.01) [b]	0.13	(0.01) [a]	0.00	(0.00) [b]	0.23	(0.02) [f]	1.37	(0.22) [e]	0.00	(0.00) [g]
16:0	0.76	(0.05) [b]	0.75	(0.08) [b]	3.15	(0.17) [a]	0.68	(0.05) [f]	0.72	(0.07) [f]	1.99	(0.14) [e]
18:0	0.99	(0.02) [b]	0.92	(0.11) [b]	2.43	(0.08) [a]	0.50	(0.07) [f]	0.49	(0.07) [f]	1.14	(0.47) [e]
20:0	0.03	(0.01) [b]	0.05	(0.04) [b]	0.19	(0.06) [a]	0.04	(0.01) [f]	0.08	(0.02) [e]	0.03	(0.02) [f]
22:0	0.09	(0.06) [b]	0.14	(0.12) [ab]	0.24	(0.00) [a]	0.10	(0.04) [f]	0.12	(0.02) [ef]	0.16	(0.02) [e]

Table 2. Cont.

	MAGE						DAGE					
	Winter		Spring		Summer		Winter		Spring		Summer	
16:1n-9	1.19	(0.45) ab	1.39	(0.29) a	0.90	(0.06) b	0.15	(0.03) f	0.17	(0.03) f	0.27	(0.02) e
16:1n-7	11.16	(0.32) b	11.20	(0.32) b	13.00	(0.47) a	20.65	(0.51) e	20.85	(0.30) e	19.54	(0.82) f
18:1n-9	0.48	(0.03) b	0.44	(0.05) b	1.02	(0.01) a	0.86	(0.04) f	0.96	(0.14) f	2.16	(0.12) e
18:1n-7	2.50	(0.14) b	2.41	(0.29) b	3.11	(0.08) a	2.74	(0.06) e	2.84	(0.17) e	2.77	(0.11) e
20:1n-11	0.21	(0.02) a	0.22	(0.02) ab	0.19	(0.01) b	0.20	(0.01) g	0.26	(0.03) f	0.32	(0.01) e
20:1n-9	0.44	(0.01) a	0.43	(0.05) a	0.53	(0.02) a	0.29	(0.00) g	0.40	(0.04) f	0.53	(0.03) e
20:1n-7	0.08	(0.01) b	0.01	(0.01) c	0.37	(0.01) a	0.07	(0.01) f	0.04	(0.00) g	1.42	(0.51) e
22:1n-9	0.14	(0.05) a	0.12	(0.03) a	0.19	(0.00) a	0.09	(0.02) f	0.14	(0.03) f	0.26	(0.03) e
22:1n-7	0.11	(0.04) a	0.10	(0.02) a	0.15	(0.00) a	0.13	(0.02) f	0.15	(0.02) ef	0.19	(0.01) e
24:1	1.29	(0.08) a	1.32	(0.48) a	1.06	(0.02) a	0.62	(0.04) e	0.65	(0.07) e	0.62	(0.07) e
EPA	61.79	(0.32) a	62.26	(0.22) a	53.17	(0.71) b	5.27	(0.28) g	6.29	(0.85) f	9.10	(0.22) e
DHA	1.06	(0.02) a	1.12	(0.06) a	1.08	(0.05) b	0.30	(0.02) f	0.39	(0.08) e	0.43	(0.01) e
Others	7.81	(0.43) a	7.07	(0.44) a	4.91	(0.69) b	5.36	(0.15) e	5.32	(0.22) e	5.22	(0.37) e
Sum	100		100		100		100		100		100	

* Me-14:0a, b and c are branched isomers; positions of the methyl branches were not determined. Note: 20:4n-6 was not reported because it could not be accurately quantified due to co-elution with an unidentified peak; total mass percent of the two co-eluting peaks was <2% in all lipid classes.

Prominent FA in TAG were similar to those of DAGE with 12-MTA present at 10–20% with highest levels in winter/spring and total branched chain FA at 17–31%, also with the highest amount in winter/spring (Table 3). Both 16:1n-7 (24–28%) and EPA (14–20%) had greatest levels in summer. Proportions of FA in PL were different than the other three lipid classes. Branched chains FA were only present at 1–5% with 12-MTA < 1%. Instead, straight chain saturates, 16:0, 18:0 and 20:0, became much more important with total saturated FA at 11–19% with highest levels in winter. For the monounsaturates, 18, 20, 22 and 24 carbon FA were present at 1–4% each so that the total for the group ranged from 16–20% (highest in summer); 16:1n-7 only represented ≤ 3% total FA. EPA was the dominant FA at 43–55% with a maximum in winter/spring and DHA was present at highest proportions in all lipid classes at ~1.5%, also with a high in winter/spring.

Table 3. Proportions of FA (mass% total FA identified) in PL and TAG isolated from *C. frondosa* viscera ($n = 3$; mean ± (SD)). Values with different letters (e.g., a–c for PL; e–g for TAG) within a FA and lipid class are significantly different (ANOVA, Tukey's test; $p < 0.05$). The PL proportion included a small contribution from MAG.

	PL						TAG					
	Winter		Spring		Summer		Winter		Spring		Summer	
4,8,12-Me-13:0	0.08	(0.01) a	0.06	(0.01) a	0.10	(0.04) a	3.98	(0.21) e	4.11	(0.53) e	2.87	(0.37) f
Me-14:0(a) *	0.00	(0.00) b	0.00	(0.00) b	0.44	(0.03) a	0.57	(0.04) e	0.61	(0.03) e	0.29	(0.03) f
Me-14:0(b) *	0.14	(0.01) a	0.14	(0.01) a	0.06	(0.04) b	0.52	(0.02) e	0.55	(0.02) e	0.42	(0.13) e
Me-14:0(c)	0.02	(0.01) a	0.00	(0.00) a	0.03	(0.01) a	0.30	(0.02) e	0.28	(0.05) e	0.12	(0.02) f
12-MTA	0.46	(0.03) a	0.32	(0.04) b	0.45	(0.14) b	19.15	(0.81) e	19.87	(0.92) e	9.99	(0.74) f
8,12-Me-14:0	0.04	(0.02) b	0.02	(0.01) b	0.17	(0.06) a	1.75	(0.25) e	1.27	(0.12) f	1.04	(0.08) g
12-Me-15:0	0.21	(0.03) b	2.39	(0.88) a	3.58	(0.30) a	2.56	(0.29) e	2.51	(0.30) e	1.33	(0.01) f
8,12-Me-15:0	0.00	(0.00) b	0.04	(0.01) a	0.03	(0.00) ab	0.18	(0.04) e	0.17	(0.04) e	0.06	(0.02) f
ai-17:0	0.44	(0.09) a	0.38	(0.00) a	0.43	(0.21) a	1.25	(0.07) g	1.31	(0.01) e	0.91	(0.02) f

Table 3. Cont.

	PL						TAG					
	Winter		Spring		Summer		Winter		Spring		Summer	
14:0	0.25	(0.11) a	0.16	(0.02) b	0.28	(0.11) ab	3.43	(0.07) g	3.82	(0.10) f	5.94	(0.25) e
15:0	0.03	(0.02) a	0.04	(0.01) a	0.00	(0.00) b	0.45	(0.24) f	0.91	(0.28) e	0.00	(0.00) g
16:0	5.06	(0.24) b	2.09	(0.31) c	5.18	(1.06) a	3.11	(0.07) g	3.43	(0.13) f	4.35	(0.32) e
18:0	12.14	(0.65) a	6.43	(0.13) b	7.99	(1.11) b	3.00	(0.06) f	2.97	(0.10) f	3.71	(0.44) e
20:0	1.03	(0.09) a	1.21	(0.02) a	0.23	(0.07) b	0.26	(0.02) f	0.36	(0.01) e	0.26	(0.02) f
22:0	0.96	(0.05) b	1.08	(0.04) b	1.65	(0.24) a	0.31	(0.01) ef	0.35	(0.09) e	0.25	(0.02) f
16:1n-9	0.27	(0.08) c	2.96	(0.85) a	1.93	(0.26) b	0.14	(0.01) f	0.15	(0.01) ef	0.17	(0.00) e
16:1n-7	1.85	(0.24) b	1.51	(0.06) c	3.08	(0.07) a	23.73	(0.41) f	24.15	(0.31) f	27.61	(0.62) e
18:1n-9	1.17	(0.04) a	1.31	(0.06) a	1.77	(0.62) a	1.99	(0.05) g	2.18	(0.07) f	2.75	(0.17) e
18:1n-7	4.21	(0.42) a	4.16	(0.25) a	3.38	(0.24) b	2.50	(0.04) ef	2.79	(0.14) e	2.34	(0.27) f
20:1n-11	2.30	(0.08) a	2.74	(0.06) a	1.90	(0.47) b	0.65	(0.05) f	0.85	(0.04) e	0.38	(0.04) g
20:1n-9	1.03	(0.10) a	1.02	(0.04) a	1.77	(0.58) a	0.60	(0.01) e	0.70	(0.04) e	0.63	(0.08) e
20:1n-7	1.18	(0.18) a	0.60	(0.13) b	0.98	(0.33) b	0.20	(0.08) f	0.12	(0.01) f	1.06	(0.23) e
22:1n-9	1.20	(0.35) a	1.20	(0.04) a	1.16	(0.37) a	0.47	(0.03) f	0.57	(0.03) e	0.48	(0.01) f
22:1n-7	1.38	(0.17) b	1.46	(0.04) b	2.07	(0.06) a	0.50	(0.03) f	0.56	(0.03) e	0.38	(0.02) g
24:1	1.80	(0.15) a	1.50	(0.12) c	2.09	(0.04) b	0.90	(0.07) e	0.96	(0.05) e	0.62	(0.19) f
EPA	51.79	(2.82) a	55.20	(0.72) a	43.45	(0.43) b	16.71	(0.20) f	14.06	(0.82) g	20.06	(0.41) e
DHA	1.66	(0.24) a	1.73	(0.11) a	1.38	(0.33) b	0.92	(0.07) e	0.86	(0.03) e	0.79	(0.02) f
Others	8.04	(0.57) a	9.01	(0.68) a	11.57	(0.72) a	5.76	(0.16) f	5.73	(0.14) f	6.22	(0.29) e
Sum	100		100		100		100		100		100	

* Me-14:0a, b and c are branched isomers; positions of the methyl branches were not determined. Note: 20:4n-6 was not reported because it could not be accurately quantified due to co-elution with an unidentified peak; total mass percent of the two co-eluting peaks was <2% in all lipid classes.

3. Discussion

The presence of ether lipids in *C. frondosa* viscera was expected as alkyl structures including saturated (branched and unbranched) and monounsaturated alkyl chains associated with an ether bond in glycerol ethers have been previously identified in Holothurians [5,6,18]. High levels of α-glyceryl ethers have been reported in lipid extracts of *Stichopus japonicas* (18%), *C. fraudatrix* (9.3%), and *C. japonica* and *C. okhotensis* (25–27%) [5,6]. The presence of DAGE ether lipids in other marine species including, for example, dogfish, shark, deep-sea squids, elasmobranch fish, oysters, sponges, snails and corals [7,8,19–24] suggests that they are ubiquitous in marine animals and therefore their presence in sea cucumber species such as *C. frondosa* is not surprising; however, total DAGE and MAGE detected here in winter was >55%, exceeding even that reported in some species of shark liver oil [25] and representing a valuable source of non-polar ether lipids. Notably, the total ether lipid level is likely even higher than we have reported since we did not attempt to quantify polar ether lipids.

Analysis of the components of glyceryl ethers derived from both DAGE and MAGE revealed unique alkyl chain structures that were characteristically rich in 16:0 and 18:0 (Figure 2). Other studies have found a similar dominance of 16 and 18 carbon O-alkyl chains in DAGE and MAGE of *C. japonica*, *C. okhotensis* and *Oneirophanta mutabilis* [5,18]. This narrow range of alkyl structures indicates a high specificity for particular substrates in the pathways responsible for the biosynthesis of alkylglycerols [26]. Rybin et al. [5] and Santos et al. [18] had suggested that the specificity might be due to two acyl-CoA reductase isoenzymes (FAR1 and FAR2) [27,28]. Both reductase isoenzymes select fatty acyl-CoA of 16 and 18 carbon chains; FAR2 is specific for palmityl-and stearyl-CoA substrates, while FAR1 targets monounsaturated palmitoleyl- and oleyl-CoA and polyunsaturated linoleyl-CoA [29]. The specificity of these enzymes was first identified in mammalian cells, but our data suggest that they likely exist in sea cucumbers as well.

The FA profile for DAGE and MAGE were characterized by the presence of high concentrations of 12-MTA and EPA, respectively (Table 2). The patterns between the alkyl groups and FA associated with DAGE and MAGE were therefore quite different. In the biosynthesis of ether lipids, 1-*O*-alkyl-*sn*-glycero-3-phosphate has been reported to be a glycerol-based intermediate found mostly in mammalian cells [30]. Esterification of this intermediate with acyl-CoA at the *sn*-2 position in the presence of alkyl-acyl-glycero-3-phosphate acyltransferase results in the formation of 1-*O*-alkyl, 2-acyl-*sn*-glycero-3-phosphate. Removal of the phosphate group from the sn-3 position of that structure by phosphohydrolase results in the formation of 1-*O*-alkyl-2-acyl-*sn*-glycerol (MAGE). DAGE is then synthesized when 1-*O*-alkyl-2-acyl-*sn*-glycerol is esterified with a long-chain acyl-CoA ester by an acyltransferase. Thus, the high concentration of EPA in MAGE is likely due to a high specificity of alkyl-acyl-glycero-3-phosphate acyltransferase in positioning long chain FA (EPA) at *sn*-2 position. Since an elevated level of EPA is not observed in DAGE, that lipid cannot be derived from simple acylation of MAGE; another mechanism must be involved and responsible for the hydrolysis of EPA in MAGE and replacement with 12-MTA in DAGE. It may be that the MAGE we found represent a deacylation product of DAGE, rather than an intermediate in DAGE synthesis. In that scenario, the prominence of EPA would suggest that DAGE containing EPA in the *sn*-2 position are the primary substrates for diacylation at the sn-3 position. Given the similarly high levels of EPA in the PL, it could also be that MAGE containing EPA in the *sn*-2 position are destined for PL synthesis while those species without are preferentially converted to DAGE. Regrettably, we did not carry out a detailed analysis of the PL composition to evaluate its ether lipid structures.

The high EPA levels we found in MAGE could also be due to contamination of the MAGE bands with another lipid class, such as DAG, since a peak with the same retention time as DAG was found in HPLC analysis; however, given the similarity in retention time of DAGE and TAG, it is possible that the peak with the same retention time as DAG was MAGE. The TLC analysis supported this, indicating that DAG was not present in our sample, since its R_f did not coincide with any bands, including MAGE. We are also confident that the MAGE band recovered from the TLC plate did contain glyceryl ethers since we identified alkyl structures within it. Thus, we believe that we have isolated a relatively pure MAGE band that did not contain contribution from DAG.

Different species of branched chain FA were identified in both DAGE and MAGE lipid classes. *Iso-* and *anteiso* branched chain FA were the most abundant monomethyl branched chain FA. Zhong et al. [13] quantified *ai*-15:0 in fresh and dried *C. frondosa* harvested near Newfoundland but no other branched chain FA were identified. *Iso-* and *anteiso-* branched FA with carbon numbers from 14–18 have been reported in small amounts in lipids extracted from many types of marine fish [31,32]; 4,8,12-Me-13:0, generally assumed to be derived from phytanic acid sourced from phytoplankton, has also been reported in many marine organisms [33]. However, a number of other single- and multi-methylated branched FA, such as 12-Me-15:0, 8,12-Me-14:0, and 8,12-Me-15:0, have not been commonly reported in lipid extracts of marine species in general, and have never been identified in sea cucumber. While 4,8,12-Me-13:0 can be derived from phytol, a product of photosynthesis, the presence of the other FA with methyl branches in the same position on different carbon numbered backbones suggests that it and the other branched chain FA are products of de novo synthesis.

The synthesis of branched chain FA in mammals has been recently described [34] and it was found to follow similar pathways as used by bacteria [35]. For instance, *iso-* and *anteiso*-branched FA can be produced biosynthetically through regular mechanisms for the synthesis of saturated FA (including involvement of acyl carrier protein) with the substitution of different primer molecules (2-methylpropanyl-CoA, 3-methylbutyryl-CoA, and 2-methylbutyryl-CoA) for acetyl-CoA with activation by the same enzyme (FA synthase) [35]. For example, the initial step for the syntheses of 12-MTA (*anteiso*-branched FA) would involve the use of one 2-methylbutyryl-CoA and 5 acetyl-CoA additions. Similarly, 4,8,12-Me-13:0 branched chain FA (an *iso*-branched FA) would involve the use of

2-methylpropanyl-CoA as a primer molecule followed by a combination of two successive 2-methylbutyryl-CoA and one acetyl-CoA additions. Branched chain FA and specifically 12-MTA have been shown to exhibit promising health benefits including anti-inflammatory, anti-cancer activity and wound healing activity [15]. Thus, their de novo synthesis in *C. frondosa* could represent an underutilized source of 12-MTA for applications in medical treatments.

Viscera lipid and FA composition varied with collection season, as commonly found with many other fish and invertebrate species [36,37], likely due to variation in diet. With the seasonal data presented here, it becomes possible to target specific harvests to maximize the yield of particular lipids or FA. For instance, the overall yield of EPA was higher in viscera in sea cucumbers harvested in summer, likely because TAG was the dominate lipid class in that season and contained ~20% EPA, so that if an omega-3 product was desired, viscera from summer harvest would be a better source. However, the more novel characteristics of the viscera are the ether lipids and 12-MTA. Those would be better targeted with a winter harvest when overall lipid yields are highest and DAGE comprising some 55% of total lipids. It is also the viscera from winter harvest that has highest 12-MTA, so its recovery would also be maximized at that time. In the production of nutraceutical oils, PL are often removed through degumming as part of the refining process [38]. By considering the FA composition within lipid classes, it is also possible to predict the effect of degumming on final lipid composition. One would anticipate, for example, that PL removal would result in an oil that would be lower overall in EPA content, but 12-MTA and ether lipids would comprise a greater proportion of the final product, with this effect being greatest in winter harvested animals. Thus, the data presented here can aid in production of both crude lipid from sea cucumber viscera with preferred lipid characteristics and the final purified product.

4. Materials and Methods

Sea cucumber viscera were donated by Ocean Pride Fisheries Limited (Lower Wedgeport, NS, Canada) from harvests conducted in January 2015 (winter; latitude 4439/longitude 6041), March 2015 (spring; latitude 4439 longitude 6040) and July 2015 (summer; latitude 4439/longitude 6041) from the Sable Island Banks off Nova Scotia, Canada. Fall harvests were not carried out. Viscera was stored frozen at -30 °C prior to evaluation.

4.1. Moisture and Lipid Content

Portions of frozen *C. frondosa* viscera were homogenized using a food processor. The moisture content was determined by drying ~25 g of homogenized viscera at 100 °C [39] to a constant mass. Lipids were determined gravimetrically after extraction following the Bligh and Dyer method [40] with slight modification. Briefly, 200 g of ground viscera were blended with 200 mL of chloroform and 400 mL of methanol. The mixture was filtered and the residual material was placed in a blender, re-extracted with 200 mL chloroform and filtered again. The combined chloroform/methanol extracts were then mixed with 200 mL of aqueous 0.88% potassium chloride and allowed to separate in a separatory funnel. The lower organic layer was filtered through a bed of anhydrous sodium sulfate to remove the residual water in the lipid. The solvent was removed using a rotator evaporator at 40 °C.

4.2. Lipid Class Analysis

Samples for lipid class profiling using HPLC were prepared by dissolving 30–35 mg of lipids in 1.0 mL of dichloromethane. A 1.0 µL aliquot of the lipid (30 mg mL^{-1} dichlormethane) was injected into an Agilent 1100 HPLC equipped with an YMC PAK-PVA-SIL-NP column (250 × 4.6 mm I.D.; 5 µm) and an ESA Corona Charged Aerosol Detector (CAD). The column was eluted with a gradient containing 0.2% v/v ethyl acetate in isooctane (solvent A), 0.02% v/v acetic acid in 2:1 acetone: ethyl acetate (solvent B) and 0.1% acetic acid in 3:3:1 $v/v/v$ isopropyl alcohol: methanol: water (solvent C), at a flow rate of 1.5 mL min^{-1} over a run time of 77 min with a post-run time of 12 min (see

Supplementary Table S1 for full details). Lipid standards (free fatty acid (FFA), monoacylglycerol (MAG), diacylglycerol (DAG), triacylglycerol (TAG), diacylglyceryl ether (DAGE), phospholipids (PL); see Supplementary Materials for identities) prepared at a concentration 1 mg mL^{-1} in dichloromethane were injected to determine retention times of each lipid component.

4.3. Isolation of Lipid Classes by TLC

Lipids (100 µL at 250 mg mL^{-1}) were streaked using capillary tubes onto a pre-coated silica gel TLC plate (20 × 20 cm, layer thickness 0.25 mm) which had been previously developed in ethyl acetate and activated in an oven for one hour at 100 °C. The streaked plate was developed in hexane: diethyl ether: acetic acid (80:20:1 by volume) and sprayed with 0.2% methanolic 2,7-dichloroflourescein for visualization of the bands upon exposure to ultraviolet light (360 nm). Lipid standards (wax ester (WE), DAGE, TAG, DAG, MAG, FFA, Phosphatidyl choline and cholesterol) were used to tentatively identify the lipid present by comparison of R_f values. Non-polar lipid (DAGE, TAG, FFA) bands were scraped off the plate and extracted three times with 3 mL of 1:1 (v/v) hexane: chloroform. Polar lipids (MAGE, PL) were recovered similarly using 2:1 methanol: chloroform (v/v). The solvent was evaporated using a stream of nitrogen and the weight of lipid in each band was determined. Recovered simple lipids (MAGE, DAGE, TAG and FFA) were dissolved in hexane, while PL was dissolved in methanol.

4.4. ^{1}H NMR and ^{13}C NMR Analysis

The NMR spectra of lipid classes identified as DAGE and MAGE using TLC were recorded on a Bruker Avance 500 MHz spectrometer. The recovered bands were dissolved in deuterated chloroform (CDCl$_3$) at 16 mg mL^{-1} for ^{1}H NMR, and 73 mg mL^{-1} for ^{13}C NMR analysis before being transferred to NMR tubes (5 mm diameter, 8 in. in length, Wilmad-LabGlass, Vineland, NJ, USA). The solvent residual signal in the CDCl$_3$ was used as a reference for chemical shift assignments. Its ^{1}H NMR shift was 7.2–7.3 ppm and ^{13}C NMR shift is ~77 ppm. The ^{1}H NMR acquisition parameters were modified from a previous study [41]: spectral width, 10,080 Hz; relaxation delay, 3 s; number of scans, 32; acquisition time, 3.25 s; total acquisition time of 6.9 min. The ^{13}C NMR acquisition parameters were as follows: spectral width, 33,333 Hz; number of scans, 512; acquisition time, 0.81 s; with a total acquisition time of 16.07 min.

4.5. Ether Lipid Identification Using GC-MS

DAGE and MAGE bands were saponified to yield glyceryl ether diols according to Christie [42] with slight modifications. The lipid was suspended in 5 mL of 2 M ethanolic potassium hydroxide and the mixture was flushed with nitrogen, sealed and heated at 100 °C for one hour. It was then cooled to room temperature, and 16 mL water and 8 mL of 1:1 hexane: diethyl ether were added to the test tube. The mixture was vortexed and, after separation of layers, the top organic layer containing unsaponifiable material was recovered. The isolated organic layer was washed with 8 mL RO water and evaporated under a stream of nitrogen. The resulting diols were then acetylated by adding 0.5 mL of acetic anhydride and pyridine (5:1) and allowing the mixture to sit overnight at room temperature [43]. The solvent was then evaporated, the remaining acetylated material was dissolved in hexane. The DAGE standard was similarly saponified and acetylated.

Saponified and acetylated recovered MAGE and DAGE were analyzed using a GC Ultra gas chromatograph coupled with a PolarisQ mass spectrometer (Thermo Fisher Scientific Inc., Waltham, MA, USA). The analysis was performed using electron ionization (EI) and chemical ionization (CI) modes with split-injection (1/100) at 250 °C. The separation was performed on a ZB-35 capillary column (35%-phenyl)-methyl polysiloxane; 30 m × 0.25 mm i.d × 0.25 µm film thickness) with helium as the carrier gas at 1.2 mL min^{-1}. The initial temperature for the program was held at 180 °C for 1 min, then increased to 350 °C at 5 °C min^{-1} and held for 3 min. The ionization energy used was 70 eV, with a multiplier voltage of 1643 V, source temperature at 200 °C, and transfer line temperature of 350 °C. Spectral data were acquired over a mass range of m/z 60–600 in both modes and the emission current was 250 µA. In CI mode, methane was used as the reagent gas at a flow rate of 1.5 mL min^{-1}. Alkyl groups associated with an ether bond in both DAGE and MAGE lipid classes were identified by ion spectra obtained for peaks occurring at unique retention times and after subtracting 59 (acetoxy group) from the total molecular mass of DAGE and MAGE.

4.6. GC-FID Analysis of FAME

Acid catalyzed transesterification with 0.5 N H_2SO_4 in methanol was used to produce FAME of recovered lipid classes [44]. FAME were determined using a GC (Bruker, SCION 436-GC) fitted with a DB-23 column ((50%-cyanopropyl)-methylpolysiloxane) (30 m × 0.25 m × 0.25 µm film thickness, Agilent Technologies, Santa Clara, CA, USA) and a flame ionization detector (FID). Splitless injection was used with an injector temperature of 250 °C. FAME samples were separated using the following temperature program: the initial temperature was held at 60 °C for 1 min, then increased to 153 °C at 45 °C min^{-1}, held for 2 min, then increased to 174 °C at 2.3 °C min^{-1} and held for 0.2 min, increased to 205 °C at 2.5 °C min^{-1} and held for 2.5 min for a total run time of 41 min.

4.7. Analysis of 3-Ppyridylcarbinol Ester Derivatives

Direct transesterification can be used to prepare 3-pyridylcarbinol ester derivatives from lipid samples [45,46]. Potassium *tert*-butoxide in tetrahydrofuran (0.1 mL, 1.0 M) was first mixed with 3-pyridylcarbinol (0.2 mL), and the mixture was added to 10 mg of lipid in 1 mL dry dichloromethane. After mixing, the sample was incubated at 40 °C for 30 min and then allowed to cool. Water (2 mL) and hexane (4 mL) were added, and the contents of the tube were mixed. The upper organic layer was collected, dried over anhydrous sodium sulfate, and evaporated to dryness using a flow of nitrogen. The resulting 3-pyridylcarbinol esters were dissolved in hexane (0.4 mg mL^{-1}) and analyzed by GCMS on a DB-1 DB-1ms capillary column (100% dimethylpolysiloxane, 30 m × 0.25 mm i.d. × 0.25 um film thickness) using the same system as described above. Helium was the carrier gas at a flow rate of 1 mL/min with splitless injection (280 °C). The initial oven temperature was held at 60 °C for 2 min, then increased to 235 °C at 20 °C min^{-1}, followed by increasing to 280 °C at 2 °C min^{-1} and holding for 10 min. The ionization energy was 70 eV, with multiplier voltage of 1643 V, source temperature at 200 °C, and transfer line at 280 °C. Spectral data were acquired over a mass range of m/z 60–500. The molecular weight of a 3-pyridylcarbinol ester derivative was determined by the molecular ion, while a 28 amu gap in the EI spectra indicated the location of the methyl branch.

4.8. Statistical Analysis

All samples were run in triplicate and all data were analyzed using one-way analysis of variance (ANOVA) with an α level of 0.05 (Minitab 17). Tukey's multiple comparison test was used when ANOVA indicated there were significant differences in the means of the three harvests (α level of 0.05).

5. Conclusions

Five lipid species were identified in *C. frondosa* using HPLC and TLC with structural identification by GCMS when necessary, and included DAGE, TAG, FFA, MAGE and PL. All except FFA were present in sufficient quantities to characterize their acyl and alkyl structures. In winter, DAGE dominated, contributing ~55% of total mass of the lipid extract; 12-MTA comprised 42% of total FA within DAGE. In summer, TAG was present in the greatest amounts at 44% with lower 12-MTA amounts but EPA was more abundant (20% of total FA). Proportions of PL and MAGE showed little variation by season, in comparison to DAGE and TAG. These results will aide in the production and marketing of nutraceutical products based on *C. frondosa* viscera lipids.

Supplementary Materials: The following supporting information can be downloaded at: https://www.mdpi.com/article/10.3390/md20070435/s1, Standards for HPLC and TLC; Table S1: Gradient elution system for lipid class profiling; Figure S1: Lipid class profiling of *C. frondosa* lipids by HPLC: (a) DAGE; (b) TAG; (c) FFA; (d) DAG; (e) MAG; and (f) PL. Figure S2: ^{13}C-NMR (A) and ^{1}H NMR (B) of recovered the MAGE band from *C. frondosa* viscera in CDCl$_3$.

Author Contributions: Conceptualization, S.M.B., R.A. and S.M.; formal analysis R.A. and W.X.; investigation, R.A. and W.X.; writing—original draft preparation, S.M.B., R.A. and S.M.; writing—review and editing, S.M.B., R.A., W.X. and S.M.; supervision, S.M.B. and S.M.; funding acquisition, S.M.B. All authors have read and agreed to the published version of the manuscript.

Funding: This research was funded by Natural Sciences and Engineering Research Council of Canada, Discovery Grant Program.

Data Availability Statement: Full data is available from the authors on request.

Acknowledgments: Thanks to J. D'Entremont of Ocean Leader Fisheries for providing raw material analyzed in this work.

Conflicts of Interest: The authors declare no conflict of interest.

References

1. Department of Fisheries and Aquaculture (DFA). *Sea Cucumber Survey Conducted*; Project Report FDP 358-4; Fisheries Diversification Program, Department of Fisheries and Aquaculture: St. John's, NL, Canada, 2002.
2. Mamelona, J.; Saint-Louis, R.; Pelletier, E. Proximate composition and nutritional profile of by-products from green urchin and Atlantic sea cucumber processing plants. *Int. J. Food Sci. Technol.* **2010**, *45*, 2119–2126. [CrossRef]
3. Department of Fisheries and Oceans (DFO). *Integrated Fisheries Management Plan Summary: Sea Cucumber (Apostichopus californicus) by Dive Pacific Region 2021/2022*; Department of Fisheries and Oceans (DFO): Ottawa, ON, Canada, 2022.
4. Vaidya, H.; Cheema, S.K. Sea cucumber and blue mussel: New sources of phospholipid enriched omega-3 fatty acids with a potential role in 3T3-L1 adipocyte metabolism. *Food Funct.* **2014**, *5*, 3287–3295. [CrossRef] [PubMed]
5. Rybin, V.; Pavel, K.; Mitrofanov, D. 1-*O*-Alkylglycerol ether lipids in two Holothurian species: *Cucumaria japonica* and *C. okhotensis*. *Nat. Prod. Commun.* **2007**, *2*, 1934578X0700200913. [CrossRef]
6. Isay, S.V.; Makarchenko, M.A.; Vaskovsky, V.E. A study of glyceryl ethers—I. content of α-glyceryl ethers in marine invertebrates from the sea of Japan and tropical regions of the Pacific Ocean. *Comp. Biochem. Physiol.* **1976**, *55B*, 301–305. [CrossRef]
7. Haraldsson, G.; Kristinsson, B. Separation of eicosapentaenoic acid and docosahexaenoic acid in fish oil by kinetic resolution using lipase. *J. Am. Oil Chem. Soc.* **1998**, *75*, 1551–1556. [CrossRef]
8. Hayashi, K.; Kishimura, H. Amount and composition of diacyl glyceryl ethers in various tissue lipids of the deep-sea squid *Berryteuthis magister*. *J. Oleo Sci.* **2002**, *51*, 523–530. [CrossRef]
9. Mollinedo, F. Antitumour ether lipids: Proapoptotic agents with multiple therapeutic indications. *Expert Opin. Ther. Pat.* **2007**, *17*, 385–405. [CrossRef]
10. Jaffrès, P.A.; Gajate, C.; Bouchet, A.M.; Couthon-Gourvès, H.; Chantôme, A.; Potier-Cartereau, M.; Besson, P.; Bougnoux, P.; Mollinedo, F.; Vandier, C. Alkyl ether lipids, ion channels and lipid raft reorganization in cancer therapy. *Pharmacol. Ther.* **2016**, *165*, 114–131. [CrossRef]
11. Torres, C.F.; Vázquez, L.; Señoráns, F.J.; Reglero, G. Enzymatic synthesis of short-chain diacylated alkylglycerols: A kinetic study. *Process Biochem.* **2009**, *44*, 1025–1031. [CrossRef]
12. Martin, D.; Morán-Valero, M.; Señoráns, F.; Reglero, G.; Torres, C. In vitro intestinal bioaccessibility of alkylglycerols versus triacylglycerols as vehicles of butyric acid. *Lipids* **2011**, *46*, 277–285. [CrossRef]
13. Zhong, Y.; Khan, M.A.; Shahidi, F. Compositional characteristics and antioxidant properties of fresh and processed sea cucumber (*Cucumaria frondosa*). *J. Agric. Food Chem.* **2007**, *55*, 1188–1192. [CrossRef] [PubMed]
14. Swanson, D.; Block, R.; Mousa, S.A. Omega-3 fatty acids EPA and DHA: Health benefits throughout life. *Adv. Nutr.* **2012**, *3*, 1–7. [CrossRef] [PubMed]
15. Collin, P.D.; Yang, P.; Newman, R. Methods and Compositions for Treating Lipoxygenase—Mediated Disease States. U.S. Patent 6,541,519, 1 April 2003.
16. Dalsgaard, J.; St John, M.; Kattner, G.; Müller-Navarra, D.; Hagen, W. Fatty acid trophic markers in the pelagic marine environment. *Adv. Mar. Biol.* **2003**, *46*, 225–340. [CrossRef] [PubMed]
17. Lambert, J.B.; Shurvell, H.F.; Lightner, D.A.; Cooks, R.G. The chemical shift. In *Introduction to Organic Spectroscopy*; Macmillan Publishing Company: New York, NY, USA, 1987; pp. 44–66.
18. Santos, V.L.C.S.; Billett, D.S.M.; Wolff, G.A. 1-*O*-alkylglyceryl ether lipids of the gut walls and contents of an Abyssal Holothurian (*Oneirophanta mutabilis*). *J. Braz. Chem. Soc.* **2002**, *13*, 653–657. [CrossRef]
19. Hallgren, B.; Larsson, S. The glyceryl ethers in the liver oils of elasmobranch fish. *J. Lipid Res.* **1962**, *3*, 31–38. [CrossRef]

20. Guella, G.; Mancini, I.; Pietra, F. (+)-Raspailyne-a, a novel, acid-sensitive acetylenic enol ether glyceride from the marine sponge *Raspialia pumila*. *J. Chem. Soc. Chem. Commun.* **1986**, *1*, 77–78. [CrossRef]
21. Myers, B.L.; Crews, P. Chiral ether glycerides from a marine sponge. *J. Organ. Chem.* **1983**, *48*, 3583–3585. [CrossRef]
22. Smith, G.M.; Djerassi, C. Phospholipid studies of marine organisms: 14. Ether lipids of the sponge *Tethya aurantia*. *Lipids* **1987**, *22*, 236–240. [CrossRef]
23. Boer, M.; Gannefors, C.; Kattner, G.; Graeve, M.; Hop, H.; Falk-Petersen, S. The arctic pteropod *Clione limacina*: Seasonal lipid dynamics and life-strategy. *Mar. Biol.* **2005**, *147*, 707–717. [CrossRef]
24. Imbs, A.; Demina, O.; Demidkova, D. Lipid class and fatty acid composition of the boreal soft coral soft coral *Gersemia rubiformis*. *Lipids* **2006**, *41*, 721–725. [CrossRef]
25. Bakes, M.J.; Nichols, P.D. Lipid, fatty acid and squalene composition of liver oil from six species of deep-sea sharks collected in southern Australian water. *Comp. Biochem. Physiol. B* **1995**, *110*, 267–275. [CrossRef]
26. Reichwald-Hacker, I. Substrate specificity of enzymes catalyzing the biosynthesis of ether lipids. In *Ether Lipids: Biochemical and Biomedical Aspects*; Mangold, H.K., Paltauf, F., Eds.; Academic Press: New York, NY, USA, 1983; pp. 129–140.
27. Cheng, J.B.; Russell, D.W. Mammalian wax biosynthesis. I. Identification of two fatty acyl-coenzyme A reductases with different substrate specificities and tissue distributions. *J. Biol. Chem.* **2004**, *279*, 37789–37797. [CrossRef] [PubMed]
28. Hartvigsen, K.; Ravandi, A.; Harkewicz, R.; Kamido, H.; Bukhave, K.; Holmer, G.; Kuksis, A. 1-*O*-alkyl-2-(-oxo)acyl-*sn*-glycerols from shark oil and human milk fat are potential precursors of PAF mimics and GHB. *Lipids* **2006**, *41*, 679–693. [CrossRef] [PubMed]
29. Magnusson, C.D.; Haraldsson, G.G. Ether lipids. *Chem. Phys. Lipids* **2011**, *164*, 315–340. [CrossRef] [PubMed]
30. Brites, P.; Waterham, H.R.; Ronald, J.A.; Wanders, R.J.A. Functions and biosynthesis of plasmalogens in health and disease. *Biochim. Biophys. Acta* **2004**, *1636*, 219–231. [CrossRef] [PubMed]
31. Ratnayake, W.M.N.; Olsson, B.; Ackman, R.G. Novel branched chain fatty acids in certain fish oils. *Lipids* **1989**, *24*, 630–637. [CrossRef]
32. Hauff, S.; Vetter, W. Quantification of branched chain fatty acids in polar and neutral lipids of cheese and fish samples. *J. Agric. Food Chem.* **2010**, *58*, 707–712. [CrossRef]
33. Ackman, R.G. Fatty acids. In *Marine Biogenic Lipids Fats and Oils*; Ackman, R.G., Ed.; CRC Press: Boca Raton, FL, USA, 1989; pp. 103–138.
34. Wallace, M.; Green, C.R.; Roberts, L.S.; Lee, Y.M.; McCarville, J.L.; Sanchez-Gurmaches, J.; Meurs, N.; Gengatharan, J.M.; Hover, J.D.; Phillips, S.A.; et al. Enzyme promiscuity drives branched-chain fatty acid synthesis in adipose tissues. *Nat. Chem. Biol.* **2018**, *14*, 1021–1031. [CrossRef]
35. Kaneda, T. *iso*-Fatty and *anteiso*-fatty acids in bacteria—Biosynthesis, function, and taxonomic significance. *Microbiol. Rev.* **1991**, *55*, 288–302. [CrossRef]
36. Budge, S.M.; Iverson, S.J.; Bowen, W.D.; Ackman, R.G. Among- and within-species variability in fatty acid signatures of marine fish and invertebrates on the Scotian Shelf, Georges Bank, and southern Gulf of St. Lawrence. *Can. J. Fish. Aquat. Sci.* **2002**, *59*, 886–898. [CrossRef]
37. Iverson, S.J.; Frost, K.J.; Lang, S.L.C. Fat content and fatty acid composition of forage fish and invertebrates in Prince William Sound, Alaska: Factors contributing to among and within species variability. *Mar. Ecol. Progr. Ser.* **2002**, *241*, 161–181. [CrossRef]
38. Bimbo, A.P. Chapter 4—Processing of marine oils. In *Long-Chain Omega-3 Specialty Oils*; Breivik, H., Ed.; The Oily Press Ltd.: Dundee, UK, 2012; pp. 77–109.
39. American Oil Chemists' Society (AOCS). *Official Methods and Recommended Practices of the American Oil Chemists' Society*, 4th ed.; AOCS Press: Champaign, IL, USA, 1990.
40. Bligh, E.G.; Dyer, W.J. A rapid method of total lipid extraction and purification. *Can. J. Biochem. Physiol.* **1959**, *37*, 911–917. [CrossRef] [PubMed]
41. Guillen, M.D.; Ruiz, A. Study of the oxidative stability of salted and unsalted salmon fillets by H nuclear magnetic resonance. *Food Chem.* **2004**, *86*, 297–304. [CrossRef]
42. Christie, W.W. *Gas Chromatography and Lipids*; The Oily Press Ltd.: Dundee, UK, 1989; p. 36.
43. Renkonen, O. Individual molecular species of phospholipids: III. Molecular species of ox-brain lecithins. *Biochim. Biophys. Acta* **1966**, *125*, 288–309. [CrossRef]
44. Budge, S.M.; Iverson, S.J.; Koopman, H.N. Studying trophic ecology in marine ecosystems using fatty acids: A primer on analysis and interpretation. *Mar. Mammal Sci.* **2006**, *22*, 759–801. [CrossRef]
45. Destaillats, F.; Angers, P. One-step methodology for the synthesis of FA picolinyl esters from intact lipids. *J. Am. Oil Chem. Soc.* **2002**, *79*, 253–256. [CrossRef]
46. Dubois, N.; Barthomeuf, C.; Bergé, J.P. Convenient preparation of picolinyl derivatives from fatty acid esters. *Eur. J. Lipid Sci. Technol.* **2006**, *108*, 28–32. [CrossRef]

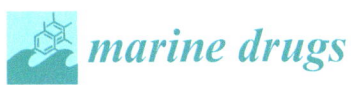

Article

Fucose-Rich Sulfated Polysaccharides from Two Vietnamese Sea Cucumbers *Bohadschia argus* and *Holothuria (Theelothuria) spinifera*: Structures and Anticoagulant Activity

Nadezhda E. Ustyuzhanina [1,*], Maria I. Bilan [1], Andrey S. Dmitrenok [1], Eugenia A. Tsvetkova [1], Sofya P. Nikogosova [1], Cao Thi Thuy Hang [2], Pham Duc Thinh [2], Dinh Thanh Trung [2], Tran Thi Thanh Van [2], Alexander S. Shashkov [1], Anatolii I. Usov [1,*] and Nikolay E. Nifantiev [1]

[1] The Laboratory of Glycoconjugate Chemistry, N.D. Zelinsky Institute of Organic Chemistry, Russian Academy of Sciences, Leninsky Prospect 47, 119991 Moscow, Russia; bilan@ioc.ac.ru (M.I.B.); dmt@ioc.ac.ru (A.S.D.); e_tsvet@ioc.ac.ru (E.A.T.); nextepwms@rambler.ru (S.P.N.); shash@ioc.ac.ru (A.S.S.); nen@ioc.ac.ru (N.E.N.)

[2] Chemical Analysis and Technology Development Department, NhaTrang Institute of Technology Research and Application, Vietnam Academy of Science and Technology, 02 Hung Vuong Street, Nhatrang 650000, Vietnam; caohang.nitra@gmail.com (C.T.T.H.); ducthinh.nitra@gmail.com (P.D.T.); dinhthanhtrung410@gmail.com (D.T.T.); tranthanhvan@nitra.vast.vn (T.T.T.V.)

* Correspondence: ustnad@gmail.com (N.E.U.); usov@ioc.ac.ru (A.I.U.); Tel.: +7-495-135-8784 (N.E.U. & A.I.U.)

Citation: Ustyuzhanina, N.E.; Bilan, M.I.; Dmitrenok, A.S.; Tsvetkova, E.A.; Nikogosova, S.P.; Hang, C.T.T.; Thinh, P.D.; Trung, D.T.; Van, T.T.T.; Shashkov, A.S.; et al. Fucose-Rich Sulfated Polysaccharides from Two Vietnamese Sea Cucumbers *Bohadschia argus* and *Holothuria (Theelothuria) spinifera*: Structures and Anticoagulant Activity. *Mar. Drugs* **2022**, *20*, 380. https://doi.org/10.3390/md20060380

Academic Editors: Vladimir I. Kalinin and Alexanra S. Silchenko

Received: 10 May 2022
Accepted: 2 June 2022
Published: 6 June 2022

Publisher's Note: MDPI stays neutral with regard to jurisdictional claims in published maps and institutional affiliations.

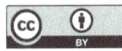

Copyright: © 2022 by the authors. Licensee MDPI, Basel, Switzerland. This article is an open access article distributed under the terms and conditions of the Creative Commons Attribution (CC BY) license (https://creativecommons.org/licenses/by/4.0/).

Abstract: Fucosylated chondroitin sulfates (FCSs) **FCS-BA** and **FCS-HS**, as well as fucan sulfates (FSs) **FS-BA-AT** and **FS-HS-AT** were isolated from the sea cucumbers *Bohadschia argus* and *Holothuria (Theelothuria) spinifera*, respectively. Purification of the polysaccharides was carried out by anion-exchange chromatography on DEAE-Sephacel column. Structural characterization of polysaccharides was performed in terms of monosaccharide and sulfate content, as well as using a series of non-destructive NMR spectroscopic methods. Both FCSs were shown to contain a chondroitin core [→3)-β-D-GalNAc-(1→4)-β-D-GlcA-(1→]$_n$ bearing sulfated fucosyl branches at O-3 of every GlcA residue in the chain. These fucosyl residues were different in pattern of sulfation: **FCS-BA** contained Fuc2*S*4*S*, Fuc3*S*4*S* and Fuc4*S* at a ratio of 1:8:2, while **FCS-HS** contained these residues at a ratio of 2:2:1. Polysaccharides differed also in content of GalNAc4*S*6*S* and GalNAc4*S* units, the ratios being 14:1 for **FCS-BA** and 4:1 for **FCS-HS**. Both FCSs demonstrated significant anticoagulant activity in clotting time assay and potentiated inhibition of thrombin, but not of factor Xa. **FS-BA-AT** was shown to be a regular linear polymer of 4-linked α-L-fucopyranose 3-sulfate, the structure being confirmed by NMR spectra of desulfated polysaccharide. In spite of considerable sulfate content, **FS-BA-AT** was practically devoid of anticoagulant activity. **FS-HS-AT** cannot be purified completely from contamination of some FCS. Its structure was tentatively represented as a mixture of chains identical with **FS-BA-AT** and other chains built up of randomly sulfated alternating 4- and 3-linked α-L-fucopyranose residues.

Keywords: sea cucumber; *Bohadschia argus*; *Holothuria (Theelothuria) spinifera*; fucosylated chondroitin sulfates; fucan sulfates; anticoagulant activity

1. Introduction

Two types of fucose-rich sulfated polysaccharides are known as components of marine invertebrates belonging to the class Holothuroidea (sea cucumbers). Unique fucosylated chondroitin sulfates (FCSs) have been found exclusively in the body walls of sea cucumbers. Molecules of these biopolymers have been shown to contain a linear core [→3)-β-D-GalNAc-(1→4)-β-D-GlcA-(1→]$_n$ identical to the backbone of vertebrate chondroitin sulfates [1,2]. This chondroitin core usually contains α-L-fucosyl branches attached to O-3 of GlcA. Depending on the species of sea cucumber, FCSs may contain four types of GalNAc units (non-sulfated and sulfated at O-4, at O-6, or both at O-4 and O-6) [3], as well as GlcA, not only fucosylated at O-3, but also sulfated at O-3 or both at O-2 and O-3 [4,5]. In addition, disaccharide branches attached to O-3 of GlcA were found side by side with monofucosyl branches in several FCSs. Thus, FCS from *Holothuria (Ludwigothuria) grisea* was shown to contain the branch α-L-Fuc-(1→2)-α-L-Fuc3S-(1→ [6]. It should be noted that this structure was suggested after reinvestigation and correction of data described previously [7,8]. Similar difucoside branches were detected in other FCSs, examples are α-L-Fuc-(1→2)-α-L-Fuc3S4S-(1→ in FCS from *Eupentacta fraudatrix* [5], α-L-Fuc2S4S-(1→3)-α-L-Fuc4S-(1→ in FCS from *Stichopus japonicas* [3] and α-L-Fuc-(1→3)-α-L-Fuc4S-(1→ in FCS from *Holothuria lentiginosa* [9]. Recently more complex branches containing galactose or galactosamine residues have been found in several FCSs, examples are α-D-Gal4S(6S)-(1→2)-α-L-Fuc3S-(1→ in FCS from *Thelenota ananas* [10], α-D-GalNAc-(1→2)-α-L-Fuc3S4S-(1→ in FCS from *Acaudina molpadioides* [11] and α-D-GalNAcS-(1→2)-α-L-Fuc3S-(1→ in FCS from *Holothuria nobilis* [12]. There is some evidence that branches may be attached not only to O-3 of GlcA, but also to O-4 or O-6 of GalNAc residues of the backbone [13–15]. These examples demonstrate high structural diversity of FCSs. Since investigation of FCSs is connected with their promising biological activities [16–19], it is clear that different biological properties of FCS should depend on their fine structural characteristics, such as degree and position of sulfation, nature and position of branches and molecular mass distribution.

Another type of fucose-rich sulfated polysaccharides of sea cucumbers is represented by fucan sulfates (FSs), which are similar in many respects to FSs of sea urchins, but differ considerably from much more complex fucoidans of brown algae [20]. The simplest structures are polymers of 3- or 4-linked monosulfated α-L-fucose residues, examples being highly regular polysaccharides [-3)-α-L-Fuc2S-(1-]$_n$ from *Stichopus horrens* [21,22] and *Stichopus herrmanni* [23]. Similar 3-linked FS, with a non-regular distribution of sulfate groups, was isolated from *Acaudina leicoprocta* [24], whereas 4-linked FSs, namely, [-4)-α-L-Fuc3S-(1-]$_n$ and [-4)-α-L-Fuc2S-(1-]$_n$, were found in *Holothuria fuscopunctata* and *Thelenota ananas*, respectively [22]. Structures of linear FSs are often represented as regular molecules built up of differently sulfated tetrasaccharide repeating units. Such polysaccharides, containing 3-linked backbone, were isolated from *Isostichopus badionotus* [25], *Acaudina molpadioides* [26], *Thelenota ananas* [27], *Pearsonothuria graeffei* [28], *Holothuria tubulosa* [29], *Holothuria polii* [30] and *Holothuria hilla* [31]. The structure of FS from *Holothuria albiventer* was shown to have a sulfated hexasaccharide repeating units [32], whereas sulfation pattern in FS from *Holothuria floridana* deviates considerably from the norm [33]. More complicated FSs contain other interfucoside linkages and/or branched carbohydrate chains. Thus, polysaccharides from *Holothuria edulis* and *Ludwigothurea grisea* contain backbones of 3-linked tetrafucosides connected by 1-2-linkages, where 2-substituted residues are additionally fucosylated (partially, as in *Ludwigothurea grisea*, or completely, as in *Holothuria edulis*) at position 4 [34]. Branched FS from *Apostichopus japonicus* contains a backbone of 3-linked α-L-Fuc2S, where every trisaccharide carries a non-sulfated 3-linked difucoside branch at-O-4 [35]. Recently some evidence has appeared on the possible presence of several structurally different FS in the same holothurian species. Thus, *Holothuria fuscopunctata* contains, in addition to 4-linked polymer of α-L-fucose 3-sulfate, another FS with tetrasaccharide repeating units -3)-α-L-Fuc2S,4S-(1-4)-α-L-Fuc-(1-3)-α-L-Fuc2S-(1-4)-α-L-Fuc-(1- with alternating 1-3 and 1-4 interfucoside linkages [36]. A new branched FS was isolated from *Pattalus mollis*. The polysaccharide contained a backbone of 4-linked α-L-Fuc2S, where every third residue was glycosylated at O-3 by α-L-Fuc4S or α-L-Fuc3S [37]. Further investigation of the same species made it possible to find, in addition to branched FS, the simultaneous presence of linear components, namely, randomly sulfated 3-linked fucan together with two differently sulfated 4-linked FS [38].

Natural fucose-enriched sulfated polysaccharides exerted excellent anticoagulant, antithrombotic, antivirus and anticancer activity together with many other biological actions [15–19]. Holothurian FCSs and FSs are isolated and characterized in order to find new biopolymers of practical importance and to establish distinct structure–activity correlations in these unique biologically active biopolymers. The Vietnamese coastal waters may be regarded as a rich source of marine invertebrates, including sea cucumbers, which contain both FCSs and FSs. For example, a novel FS with anticancer activity has been isolated from the Vietnamese sea cucumber *Stichopus variegatus* [39]. In the present communication we describe the isolation and structural characterization of sulfated polysaccharides from two Vietnamese holothurian species, *Bohadschia argus* and *Holothuria spinifera* (Figure S1). Some preliminary data on anticoagulant activity of these polysaccharides were obtained as well. It should be noted that FCS from *Bohadschia argus* has been carefully investigated previously [40], whereas accompanying FS and both FCS and FS of *Holothuria spinifera* have not been described in the literature. FCS isolated from *H. spinifera* was structurally similar to the corresponding FCS of *B. argus*. Both polysaccharides demonstrated anticoagulant activity *in vitro*, comparable with that of LMWH (enoxaparin). Surprisingly FS, isolated from *H. spinifera*, was practically inactive in these tests, in spite of its rather high sulfate content.

2. Results and Discussion

Crude extracts of sulfated polysaccharides were obtained from the body walls of sea cucumbers *Bohadschia argus* and *Holothuria spinifera* (Figure S2) by conventional solubilization of biomass in the presence of papain [8] followed by treatment of the extract with hexadecyltrimethylammonium bromide to precipitate the sulfated components, which were then transformed into water-soluble sodium salts by dissolving in 2 M NaCl and precipitation with ethanol, giving rise to crude sulfated polysaccharides **SP-BA** and **SP-HS**, respectively. Both crude extracts were subjected to anion-exchange chromatography on DEAE-Sephacel column. The fractions obtained as the result of chromatographic resolution are listed in Table 1.

Table 1. Characteristics of crude polysaccharide preparations **SP-BA** and **SP-HS** and the fractions obtained by their chromatography on DEAE-Sephacel and then used for structural analysis (composition in molar ratios relative to fucose).

Sample	Fuc	Gal	GlcNAc	GalNAc	UA, Na-salt	SO_3Na	Molecular Weight, kDa (Dispercity)
SP-BA	1.00	0.14	0.07	0.30	0.30	2.05	
FCS-BA	1.00	0.09	n.d.	0.78	0.83	4.04	32 (1.55)
FS-BA-AT	1.00	0.09	0.04	0.06	0.04	1.28	55 (1.35)
SP-HS	1.00	0.12	0.08	0.3	0.21	2.44	
FCS-HS	1.00	0.12	0.04	0.74	1.10	3.44	30 (1.62)
FS-HS-AT	1.00	0.09	0.04	0.18	0.18	1.69	

Isolation of FCS from *Bohadschia argus* has been described previously, and the polysaccharide was used to obtain oligosaccharides acting as anticoagulants by intrinsic factor Xase complex inhibition [40]. According primarily to NMR spectral data, this polysaccharide had a typical FCS structure that was wholly 3-O-fucosylated GlcA and 4,6-disulfated GalNAc in the core with Fuc3S4S (~95%) and Fuc2S4S (~5%) as branches. In our work three fractions appeared (**FCS-BA1**, **FCS-BA2**, and **FCS-BA3**) by elution with water, 0.75 M and 1.0 M NaCl, respectively. These preparations were obtained in comparable yields of about 10% and contained GlcA, GalNAc, Fuc and sulfate in ratios near to the majority of known holothurian FCSs. Detection of minor Gal and GlcN in hydrolysates may be explained by the possible presence of small amounts of other GAGs, which could not be eliminated by anion-exchange chromatography. Appearance of a part of FCS eluted with water, and hence not absorbed on anion-exchanger, may probably be explained by the high molecular weight of **FCS-BA1** (cf. [38]), whereas **FCS-BA2** and **FCS-BA3**, having similar NMR spectra, were eluted separately, probably due to slightly different position of sulfation. All three FCS fractions had similar behavior in agarose gel electrophoresis

(Figure S3). Fraction eluted with 1.0 M NaCl and designated as **FCS-BA** (Table 1) was used further for structural analysis.

The structure of **FCS-BA** was characterized using 1D and 2D NMR spectroscopy (Figures 1, 2, and S4, Table S1). The presence of Fuc, GalNAc and GlcA units in both polysaccharides was confirmed by the characteristic values of chemical shifts of C-6 for Fuc (δ 17.2 ppm) and GlcA (δ 176.0 ppm), as well as of C-2 for GalNAc (δ 52.7 ppm) in ^{13}C NMR spectrum (Figure 1). The anomeric region in ^{1}H NMR spectrum contained several low-field signals indicating the presence of different fucosyl branches (Figure 2). These spectra gave no doubts that **FCS-BA** belongs to the well-known class of holothurian FCSs [1,2,41,42]. It should be emphasized that very small intensity of C-6 signal in ^{13}C NMR spectrum (δ 62.3 ppm, Figure 1) means that practically all the GalNAc residues are 4,6-disulfated. The ratio between residues **B** and **C** (Figure 3) was found to be 14:1. According to intensities of anomeric signals of sulfated Fuc residues it is possible to conclude that Fuc3S,4S (**E**, δ 5.34 ppm) predominates considerably over the two other branches (**D**, δ 5.68 ppm, and **F**, δ 5.40 ppm) in the polysaccharide molecule (Figure 3, the calculated ratio **D:E:F** = 1:8:2).

Chromatography of **SP-HS** gave rise to **FCS-HS**, which was eluted, as expected, with 1.0 M NaCl. Its electrophoretic mobility in agarose gel was identical to **FCS-BA** (Figure S3). According to NMR spectra (Figures 1 and 2), which are very similar to those of **FCS-BA**, the polysaccharide undoubtedly belongs to FCSs. There are some minor structural differences between these two samples. Thus, the more intense signal at δ 62.3 ppm (Figure 1) corresponds to more substantial content of GalNAc residues non-sulfated at C-6 (the ratio between residues **B** and **C**, Figure 3, was found to be 4:1), whereas signals at δ 5.68 ppm and δ 5.34 ppm, having practically equal intensities (Figure 2), show the more substantial content of Fuc2S,4S in **FCS-HS**. The molar ratio between differently sulfated fucose residues **D:E:F** (Figure 3) was calculated as 2:2:1.

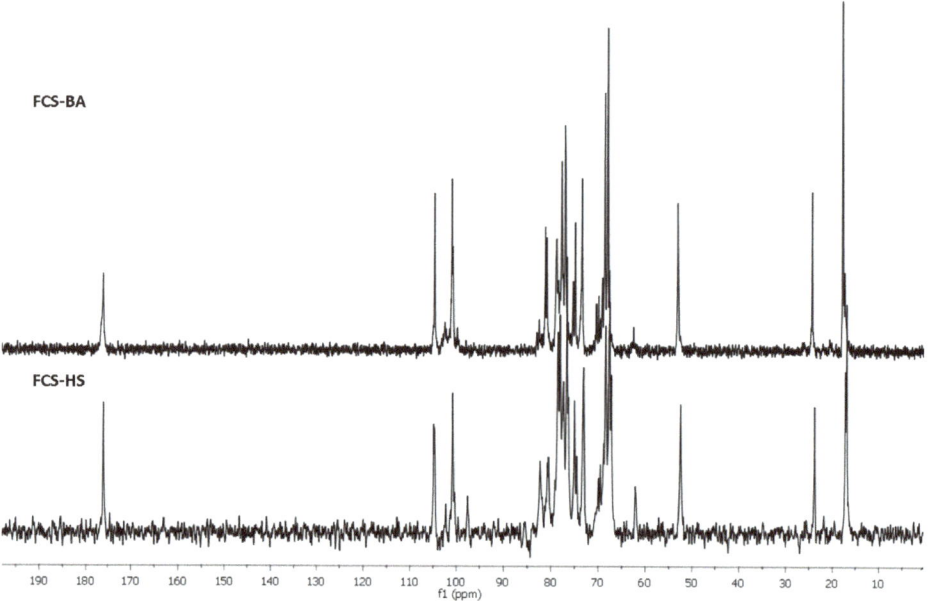

Figure 1. The ^{13}C NMR spectra of fucosylated chondroitin sulfates **FCS-BA** and **FCS-HS**.

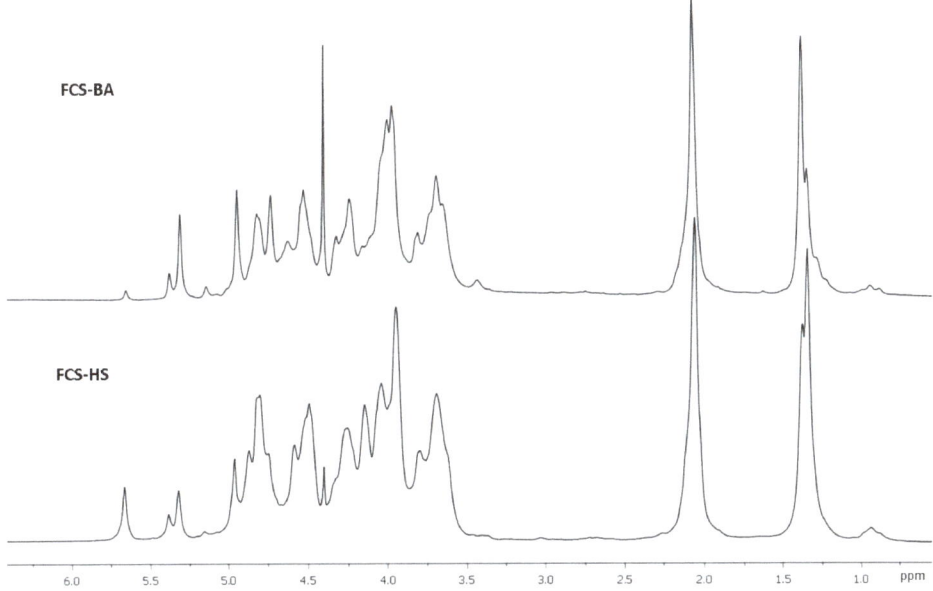

Figure 2. Fragments of ^{1}H NMR spectra of fucosylated chondroitin sulfates **FCS-BA** and **FCS-HS**.

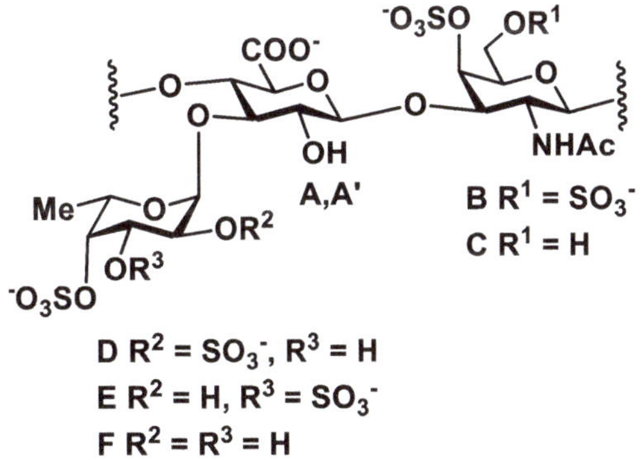

Figure 3. Repeating blocks of fucosylated chondroitin sulfates **FCS-BA** and **FCS-HS**. Unit **A** bears Fuc2S4S (**D**), whereas unit **A'** bears Fuc3S4S (**E**) or Fuc4S (**F**).

A rather unusual property of **SP-BA** is its incomplete solubility in water. The non-soluble gel-like fraction separated by centrifugation was treated with dilute acid in very mild conditions, giving rise to precipitate, which was shown to be mainly a protein. Neutralization of mother liquor followed by gel chromatography afforded **FS-BA-AT** (Table 1). Application of 1D and 2D NMR experiments (COSY, HSQC, and ROESY) led to assigning all the signals in NMR spectra (Figures 4, 5, and S5, Table S2) and to establish the structure of **FS-BA-AT** as a regular linear polymer of 4-linked fucose 3-sulfate (Figure 6). As mentioned above, similar polysaccharide was isolated previously from *Holothuria fuscopunctata* [22]. The signal assignments presented in [22] and our data are given in Table S2 for comparison. The systematic differences up to 2 ppm in carbon chemical shifts between spectra of two polymers probably arise due to alternative conditions of signal registration used in these two works. The structure of linear backbone built up of 4-linked α-L-fucopyranose in

FS-BA-AT was confirmed by NMR spectra of its desulfated preparation **FS-BA-AT-DS** (Table S2).

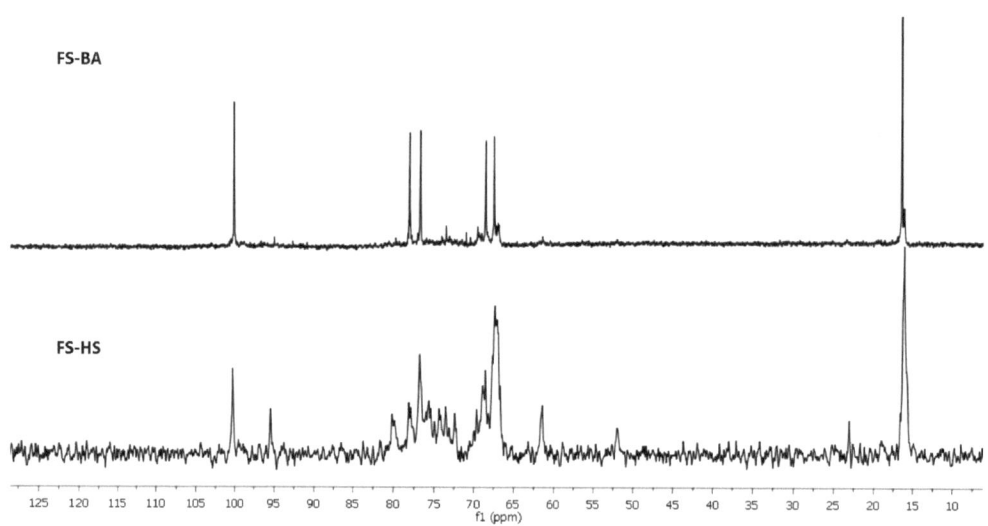

Figure 4. The ^{13}C NMR spectra of sulfated fucans **FS-BA** and **FS-HS**.

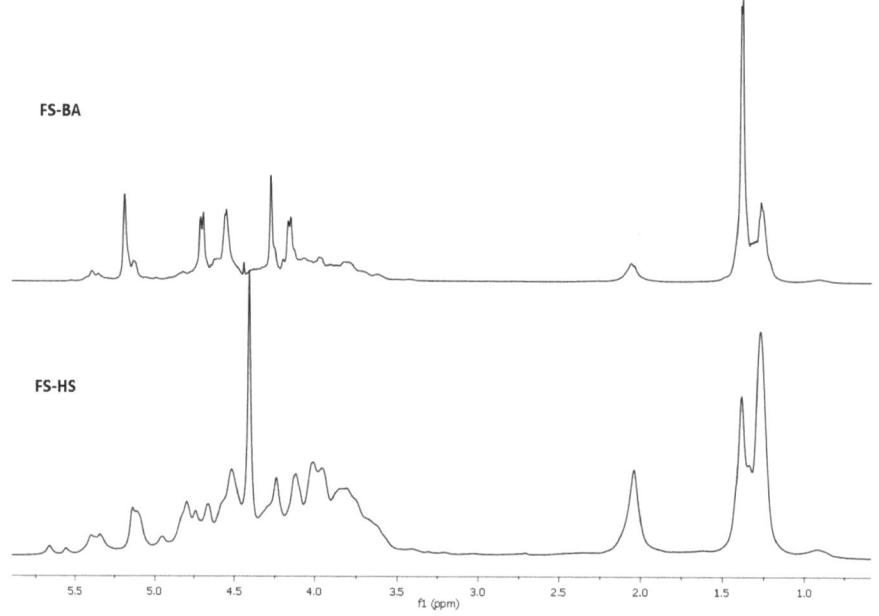

Figure 5. The ^{1}H NMR spectra of sulfated fucans **FS-BA** and **FS-HS**.

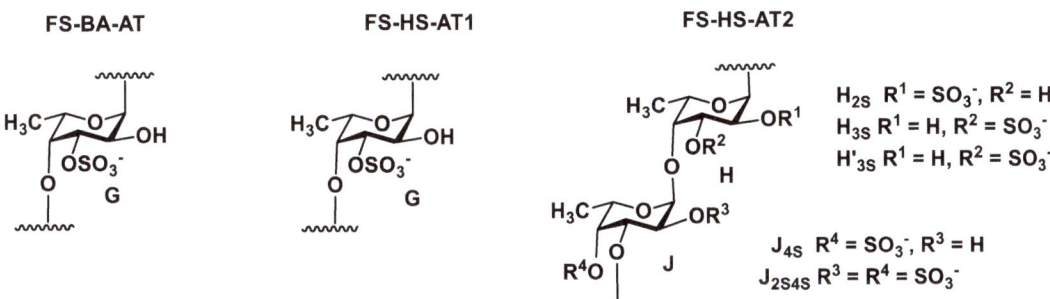

Figure 6. Repeating blocks of fucans **FS-BA-AT** and **FS-HS-AT**.

Preparation **SP-HS** was also partially soluble in water, but in this case a rather small insoluble fraction (12%) was not investigated further. Anion-exchange chromatography afforded the main fraction **FS-HS**, not absorbed on the column and eluted with water. To improve the resolution of spectral signals, this fraction was treated with dilute acid, as above, to give **FS-HS-AT**. The NMR spectra of **FS-HS-AT** were shown to be rather complicated for detailed analysis due to overlapping of many important signals (Figures 4, 5, and S6). This complexity may be explained by the random distribution of sulfates along the polymeric chains, since sulfation at every position causes a change in chemical shifts not only in its own residue, but also in both neighboring glycosylated and glycosylating residues. Nevertheless, the assignment of many signals and the corresponding correlations in the anomeric region of the spectra has been suggested (Table S3) based on the assumption about the simultaneous presence of two types of polymers containing randomly sulfated repeating units shown in Figure 6. Further attempts to resolve the complex preparation **FS-HS-AT** are now in progress.

Since FCSs and FSs are known to demonstrate anticoagulant and antithrombotic activities [16,43], we have studied three isolated samples **FCS-BA**, **FCS-HS** and **FS-BA-AT** as anticoagulant agents in vitro. Low molecular weight heparin (enoxaparin) was used as standard (Figure 7). In the clotting time assay (APTT-test) the effects of branched **FCS-BA** and **FCS-HS** were higher than that of enoxaparin, while linear **FS-BA-AT** was almost inactive at the same concentrations (Figure 7A). The values of 2APTT (the concentrations that led to two-time increasing of clot formation) were 2.6 ± 0.1 μg/mL for **FCS-HS**, 3.1 ± 0.1 μg/mL for **FCS-BA**, and 3.8 ± 0.2 μg/mL for enoxaparin. The active samples **FCS-BA** and **FCS-HS** were studied further in the experiments with purified proteins thrombin and factor Xa (Figure 7B,C). It was shown that in the presence of anti-thrombin III (ATIII) **FCS-BA** and **FCS-HS** potentiate the inhibition of thrombin, although their effect was slightly lower than that of enoxaparin (Figure 7B). This activity may be explained by specific formation of the ternary complex between thrombin, antithrombin III and FCS. The possibility of such complexation was demonstrated by computer docking studies in one of our previous works [44]. At the same time both samples had very low activity against factor Xa (Figure 7C).

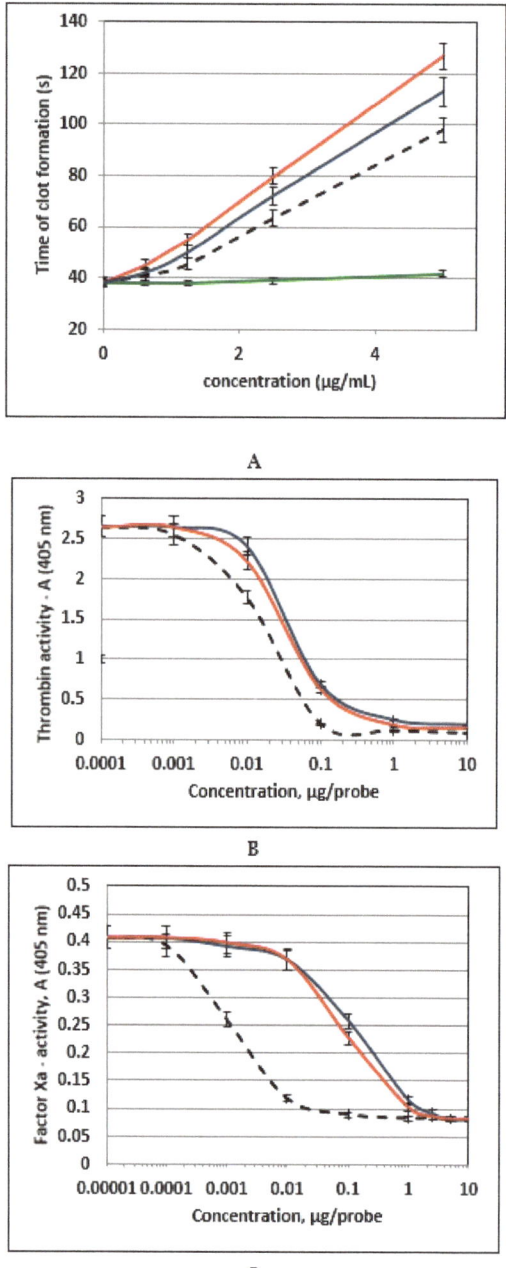

Figure 7. Anticoagulant activity of polysaccharides **FCS-BA** (blue), **FCS-HS** (red), **FS-BA-AT** (green) and enoxaparin (dotted line). (**A**) APTT assay, (**B**) Anti-IIa-activity in the presence of ATIII, (**C**) Anti-Xa-activity in the presence of ATIII. $n = 4$, $p < 0.05$.

3. Materials and Methods

3.1. General Methods

Procedures for determination of neutral monosaccharides, amino sugars, uronic acids and sulfate content of polysaccharides have been described previously [45–47]. Solvolytic desulfation [45] was used to prepare **FS-HS-AT-DS** from **FS-HS-AT**. Molecular weights of polysaccharides were evaluated by chromatographic comparison with standard pullulans [48].

3.2. Isolation of Polysaccharides

Wild sea cucumbers *Holothuria (Theelothuria) spinifera* (Theel, 1886) and *Bohadschia argus* (Jaeger, 1833) with size range of 20–30 cm in length and 300–500 g in weight were collected in October 2020 at the coast-line of Nhatrang Bay, Vietnam. The samples were stored in sea water and transported to the laboratory in a day. After removing the viscera and washing, the fresh sea cucumber body walls were treated with 96% ethanol for 3 to 5 days, followed by soaking in acetone overnight at room temperature. Finally, the defatted samples were chopped and air-dried. Sulfated polysaccharides were isolated from the body wall of the sea cucumber using a method of Pham Duc Thinh et al., 2018 [39] (Figure 2). The defatted residue (50 g) was incubated with papain (10 g) in 1 L of 0.1 M sodium acetate buffer (pH 6) containing 5 mM EDTA and 5 mM cysteine at 60 °C for 24 h. The obtained mixture was heated at 100 °C for 20 min to inactivate the enzyme and to remove a small precipitate. The supernatant was treated with aqueous 10% hexadecyltrimethylammonium bromide solution (Cetavlon) up to complete precipitation of sulfated polysaccharides and left overnight at 4 °C. The resulting precipitate was centrifuged, washed with distilled water, dissolved in a mixture of 2 M NaCl and EtOH (4:1), precipitated with 3 volumes of 96% ethanol, and left at 4 °C for 24 h. The precipitate was centrifuged, washed with ethanol, dissolved in water, dialyzed, concentrated under a vacuum, and lyophilized to obtain crude sulfated polysaccharide **SP-HS** from *Holothuria spinifera* (yield 3,63%) and **SP-BA** from *Bohadschia argus* (yield 3,57%). Composition of crude polysaccharides is given in Table 1.

A suspension of 400 mg of **SP-BA** in 90 mL of water was stirred at room temperature for several hours and centrifuged at 6.000 rpm for 30 min. The gel-like precipitate was washed several times with water and lyophilized to give **FS-BA-ins**. The supernatant was placed on a column (3 × 10 cm) with DEAE-Sephacel (Saint Louis, MO, USA) in Cl$^-$-form and eluted with water followed by NaCl solution of increasing concentration (0.5, 0.75, 1.0 and 1.5 M), each time up to the absence of a positive reaction of eluate for carbohydrates [49]. Fractions were desalted on Sephadex G-15 (Saint Louis, MO, USA) column and lyophilized. Fractions eluted with water, 0.75 M NaCl and 1.0 M NaCl with the yields of 7.3, 11.8 and 11.8%, respectively, had similar composition and NMR spectra. The latter fraction was designated as **FCS-BA** and used further for structural analysis. Similar treatment of **SP-HS** gave rise to a rather small water-insoluble fraction (yield 12%), which was not investigated further. Chromatography of the water-soluble part of a sample on DEAE-Sephacel afforded the main fraction **FS-HS** eluted with water (yield 34.7%) and the second considerable fraction **FCS-HS** eluted with 1.0 M NaCl (yield 24.5%, Table 1).

3.3. Dilute Acid Treatment of Samples

A suspension of 170 mg of **FS-BA-ins** in 20 mL of 0.1 M HCl was stirred at 50 °C for 3 h, the insoluble material was centrifuged, washed and lyophilized to give a preparation (35.3%) containing 77.6% of protein and no carbohydrates. A viscous supernatant was neutralized by NaHCO$_3$, desalted on Sephadex G-15 and chromatographed on DEAE-Sephacel, as above. The main polysaccharide fraction eluted with 1 M NaCl was desalted and lyophilized to afford **FS-BA-AT** (Table 1). Preparation **FS-HS-AT** was obtained after similar mild acid treatment of **FS-HS** (Table 1).

3.4. Agarose Gel Electrophoresis (PAGE)

Polysaccharides, heparin and enoxaparin (Clexan, Sanofi, Paris, France) (15 µg) were applied to 0.6% agarose gel prepared in 60 mM 1,3 diaminopropan-acetate buffer pH 9.0. Electrophoresis was run at 100 V in 60 mM 1,3 diaminopropan-acetate buffer pH 9.0 for 120 min. After migration gel was soaked in 0.1% cetyltrimethylammonium bromide for 30 min, dried, stained with 0.003% Stains-all in formamide-isopropanol-water (5:25:70) overnight in the dark and destained with water.

3.5. NMR Spectroscopy

The NMR spectra were recorded using the facilities of Zelinsky Institute Shared Center. Sample preparation and the conditions of experiments were described previously [50].

3.6. Anticoagulant Activity Measured in Clotting Time Test

The activated partial thromboplastin time assay for samples **FCS-BA**, **FCS-HS**, **FS-BA** and enoxaparin (Clexane®, Sanofi, Paris, France) was performed using Coatron®M2 coagulation analyzer (TECO, Munich, Germany) as described previously [4,51]. Briefly, a solution (10 µL) with concentration of 75 µg/mL, 37.5 µg/mL or 19.0 µg/mL of a polysaccharide sample (**FCS-BA**, **FCS-HS**, **FS-BA**, or enoxaparin) in purified water was added to 50 µL of normal plasma (Cormay, Poland). The mixture was incubated for 2 min at 37 °C, then 50 µL of APTT reagent (Cormay, Poland) was added, and the mixture was incubated again for 3 min at 37 °C. Then 50 µL of $CaCl_2$ solution (0.025M) was added, and the time of clot formation was recorded. Purified water instead of a saccharide solution was used as a control.

3.7. Effect of Polysaccharides on Thrombin or Factor Xa Inactivation by Antithrombin III

Both experiments were carried out for samples **FCS-BA**, **FCS-HS**, and enoxaparin (Clexane®, Sanofi) at 37 °C in a 96-well plate using MultiscanGo (Thermo, Stockholm, Sweden) as described previously [15]. Briefly, a solution of polysaccharide sample (**FCS-BA**, **FCS-HS**, or enoxaparin) (20 µL) with concentrations of 500, 50, 5, 0.5, 0.05 µg/mL in Tris-HCl buffer (0.15 µM, pH 8.4) was added to 50 µL of a solution of ATIII (0.2 U/mL, Renam, Moscow, Russia) in Tris-HCl buffer. After 3 min incubation an aqueous solution of thrombin (50 µL, 20 U/mL, Renam, Russia) was added, and the mixture was incubated for 2 min. Then a chromogenic substrate (50 µL, 2 mM, Renam, Russia) was added, and the mixture was kept for 2 min. Absorbance of p-nitroaniline (405 nm) was measured.

To 50 µL of a solution of ATIII (0.5 U/mL) in Tris-HCl buffer a solution of a polysaccharide sample (**FCS-BA**, **FCS-HS** or enoxaparin) (20 µL) with concentrations of 500, 50, 5, 0.5, 0.05 µg/mL in Tris-HCl buffer was added. After 3 min incubation an aqueous solution of factor Xa (50 µL, 2 U/mL, Renam, Russia) was added, and the mixture was incubated for 2 min. Then a chromogenic substrate (50 µL, 2 mM, Renam, Russia) was added, and the mixture was kept for 2 min. Absorbance of p-nitroaniline (405 nm) was measured.

3.8. Statistical Analysis

All biological experiments were performed in quadruplicate (n = 4). The results are presented as Mean ± SD. Statistical significance was determined with Student's *t* test. The *p* values less than 0.05 were considered as significant.

4. Conclusions

Fucosylated chondroitin sulfate **FCS-BA** and fucan sulfate **FS-BA** were isolated from the sea cucumber *Bohadschia argus*. Similar preparations **FCS-HS** and **FS-HS** were obtained from *Holothuria (Theelothuria) spinifera*. The main components of both FCSs were GlcA, GalNAc, Fuc and sulfate. Based on the data of NMR spectroscopy, both polysaccharides were shown to contain chondroitin core [→3)-β-D-GalNAc-(1→4)-β-D-GlcA-(1→]$_n$ bearing sulfated fucosyl branches at O-3 of every GlcA residue in the chain. These fucosyl residues were different in pattern of sulfation: **FCS-BA** contained Fuc2S4S, Fuc3S4S and Fuc4S in a ratio of 1:8:2, while **FCS-HS** included Fuc2*S*4*S*, Fuc3*S*4*S* and Fuc4*S* in a ratio of 2:2:1. Moreover, the polysaccharides differ also in GalNAc4*S*6*S* and GalNAc4*S* units content, the ratios being 14:1 for **FCS-BA** and 4:1 for **FCS-HS**. Both polysaccharides demonstrated significant anticoagulant activity in clotting time assay. This activity is probably connected with the ability of these FCSs to potentiate inhibition of thrombin by formation of ternary complex with thrombin and antithrombin III. Such complexation was confirmed previously by computer docking experiments [44]. At the same time activity of these FCSs as inhibitors of Xa was rather low. Fucan sulfate **FS-BA** was shown to be a linear polymer of 4-linked α-L-fucopyranose 3-sulfate, structure being confirmed by NMR spectra of the native polysaccharide and its desulfated derivative. It is interesting to mention that **FS-BA**, despite its rather substantial sulfate content, was practically devoid of anticoagulant activity. **FS-HS** had much more complex NMR spectra, and its structure was tentatively represented as a polysaccharide containing fragments which coincide with **FS-BA**, together with other fragments built up of randomly sulfated alternating 4- and 3-linked α-L-fucopyranose residues.

Supplementary Materials: The following are available online at https://www.mdpi.com/article/10.3390/md20060380/s1, Figure S1: Sea cucumbers (A) *Bohadschia argus* (Jaeger, 1833) and (B) *Holothuria (Theelothuria) spinifera* (Theel, 1886). Figure S2: Agarose gel electrophoresis of polysaccharides. Figure S3. The HSQC NMR spectrum of FCS-BA. Table S1. The data of the 1H and 13C NMR spectra (chemical shifts, ppm) of fucosylated chondroitin sulfates. Figure S4. The HSQC NMR spectrum of FS-BA-AT. Table S2. The data of 1H and 13C NMR spectra (chemical shifts, ppm) of sulfated fucan FS-BA-AT and its desulfated derivative FS-BA-AT-DS. Figure S5. The HSQC NMR spectrum of FS-HS-AT. Table S3. ^{13}C and ^{1}H chemical shifts (δ, ppm) of anomeric atoms in the NMR spectra of fucan sulfate FS-HS-AT (see Figure 6).

Author Contributions: Conceptualization, A.I.U., N.E.N., P.D.T., T.T.T.V. and N.E.U.; methodology, A.I.U., M.I.B. and N.E.U.; analysis, M.I.B., E.A.T., N.E.U., D.T.T., C.T.T.H., A.S.D. and A.S.S.; investigation, M.I.B., N.E.U., S.P.N., A.S.D., A.S.S., T.T.T.V. and A.I.U.; resources, D.T.T. and C.T.T.H.; writing—original draft preparation, N.E.U. and A.I.U.; writing—review and editing, all authors; supervision, A.I.U., N.E.N. and P.D.T. All authors have read and agreed to the published version of the manuscript.

Funding: This work was supported by the Russian Foundation for Basic Research, Russia (Project 21-53-54004 Viet_a) and the Vietnam Academy of Science and Technology (Grant number QTRU01.07/21-22).

Conflicts of Interest: The authors declare no conflict of interest. The funders had no role in the design of the study; in the collection, analyses, or interpretation of data; in the writing of the manuscript, or in the decision to publish the results.

References

1. Pomin, V.H. Holothurian fucosylated chondroitin sulfates. *Mar. Drugs* **2014**, *12*, 232–254. [CrossRef] [PubMed]
2. Ustyuzhanina, N.E.; Bilan, M.I.; Nifantiev, N.E.; Usov, A.I. New insight on the structural diversity of holothurian fucosylated chondroitin sulfates. *Pure Appl. Chem.* **2019**, *91*, 1065–1071. [CrossRef]
3. Gong, P.-X.; Li, Q.-Y.; Wu, Y.-C.; Lu, W.-Y.; Zeng, J.; Li, H.-J. Structural elucidation and antidiabetic activity of fucosylated chondroitin sulfate from sea cucumber *Stichopus japonicas*. *Carbohydr. Polym.* **2021**, *262*, 117969. [CrossRef] [PubMed]
4. Ustyuzhanina, N.E.; Bilan, M.I.; Dmitrenok, A.S.; Shashkov, A.S.; Kusaykin, M.I.; Stonik, V.A.; Nifantiev, N.E.; Usov, A.I. Structure and biological activity of a fucosylated chondroitin sulfate from the sea cucumber *Cucumaria japonica*. *Glycobiology* **2016**, *26*, 449–459. [CrossRef]
5. Ustyuzhanina, N.E.; Bilan, M.I.; Dmitrenok, A.S.; Nifantiev, N.E.; Usov, A.I. Two fucosylated chondroitin sulfates from the sea cucumber *Eupentacta fraudatrix*. *Carbohydr. Polym.* **2017**, *164*, 8–12. [CrossRef]
6. Santos, G.R.C.; Porto, A.C.O.; Soares, P.A.G.; Vilanova, E.; Mourão, P.A.S. Exploring the structure of fucosylated chondroitin sulfate through bottom-up nuclear magnetic resonance and electrospray ionization-high-resolution mass spectrometry approach. *Glycobiology* **2017**, *27*, 625–634. [CrossRef]
7. Vieira, R.P.; Mourão, P.A.S. Occurrence of a unique fucose-branched chondroitin sulfate in the body wall of a sea cucumber. *J. Biol. Chem.* **1988**, *263*, 18176–18183. [CrossRef]
8. Vieira, R.P.; Mulloy, B.; Mourão, P.A.S. Structure of a fucose-branched chondroitin sulfate from sea cucumber. Evidence for the presence of 3-O-sulfo-β-D-glucuronosyl residues. *J. Biol. Chem.* **1991**, *266*, 13530–13536. [CrossRef]

9. Soares, P.A.G.; Ribeiro, K.A.; Valente, A.P.; Capillé, N.V.; Oliveira, S.-N.M.C.G.; Tovar, A.M.F.; Pereira, M.S.; Vilanova, E.; Mourão, P.A.S. A unique fucosylated chondroitin sulfate type II with strikingly homogeneous and neatly distributed α-fucose branches. *Glycobiology* **2018**, *28*, 565–579. [CrossRef] [PubMed]
10. Yin, R.; Zhou, L.; Gao, N.; Lin, L.; Sun, H.; Chen, D.; Cai, Y.; Zuo, Z.; Hu, K.; Huang, S.; et al. Unveiling the disaccharide-branched glycosaminoglycan and anticoagulant potential of its derivatives. *Biomacromolecules* **2021**, *22*, 1244–1255. [CrossRef]
11. Mao, H.; Cai, Y.; Li, S.; Sun, H.; Lin, L.; Pan, Y.; Yang, W.; He, Z.; Chen, R.; Zhou, L.; et al. A new fucosylated glycosaminoglycan containing disaccharide branches from *Acaudina molpadioides*: Unusual structure and anti-intrinsic tenase activity. *Carbohydr. Polym.* **2020**, *245*, 116503. [CrossRef]
12. Li, S.; Zhong, W.; Pan, Y.; Lin, L.; Cai, Y.; Mao, H.; Zhang, T.; Li, S.; Chen, R.; Zhou, L.; et al. Structural characterization and anticoagulant analysis of the novel branched fucosylated glycosaminoglycan from the sea cucumber *Holothuria nobilis*. *Carbohydr. Polym.* **2021**, *269*, 118290. [CrossRef]
13. Yang, J.; Wang, Y.; Jiang, T.; Lv, Z. Novel branch patterns and anticoagulant activity of glycosaminoglycan from sea cucumber *Apostichopus japonicus*. *Int. J. Biol. Macromol.* **2015**, *72*, 911–918. [CrossRef]
14. Ustyuzhanina, N.E.; Bilan, M.I.; Dmitrenok, A.S.; Shashkov, A.S.; Nifantiev, N.E.; Usov, A.I. The structure of a fucosylated chondroitin sulfate from the sea cucumber *Cucumaria frondosa*. *Carbohydr. Polym.* **2017**, *165*, 7–12. [CrossRef]
15. Ustyuzhanina, N.E.; Bilan, M.I.; Dmitrenok, A.S.; Silchenko, A.S.; Grebnev, B.B.; Stonik, V.A.; Nifantiev, N.E.; Usov, A.I. Fucosylated chondroitin sulfates from the sea cucumbers *Paracaudina chilensis* and *Holothuria hilla*: Structures and anticoagulant activity. *Mar. Drugs* **2020**, *18*, 540. [CrossRef]
16. Li, H.; Yuan, Q.; Lv, K.; Ma, H.; Gao, C.; Liu, Y.; Zhang, S.; Zhao, L. Low-molecular-weight fucosylated glycosaminoglycan and its oligosaccharides from sea cucumber as novel anticoagulants: A review. *Carbohydr. Polym.* **2021**, *251*, 117034. [CrossRef]
17. Lu, W.; Yang, Z.; Chen, J.; Wang, D.; Zhang, Y. Recent advances in antiviral activities and potential mechanisms of sulfated polysaccharides. *Carbohydr. Polym.* **2021**, *272*, 118526. [CrossRef]
18. Fonseca, R.J.C.; Mourão, P.A.S. Pharmacological activities of sulfated fucose-rich po0lysaccharides after oral administration: Perspectives for the development of new carbohydrate-based drugs. *Mar. Drugs* **2021**, *19*, 425. [CrossRef]
19. Xu, H.; Zhou, Q.; Liu, B.; Chen, F.; Wang, M. Holothurian fucosylated chondroitin sulfates and their potential benefits for human health: Structures and biological activities. *Carbohydr. Polym.* **2022**, *275*, 118691. [CrossRef]
20. Pereira, M.S.; Mulloy, D.; Mourão, P.A.S. Structure and anticoagulant activity of sulfated fucans. Comparison between the regular, repetitive, and linear fucans from echinoderms with the more heterogeneous and branched polymers from brown algae. *J. Biol. Chem.* **1999**, *274*, 7656–7667. [CrossRef]
21. Ustyuzhanina, N.E.; Bilan, M.I.; Dmitrenok, A.S.; Borodina, E.Y.; Nifantiev, N.E.; Usov, A.I. A highly regular fucan sulfate from the sea cucumber *Stichopus horrens*. *Carbohydr. Res.* **2018**, *456*, 5–9. [CrossRef]
22. Shang, S.; Mou, R.; Zhang, Z.; Gao, N.; Lin, L.; Li, Z.; Wu, M.; Zhao, J. Structural analysis and anticoagulant activities of three highly regular fucan sulfates as novel intrinsic factor Xase inhibitors. *Carbohydr. Polym.* **2018**, *195*, 257–266. [CrossRef]
23. Li, X.; Li, S.; Liu, J.; Lin, L.; Sun, H.; Yang, W.; Cai, Y.; Gao, N.; Zhou, L.; Qin, H.; et al. A regular fucan sulfate from *Stichopus herrmanni* and its peroxide depolymerization: Structure and anticoagulant activity. *Carbohydr. Polym.* **2021**, *256*, 117513. [CrossRef] [PubMed]
24. He, W.; Sun, H.; Su, L.; Zhou, D.; Zhang, X.; Shanggui, D.; Chen, Y. Structure and anticoagulant activity of a sulfated fucan from the sea cucumber *Acaudina leucoprocta*. *Int. J. Biol. Macromol.* **2020**, *164*, 87–94. [CrossRef]
25. Chen, S.; Hu, Y.; Ye, X.; Li, G.; Yu, G.; Xue, C.; Chai, W. Sequence determination and anticoagulant and antithrombotic activities of a novel sulfated fucan isolated from the sea cucumber *Isostichopus badionotus*. *Biochim. Biophys. Acta* **2012**, *1820*, 989–1000. [CrossRef]
26. Yu, L.; Ge, L.; Xue, C.; Chang, Y.; Zhang, C.; Xu, X.; Wang, Y. Structural study of fucoidan from sea cucumber *Acaudina molpadioides*: A fucoidan containing novel tetrafucose repeating unit. *Food Chem.* **2014**, *142*, 197–200. [CrossRef] [PubMed]
27. Yu, L.; Xue, C.; Chang, Y.; Xu, X.; Ge, L.; Liu, G.; Wang, Y. Structure elucidation of fucoidan composed of a novel tetrafucose repeating unit from sea cucumber *Thelenota ananas*. *Food Chem.* **2014**, *146*, 113–119. [CrossRef]
28. Hu, Y.; Li, S.; Li, J.; Ye, X.; Ding, T.; Liu, D.; Chen, J.; Ge, Z.; Chen, S. Identification of a highly sulfated fucoidan from sea cucumber *Pearsonothuria graeffei* with well-repeated tetrasaccharides units. *Carbohydr. Polym.* **2015**, *134*, 808–816. [CrossRef] [PubMed]
29. Chang, Y.; Hu, Y.; Yu, L.; McClements, D.J.; Xu, X.; Liu, G.; Xue, C. Primary structure and chain conformation of fucoidan extracted from sea cucumber *Holothuria tubulosa*. *Carbohydr. Polym.* **2016**, *136*, 1091–1097. [CrossRef] [PubMed]
30. Li, C.; Niu, Q.; Li, S.; Zhang, X.; Liu, C.; Cai, C.; Li, G.; Yu, G. Fucoidan from sea cucumber *Holothuria polii*: Structural elucidation and stimulation of hematopoietic activity. *Int. J. Biol. Macromol.* **2020**, *154*, 1123–1131. [CrossRef]
31. Chen, G.; Yu, L.; Zhang, Y.; Chang, Y.; Liu, Y.; Shen, J.; Xue, C. Utilizing heterologously overexpressed endo-1,3-fucanase to investigate the structure of sulfated fucan from sea cucumber (*Holothuria hilla*). *Carbohydr. Polym.* **2021**, *272*, 118480. [CrossRef]
32. Cai, Y.; Yang, W.; Yin, R.; Zhou, L.; Li, Z.; Wu, M.; Zhao, J. An anticoagulant fucan sulfate with hexasaccharide repeating units from the sea cucumber *Holothuria albiventer*. *Carbohydr. Res.* **2018**, *464*, 12–18. [CrossRef] [PubMed]
33. An, Z.; Zhang, Z.; Zhang, X.; Yang, H.; Li, H.; Liu, M.; Shao, Y.; Zhao, X.; Zhang, H. Oligosaccharide mapping analysis by HILIC-ESI-HCD-MS/MS for structural elucidation of fucoidan from sea cucumber *Holothuria floridana*. *Carbohydr. Polym.* **2022**, *275*, 118694. [CrossRef]

34. Wu, M.; Xu, L.; Zhao, L.; Xiao, C.; Gao, N.; Luo, L.; Yang, L.; Li, Z.; Chen, L.; Zhao, J. Structural analysis and anticoagulant activities of the novel sulfated fucan possessing a regular well-defined repeating unit from sea cucumber. *Mar. Drugs* **2015**, *13*, 2063–2084. [CrossRef]
35. Yu, L.; Xue, C.; Chang, Y.; Hu, Y.; Xu, X.; Ge, L.; Liu, G. Structure and rheological characteristics of fucoidan from sea cucumber *Apostichopus japonicus*. *Food Chem.* **2015**, *180*, 71–76. [CrossRef]
36. Gao, N.; Chen, R.; Mou, R.; Xiang, J.; Zhou, K.; Li, Z.; Zhao, J. Purification, structural characterization and anticoagulant activities of four sulfated polysaccharides from sea cucumber *Holothuria fuscopunctata*. *Int. J. Biol. Macromol.* **2020**, *164*, 3421–3428. [CrossRef] [PubMed]
37. Zheng, W.; Zhou, L.; Lin, L.; Cai, Y.; Sun, H.; Zhao, L.; Gao, N.; Yin, R.; Zhao, J. Physicochemical characteristics and anticoagulant activities of the polysaccharides from sea cucumber *Pattalus mollis*. *Mar. Drugs* **2019**, *17*, 198. [CrossRef] [PubMed]
38. Ma, Y.; Gao, N.; Zuo, Z.; Li, S.; Zheng, W.; Shi, X.; Liu, Q.; Ma, T.; Yin, R.; Li, X.; et al. Five distinct fucan sulfates from sea cucumber *Pattalus mollis*: Purification, structural characterization and anticoagulant activities. *Int. J. Biol. Macromol.* **2021**, *186*, 535–543. [CrossRef]
39. Pham Duc, T.; Ly, B.M.; Usoltseva, R.V.; Shevchenko, N.M.; Rasin, A.B.; Anastyuk, S.D.; Malyarenko, O.S.; Zvyagintseva, T.N.; San, P.T.; Ermakova, S.P. A novel sulfated fucan from Vietnamese sea cucumber *Stichopus variegatus*: Isolation, structure and anticancer activity in vitro. *Int. J. Biol. Macromol.* **2018**, *117*, 1101–1109.
40. Yin, R.; Zhou, L.; Gao, N.; Li, Z.; Zhao, L.; Shang, F.; Wu, M.; Zhao, J. Oligosaccharides from depolymerized fucosylated glycosaminoglycan: Structures and minimum size for intrinsic factor Xase complex inhibition. *J. Biol. Chem.* **2018**, *293*, 14089–14099. [CrossRef]
41. Pomin, V.H. NMR structural determination of unique invertebrate glycosaminoglycans endowed with medical properties. *Carbohydr. Res.* **2015**, *413*, 41–50. [CrossRef]
42. Ustyuzhanina, N.E.; Bilan, M.I.; Nifantiev, N.E.; Usov, A.I. Structural analysis of holothurian fucosylated chondroitin sulfates: Degradation versus non-destructive approach. *Carbohydr. Res.* **2019**, *476*, 6–11. [CrossRef]
43. Mourão, P.A.S. Perspective on the use of sulfated polysaccharides from marine organisms as a source of new antithrombotic drugs. *Mar. Drugs* **2015**, *13*, 2770–2784. [CrossRef] [PubMed]
44. Gerbst, A.G.; Ustyuzhanina, N.E.; Nifantiev, N.E. Computational study of the possible formation of the ternary complex between thrombin, antithrombin III and fucosylated chondroitin sulfates. *Mendeleev Commun.* **2015**, *25*, 420–421. [CrossRef]
45. Bilan, M.I.; Grachev, A.A.; Ustuzhanina, N.E.; Shashkov, A.S.; Nifantiev, N.E.; Usov, A.I. Structure of a fucoidan from the brown seaweed *Fucus evanescens* C.Ag. *Carbohydr. Res.* **2002**, *337*, 719–730. [CrossRef]
46. Bilan, M.I.; Zakharova, A.N.; Grachev, A.A.; Shashkov, A.S.; Nifantiev, N.E.; Usov, A.I. Polysaccharides of algae: 60. Fucoidan from the Pacific brown alga *Analipus japonicus* (Harv.) Winne (Ectocarpales, Scytosiphonaceae). *Russ. J. Bioorg. Chem.* **2007**, *33*, 38–46. [CrossRef] [PubMed]
47. Usov, A.I.; Bilan, M.I.; Klochkova, N.G. Polysaccharides of algae: 48. Polysaccharide composition of several calcareous red algae: Isolation of alginate from *Corallina pilulifera* P. et R. (Rhodophyta, Corallinaceae). *Bot. Mar.* **1995**, *38*, 43–51. [CrossRef]
48. Guo, X.; Condra, M.; Kimura, K.; Berth, G.; Dautzenberg, H.; Dubin, P.L. Determination of molecular weight of heparin by size exclusion chromatography with universal calibration. *Anal. Biochem.* **2003**, *312*, 33–39. [CrossRef]
49. Dubois, M.; Gilles, K.A.; Hamilton, J.K.; Rebers, P.A.; Smith, F. Colorimetric method for determination of sugars and related substances. *Anal Chem.* **1956**, *28*, 350–356. [CrossRef]
50. Ustyuzhanina, N.E.; Bilan, M.I.; Dmitrenok, A.S.; Tsvetkova, E.A.; Shashkov, A.S.; Stonik, V.A.; Nifantiev, N.E.; Usov, A.I. Structural characterization of fucosylated chondroitin sulfates from sea cucumbers *Apostichopus japonicus* and *Actinopyga mauritiana*. *Carbohydr. Polym.* **2016**, *153*, 399–405. [CrossRef]
51. Ustyuzhanina, N.E.; Bilan, M.I.; Dmitrenok, A.S.; Borodina, E.Y.; Stonik, V.A.; Nifantiev, N.E.; Usov, A.I. A highly regular fucosylated chondroitin sulfate from the sea cucumber *Massinium magnum*: Structure and effects on coagulation. *Carbohydr. Polym.* **2017**, *167*, 20–26. [CrossRef] [PubMed]

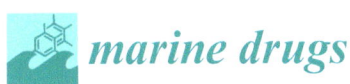

Article

Disulfated Ophiuroid Type Steroids from the Far Eastern Starfish *Pteraster marsippus* and Their Cytotoxic Activity on the Models of 2D and 3D Cultures

Alla A. Kicha *, Anatoly I. Kalinovsky, Timofey V. Malyarenko, Olesya S. Malyarenko, Svetlana P. Ermakova, Roman S. Popov, Valentin A. Stonik and Natalia V. Ivanchina

G.B. Elyakov Pacific Institute of Bioorganic Chemistry, Far Eastern Branch of the Russian Academy of Sciences, Pr. 100-let Vladivostoku 159, 690022 Vladivostok, Russia; kaaniw@piboc.dvo.ru (A.I.K.); malyarenko-tv@mail.ru (T.V.M.); malyarenko.os@gmail.com (O.S.M.); svetlana_ermakova@hotmail.com (S.P.E.); prs_90@mail.ru (R.S.P.); stonik@piboc.dvo.ru (V.A.S.); ivanchina@piboc.dvo.ru (N.V.I.)
* Correspondence: kicha@piboc.dvo.ru; Tel.: +7-423-2312-360; Fax: +7-423-2314-050

Citation: Kicha, A.A.; Kalinovsky, A.I.; Malyarenko, T.V.; Malyarenko, O.S.; Ermakova, S.P.; Popov, R.S.; Stonik, V.A.; Ivanchina, N.V. Disulfated Ophiuroid Type Steroids from the Far Eastern Starfish *Pteraster marsippus* and Their Cytotoxic Activity on the Models of 2D and 3D Cultures. *Mar. Drugs* **2022**, *20*, 164. https://doi.org/10.3390/md20030164

Academic Editor: Marie-Lise Bourguet-Kondracki

Received: 31 January 2022
Accepted: 22 February 2022
Published: 24 February 2022

Publisher's Note: MDPI stays neutral with regard to jurisdictional claims in published maps and institutional affiliations.

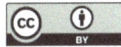

Copyright: © 2022 by the authors. Licensee MDPI, Basel, Switzerland. This article is an open access article distributed under the terms and conditions of the Creative Commons Attribution (CC BY) license (https://creativecommons.org/licenses/by/4.0/).

Abstract: New steroidal 3β,21-disulfates (**2–4**), steroidal 3β,22-disulfate (**5**), and the previously known related steroidal 3β,21-disulfate (**1**) were isolated from the ethanolic extract of the Far Eastern starfish *Pteraster marsippus*, collected off Urup Island in the Sea of Okhotsk. The structures of these compounds were determined by intensive NMR and HRESIMS techniques as well as by chemical transformations. Steroids **2** and **3** have an oxo-group in the tetracyclic nucleus at position C-7 and differ from each other by the presence of the 5(6)-double bond. The Δ^{24}-22-sulfoxycholestane side chain of the steroid **5** has not been found previously in the starfish or ophiuroid steroids. The cytotoxic activities of **1**, **4**, **5**, and the mixture of **2** and **3** were determined on the models of 2D and 3D cultures of human epithelial kidney cells (HEK293), melanoma cells (SK-MEL-28), small intestine carcinoma cells (HuTu80), and breast carcinoma cells (ZR-75-1). The mixture of **2** and **3** revealed a significant inhibitory effect on the cell viability of human breast carcinoma ZR-75-1 cells, but other tested compounds were less effective.

Keywords: disulfated steroids; NMR spectra; starfish; *Pteraster marsippus*; cytotoxic activity; 3D culture

1. Introduction

Marine sulfated steroids are often found in representatives of two classes of marine echinoderms, namely ophiuroids and particularly starfish (the phylum Echinodermata), and in sponges (the phylum Porifera) [1,2]. These compounds have been reported to exhibit various biological activities, including anticancer, antimicrobial, cardiovascular, and antifouling properties [3]. Steroidal monosulfates, encountered in different species of starfish, are represented by sterol sulfates and polyhydroxysteroids, containing from four to nine hydroxy groups and a sulfate group at different positions of the tetracyclic core and side chains. In that position, the polyhydroxysteroids were found in both free and glycosylated forms with one to three monosaccharide units and also were found in sulfated form. Moreover, the most common steroidal oligoglycosides of starfish are known as classical asterosaponins and contain an oligosaccharide chain, attached to C-6 and including five or six monosaccharide residues and a sulfate group at C-3 [4–10]. On the other hand, characteristic secondary metabolites of ophiuroids are mainly steroidal disulfates that differ from other sulfated compounds of echinoderms in some structural peculiarities, namely in the presence of sulfoxy groups at 3α and 21 positions in 5β-, or Δ^5-, and very rarely 5α-cholestane cores. It is of interest, that similar steroidal disulfates, containing sulfoxy groups at 3β (or 3α) and 21 positions in 5α-, or Δ^5-cholestane nuclei were found in some species of the Pterasteridae family belonging to the Asteroidea class. From six species of starfish belonging to the Pterasteridae family, in particular *Euretaster insignis* [11], *Pteraster* sp. and *Pteraster tessellatus* [12,13],

Diplopteraster multipes [14], *Pteraster pulvillus* [15], and *Pteraster obscurus* [16], nine new disulfated steroidal compounds and six compounds studied as desulfated derivatives, obtained after solvolytic desulfation have been structurally described. At the same time, the polyhydroxylated steroids and asterosaponins, common in starfish, were absent in the studied starfish species belonging to the family Pterasteridae. Based on the structural similarity of steroidal disulfates isolated from this family of starfish and from different ophiuroids, it was assumed that there is a closer phylogenetic relationship between the Asteroidea and Ophiuroidea classes than other classes of Echinodermata [13].

At the present time, structural studies on steroidal disulfates from starfish and ophiuroids are somewhat ahead of the investigation of their biological activities. Nevertheless, the steroidal metabolites of ophiuroids were reported to inhibit the protein tyrosine kinase (PTK) [17], to show antiviral activity against HIV-1 and HIV-2 [18], and to be potent antagonists of farnesoid-X-receptor (FXR), a ligand-regulated transcription factor involved in the supporting of the lipid and glucose homeostasis in mammals [19]. These compounds enhanced oxygen-dependent metabolism, increased adhesive and phagocytic properties, induced the expression of pro-inflammatory cytokines TNF-α and IL-8 in neutrophils, and enhanced the production of antibody-forming cells in the mouse spleen [20]. Biological activities of steroidal disulfates from Pterasteridae starfish were less studied, but hemolytic activity on mouse erythrocytes was reported [15]. Thereby, the investigation of the biological activities of steroidal disulfates of starfish and ophiuroids requires further continuation.

In the present article, we describe the results of our study on the fraction of sulfated steroids from the ethanolic extract of the Far Eastern starfish *Pteraster marsippus* Fisher, 1910 (order Velatida, family Pterasteridae) collected by trawling at a depth of 84–88 m in the Sea of Okhotsk near Urup Island. We have isolated and structurally elucidated four new disulfated steroids **2–5** along with one previously known related compound **1**. Additionally, the cytotoxic activities of **1**, **4**, **5**, and the mixture of **2** and **3** on the models of 2D and 3D cancer cell cultures have been determined.

2. Results

2.1. The Isolation and Structure Elucidation of Compounds 1–5 from P. marsippus

The ethanol extract of the starfish *P. marsippus* was separated by column chromatography on Polychrome 1, Si gel, and Florisil followed by reversed-phase HPLC on semi-preparative Discovery C18 and analytical YMC-Pack Pro C18 columns to give four new disulfated steroids **2–5** along with one previously known related compound **1** (Figure 1).

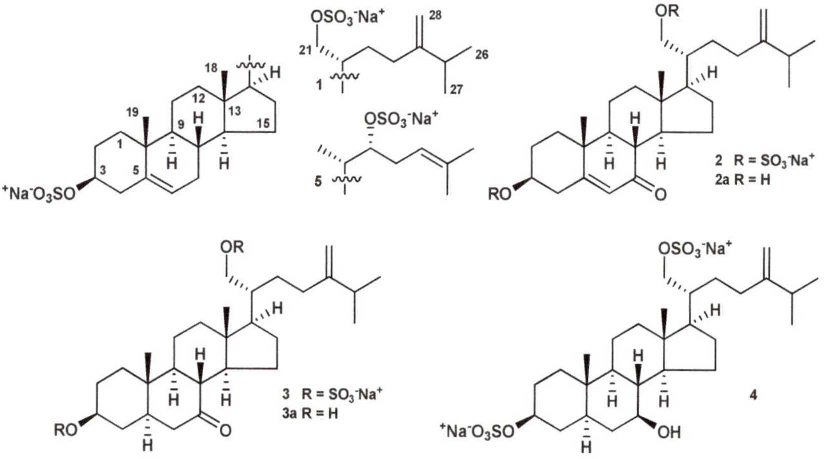

Figure 1. Structures of compounds **1–5** isolated from *P. marsippus*.

The molecular formula of steroid **1** was established to be $C_{28}H_{44}Na_2O_8S_2$ from the $[M - Na]^-$ and $[M - 2Na]^{2-}$ ion peaks at m/z 595.2388 and 286.1253 in the (−)HRESIMS, respectively, and from the $[M + Na]^+$ sodium adduct ion peak at m/z 641.2154 in the (+)HRESIMS (Figure S1). The presence of sulfate groups in **1** is confirmed by HRESIMS as well as by the presence in the (−)HRESIMS/MS spectrum of $[M-2Na]^{2-}$ ion of fragment ions at m/z 96.9610 $[HSO_4]^-$, 136.9917 $[C_3H_5O_4S]^-$, 391.1958 $[M - Na - NaHSO_4 - C_6H_{12}]^-$, 459.2584 $[M - Na - NaHSO_4 - CH_4]^-$, and 475.2898 $[M - Na - NaHSO_4]^-$. The ^1H- and ^{13}C-NMR spectroscopic data attributable to the tetracyclic nucleus of **1** revealed the proton and carbon chemical shifts of two angular methyl groups CH_3-18 (δ_H 0.75 s, δ_C 12.5) and CH_3-19 (δ_H 1.03 s, δ_C 19.7), an oxygenated methine CH-3 (δ_H 4.13 m, δ_C 79.9), and the 5(6) double bond (δ_H 5.38 m; δ_C 141.7, 123.2). The proton and carbon resonances of CH_3-18, CH_3-19, CH-3, C-5, CH-6 and the broad multiplet of H-3 (ΔW = 39.3 Hz) indicated a Δ^5-3β-sulfoxy steroidal nucleus in **1** [11].

The proton and carbon signals belonging to the side chain of **1** showed the presence of two secondary methyls CH_3-26 [δ_H 1.02 d (J = 6.8); δ_C 22.4] and CH_3-27 [δ_H 1.03 d (J = 6.8); δ_C 22.5], an distinctive oxygenated methylene CH_2-21 [δ_H 4.21 dd (J = 9.8, 3.7), 3.94 dd (J = 9.8, 6.4); δ_C 69.3], and the 24(28) double bond [δ_H 4.71 br s, 4.68 br d (J = 1.3); δ_C 157.9, 106.9]. These data testified about the $\Delta^{24(28)}$-21-sulfoxy-24-methylcholestane side chain in **1** [11,16]. An analysis of the COSY, HSQC, HMBC, and ROESY spectra supported the proposed structure of tetracyclic and side-chain moieties and allowed us to define all the proton and carbon signals in **1** (Tables 1 and 2, Figures S2–S7). The COSY and HSQC experiments showed a spin coupling system of the protons at C-1 to C-4, C-6 to C-12 through C-11, C-14 to C-17, C-17 to C-21 through C-20, C-20 to C-23, and at C-25 to C-26 and C-27 (Figures S4 and S5). The overall steroid structure of **1** was confirmed by the key HMBC correlations H_3-18/C-12, C-13, C-14, C-17; H_3-19/C-1, C-5, C-9, C-10; H_2-21/C-17, C-20; H-25/C-26, C-27; H_3-26/C-24; and H_2-28/C-25, C-26 (Figure S6). The presence of the key ROESY cross-peaks Hα-4/H-6; H-9/Hα-1, Hα-7; Hα-16/H-17; Hβ-16/H-20; H_3-18/H-8, Hβ-12, Hβ-15, Hβ-16; H_3-19/Hβ-1, Hβ-2, Hβ-4; H-28/H_2-22, H_2-23; and H'-28/H-25, H_3-26, H_3-27 exhibited the $\Delta^{5,24(28)}$-24-methylcholestane skeleton in **1** (Figure S7). The 20R configuration was determined based on the ROESY correlations of Hβ-12/H-20, H_3-18/H-20, H_2-21 [21] and the coupling constants and chemical shifts of the methylene group CH_2-21, which were close to similar values in the ^1H- and ^{13}C-NMR spectra of related previously studied (20R)-21-sulfoxysteroids from starfish and ophiuroids [11,13–16,22]. Thus, the structure (20R)-24-methylcholesta-5,24(28)-diene-3β,21-diyl disulfate disodium salt was assigned for **1**. Compound **1** was previously found in the mixture of disulfated 3β,21-dihydroxysteroids from the starfish *Euretaster insignis* [11]. Its structure was proposed on the basis of the structure definition of the desulfated derivative, (20R)-24-methylcholesta-5,24(28)-diene-3,21-diol, obtained by solvolysis of the steroid mixture followed by HPLC separation. The ^1H- and ^{13}C-NMR spectroscopic data of **1** itself are presented here for the first time.

An attempt to separate compounds **2** and **3** using repeated reversed-phase HPLC were failed. However, structures of **2** and **3** were established in the mixture by the thorough analysis of the 1D and 2D NMR spectra, including ^1H- and ^{13}C-NMR, 1D TOCSY, COSY, HSQC, HMBC, and ROESY experiments (Figures S8–S13). The molecular formula of steroid **2** was determined to be $C_{28}H_{42}Na_2O_9S_2$ from the $[M - Na]^-$ and $[M - 2Na]^{2-}$ ion peaks at m/z 609.2177 and 293.1148 in the (−)HRESIMS, respectively, and from the $[M + Na]^+$ sodium adduct ion peak at m/z 655.1943 in the (+)HRESIMS (Figure S14). The presence of sulfate groups in **2** is confirmed by HRESIMS as well as by the presence in the (−)HRESIMS/MS spectrum of $[M-2Na]^{2-}$ of fragment ions at m/z 96.9612 $[HSO_4]^-$, 136.9917 $[C_3H_5O_4S]^-$, 405.1745 $[M - Na - NaHSO_4 - C_6H_{12}]^-$ and 489.2682 $[M - Na - NaHSO_4]^-$. The molecular formula of steroid **3** was established to be $C_{28}H_{44}Na_2O_9S_2$ from the $[M - Na]^-$ and $[M - 2Na]^{2-}$ ion peaks at m/z 611.2299 and 294.1222 in the (−)HRESIMS, respectively, and from the $[M + Na]^+$ sodium adduct ion peak at m/z 657.2077 in the (+)HRESIMS (Figure S14). The presence of sulfate groups in **3** is confirmed by HRESIMS as well as by the presence in the (−)HRESIMS/MS spectrum of [M − 2Na]$^{2−}$ of fragment ions at m/z 96.9612 [HSO$_4$]$^−$, 136.9917 [C$_3$H$_5$O$_4$S]$^−$, 407.1891 [M − Na − NaHSO$_4$ − C$_6$H$_{12}$]$^−$, and 491.2825 [M − Na − NaHSO$_4$]$^−$. The detailed comparison of the ^{1}H- and ^{13}C-NMR, mass spectra of **1**, and the mixture of **2** and **3** clearly indicated that these compounds have the same Δ$^{24(28)}$-21-sulfoxy-24-methylcholestane side chain, and steroids **2** and **3** differ from **1** by the existence of an additional oxo-group in tetracyclic pattern (Tables 1 and 2). Moreover, it followed from the chemical shifts and intensities of the proton signals in the ^{1}H-NMR spectrum that **2** unlike **3** has a supplementary double bond in the steroidal nucleus, which agreed with the molecular mass difference of 2 amu between **2** and **3** in the mass-spectra.

The proton and carbon resonances of two angular methyl groups CH$_3$-18 (δ_H 0.75 s, δ_C 12.7) and CH$_3$-19 (δ_H 1.24 s, δ_C 17.6), an oxygenated methine CH-3 (δ_H 4.26 m, δ_C 78.0), a 5(6) double bond [δ_H 5.68 br d (J = 1.6); δ_C 168.3, 126.8], and a 7-oxo group (δ_C 204.4) attributable to the tetracyclic moiety of **2** were observed in the ^{1}H- and ^{13}C-NMR spectra. These values of chemical shifts allowed us to suppose a Δ^5-7-oxo-3β-sulfoxy steroidal nucleus in **2**. The COSY and HSQC experiments led to the identification of the proton sequences at C-1 to C-4, C-8 to C-12 through C-11, C-8 to C-17 through C-14, C-17 to C-21 through C-20, C-20 to C-23, and at C-25 to C-26 and C-27 (Figure 2). Since it is difficult to identify some proton signals in the ^{1}H-NMR spectrum of a mixture of two compounds only using 2D NMR experiments, the irradiation of protons Hα-2, Hβ-4, H-6, and H-8 of **2** in the 1D TOCSY experiments was additionally performed, which gave enhancing signals of the neighboring protons H$_2$-1, Hβ-2, H-3, and H$_2$-4; H$_2$-1, H$_2$-2, H-3, and Hα-4; H-3 and H$_2$-4; and H-9, H-11, H-14, and Hβ-15, respectively. The key HMBC correlations H-4/C-5, C-6; H-8/C-7, C-9; H-17/C-20, C-21, C-22; H$_3$-18/C-12, C-13, C-14, C-17; H$_3$-19/C-1, C-5, C-9, C-10; and H$_3$-26/C-24, C-25, C-28; and the key ROESY correlations Hα-1/H-9; Hα-4/H-6; Hβ-12/H$_2$-21; H-14/Hα-16; H$_3$-18/H-8, Hβ-11, H-20, H$_2$-21; H$_3$-19/Hβ-1, Hβ-2, Hβ-4, H-8, Hβ-11; H-28/H$_2$-22, H$_2$-23; and H′-28/H-25, H$_3$-26, H$_3$-27 exhibited a 3β,21-disulfoxy-7-oxo pattern in the Δ$^{5,24(28)}$-24-methylcholestane skeleton in **2** (Figures 2 and 3). Based on the above-mentioned data, the structure of **2** was defined as (20R)-7-oxo-24-methylcholesta-5,24(28)-diene-3β,21-diyl disulfate disodium salt.

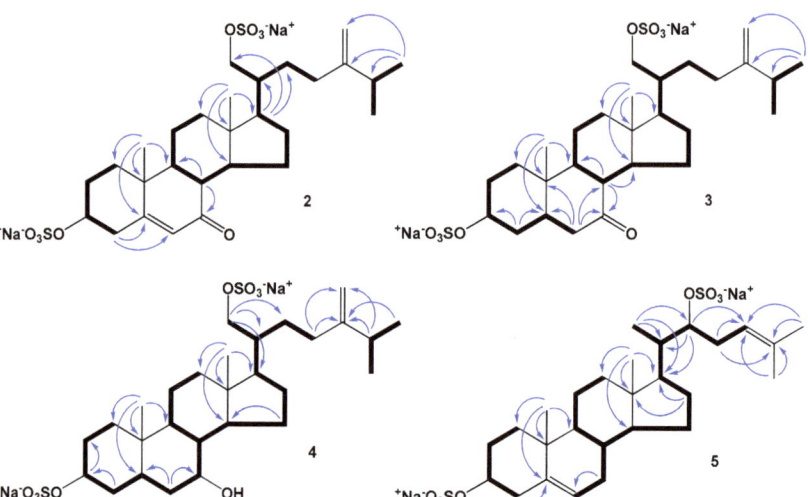

Figure 2. COSY and key HMBC correlations of compounds **2–5**.

Table 1. ^{1}H-NMR (700.13 MHz) chemical shifts of compounds **1–5** in CD$_3$OD, with δ in ppm and J values in Hz [a].

Position	1	2	3	4	5
1β α	1.89 dt (13.8, 3.7) 1.11 m	2.02 dt (13.9, 3.7) 1.26 td (13.9, 3.5)	1.81 dt (13.9, 3.5) 1.07 td (13.9, 3.7)	1.76 dt (13.8, 3.7) 0.98 td (13.8, 3.8)	1.89 dt (13.5, 3.5) 1.11 m
2α β	2.05 m 1.63 m	2.15 m 1.76 m	2.06 m 1.60 m	2.02 m 1.53 m	2.05 m 1.62 m
3	4.13 m (ΔW = 39.3 Hz)	4.26 m	4.25 m	4.24 m	4.13 m
4α β	2.53 ddd (13.2, 4.8, 2.2) 2.34 td (13.2, 2.0)	2.79 ddd (14.0, 5.0, 2.3) 2.54 ddd (14.0, 11.8, 1.9)	1.86 m 1.57 m	1.81 m 1.43 m	2.53 ddd (13.4, 4.8, 2.2) 2.33 m
5	–	–	1.52 m	1.22 m	–
6β α	5.38 m	5.68 br d (1.6)	2.46 t (12.3) 1.94 dd (12.3, 3.2)	1.33 t (12.8) 1.55 m	5.38 m
7β α	1.97 m 1.56 m	–	–	3.25 td (10.6, 5.2)	1.96 m 1.54 m
8	1.48 m	2.31 dd (12.6, 10.7)	2.47 m	1.40 m	1.47 m
9	0.97 td (11.7, 4.6)	1.53 m	1.09 m	0.71 m	0.96 m
10	–	–	–	–	–
11α β	1.57 m 1.04 m	1.63 m	1.62 m 1.55 m	1.58 m 1.35 m	1.54 m 1.05 m
12β α	2.04 m 1.25 td (13.0, 4.2)	2.07 m 1.22 m	2.02 m 1.16 m	1.99 m 1.19 m	2.01 dt (12.8, 3.5) 1.23 td (12.8, 4.2)
13	–	–	–	–	–
14	1.06 m	1.35 m	1.47 m	1.19 m	1.09 m
15α β	1.64 m 1.13 m	2.40 m 1.28 m	2.20 m 1.02 m	1.90 m 1.48 m	1.61 m 1.09 m
16α β	1.87 m 1.37 m	1.90 m 1.39 m	1.88 m 1.35 m	1.83 m 1.34 m	2.22 m 1.16 m
17	1.48 m	1.48 m	1.48 m	1.43 m	1.63 m
18	0.75 s	0.75 s	0.72 s	0.73 s	0.70 s
19	1.03 s	1.24 s	1.12 s	0.86 s	1.02 s
20	1.72 m	1.69 m	1.69 m	1.68 m	1.58 m
21	4.21 dd (9.8, 3.7) 3.94 dd (9.8, 6.4)	4.18 dd (9.6, 4.0) 3.99 dd (9.6, 5.7)	4.17 dd (9.6, 4.1) 3.96 dd (9.6, 5.7)	4.18 dd (9.7, 3.8) 3.94 dd (9.7, 6.2)	0.96 d (6.7)
22	1.64 m 1.48 m	1.64 m 1.49 m	1.64 m 1.49 m	1.64 m 1.48 m	4.36 dd (10.6, 4.5)
23	2.17 ddd (15.0, 11.1, 4.6) 2.04 m	2.19 m 2.02 m	2.19 m 2.02 m	2.17 m 2.03 m	2.66 m 2.34 m
24	–	–	–	–	5.05 t (7.7)
25	2.25 quin (6.7)	2.25 m	2.25 m	2.25 quin	–
26	1.02 d (6.8)	1.02 d (6.8)	1.02 d (6.8)	1.02 d (6.8)	1.69 s
27	1.03 d (6.8)	1.03 d (6.8)	1.03 d (6.8)	1.03 d (6.8)	1.65 s
28	4.71 br s 4.68 br d (1.3)	4.71 br d (1.2) 4.69 br d (1.2)	4.71 br d (1.2) 4.69 br d (1.2)	4.71 br s 4.68 br d (1.5)	

[a] Assignments from 700.13 MHz COSY, HSQC, HMBC (8 Hz), and ROESY (250 msec) data; s, singlet; d, doublet; t, triplet; m, multiplet; br s, broad singlet; br d, broad doublet; dd, doublet of doublets; ddd, doublet of doublet of doublets; dt, doublet of triplets; quin, quintet.

Table 2. ^{13}C-NMR (176.04 MHz) chemical shifts of compounds 1–5 in CD$_3$OD.

Position	1	2	3	4	5
1	38.5	37.4	37.1	38.1	38.4
2	30.0	29.6	29.4	29.7	30.0
3	79.9	78.0	78.8	79.4	79.9
4	40.4	40.1	36.2	35.9	40.4
5	141.7	168.3	48.2	43.6	141.6
6	123.2	126.8	46.9	39.9	123.3
7	33.0	204.4	214.3	75.7	33.0
8	33.3	46.6	51.1	44.1	33.3
9	51.7	51.4	56.7	54.0	51.6
10	37.7	39.7	37.0	36.0	37.7
11	22.1	22.2	22.9	22.6	22.1
12	40.2	39.1	39.2	40.5	41.0
13	43.4	44.2	43.6	44.5	43.3
14	58.0	51.3	50.4	57.3	58.0
15	25.2	27.3	25.9	27.9	25.4
16	28.7	28.9	28.8	29.0	29.2
17	51.8	50.7	50.7	51.2	53.2
18	12.5	12.7	12.6	12.9	12.1
19	19.7	17.6	12.0	12.7	19.7
20	41.1	41.0	41.0	41.0	39.4
21	69.3	69.2	69.2	69.4	12.8
22	29.7	29.8	29.8	29.7	82.6
23	31.6	31.8	31.8	31.8	31.7
24	157.9	157.8	157.8	157.9	121.2
25	34.9	34.8	34.8	34.9	134.8
26	22.4	22.3	22.4	22.3	26.0
27	22.5	22.5	22.5	22.5	18.1
28	106.9	107.0	107.8	106.9	

The ^{1}H- and ^{13}C-NMR spectroscopic data belonging to the steroidal nucleus of 3 displayed the proton and carbon resonances of two angular methyl groups CH$_3$-18 (δ_H 0.72 s, δ_C 12.6) and CH$_3$-19 (δ_H 1.12 s, δ_C 12.0), an oxygenated methine CH-3 (δ_H 4.25 m, δ_C 78.8), and a 7-oxo group (δ_C 214.3). These chemical resonances and the absence of a 5(6) double bond corresponded to a 7-oxo-3β-sulfoxy tetracyclic pattern in 3 (Tables 1 and 2). The COSY and HSQC experiments revealed a spin coupling system of the protons at C-1 to C-6, C-8 to C-12 through C-11, C-8 to C-17 through C-14, C-17 to C-21 through C-20, C-20 to C-23, and at C-25 to C-26 and C-27 (Figure 2). In addition, the irradiation of protons Hβ-1 and Hα-6 of 3 in the 1D TOCSY experiments gave the chemical shifts of neighboring protons: Hα-1, Hα-2, H-3, Hα-4, and H$_2$-6; H$_2$-1, Hα-2, H-3, Hα-4, and Hβ-6, respectively. In the HMBC spectrum the correlations H-4/C-3, C-5; H-6/C-5, C-7, C-8, C-10; H-8/C-9, C-14; H$_3$-18/C-12, C-13, C-14, C-17; H$_3$-19/C-1, C-5, C-9, C-10; and H$_3$-26/C-24, C-25, C-28, and, in the ROESY spectrum, the cross-peaks Hβ-12/H$_2$-21; Hβ-17/H-20; H$_3$-18/H-8, Hβ-11, H-20, H$_2$-21; H$_3$-19/Hβ-1, Hβ-2, Hβ-4, H-8; H-28/H$_2$-22, H$_2$-23; and H′-28/H-25, H$_3$-26, H$_3$-27 indicated a 3β,21-disulfoxy-7-oxo substitution in the $\Delta^{24(28)}$-24-methyl-5αcholestane skeleton in **3** (Figures 2 and 3). Thus, the structure of **3** was determined as (20*R*)-7-oxo-24-methyl-5α-cholest-24(28)-ene-3β,21-diyl disulfate disodium salt. Evaluation of the intensities of the CH$_3$-18 and CH$_3$-19 signals in the ^{1}H- and ^{13}C-NMR spectra showed a ratio **2** and **3** in the mixture of approximately 1:1 for with a slight advantage of **2**.

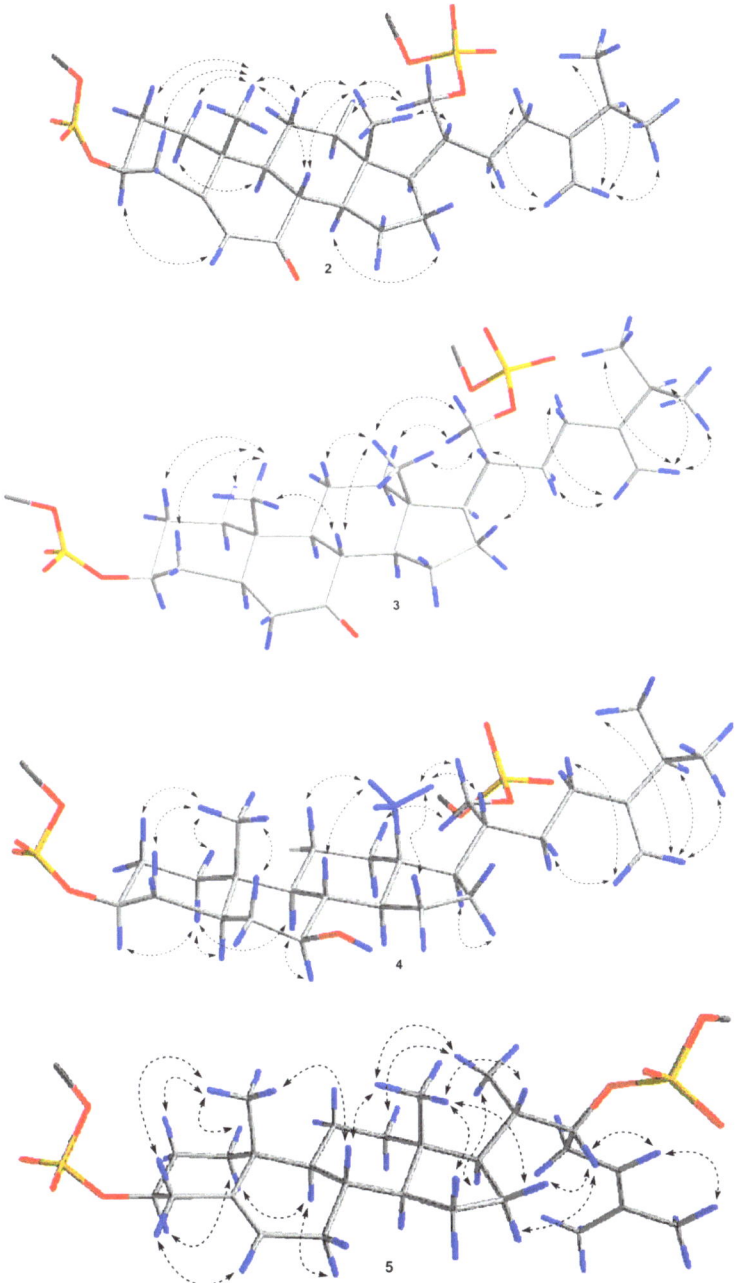

Figure 3. Key ROESY correlations for compounds **2**–**5**. Colors reveal the atoms of hydrogen (blue), oxygen (red), sulfur (yellow), and carbon (grey) and their bonds.

Solvolysis of the mixture of **2** and **3** in dioxane/pyridine afforded the mixture of desulfated derivatives **2a** and **3a**, which were separated by HPLC on YMC-Pack-Pro C18 column to give individual compounds. The molecular formula of desulfated steroid **2a** was established to be $C_{28}H_{44}O_3$ from the $[M - H]^-$ ion peak at m/z 427.3215 in the (−)HRESIMS and from the $[M + Na]^+$ sodium adduct ion peak at m/z 451.3175 in the (+)HRESIMS, respectively (Figure S15). Along with mass spectra, the presence of the proton and carbon signals characteristic of two angular methyl groups CH_3-18 (δ_H 0.73 s, δ_C 12.7) and CH_3-19 (δ_H 1.23 s, δ_C 17.8), an oxygenated methine CH-3 (δ_H 3.54 m, δ_C 71.2), a 5(6) double bond [δ_H 5.65 m; δ_C 169.1, 126.3], a 7-oxo group (δ_C 204.6), an oxygenated methylene CH_2-21 [δ_H 3.69 dd (J = 10.7, 4.2), 3.54 dd (J = 10.7, 5.5); δ_C 63.2], and a 24(28) double bond [δ_H 4.73 br s, 4.69 br d (J = 1.4); δ_C 157.8, 106.9], two secondary methyls CH_3-26 [δ_H 1.03 d (J = 6.8); δ_C 22.5] and CH_3-27 [δ_H 1.03 d (J = 6.8); δ_C 22.3] in the ^{1}H- and ^{13}C-NMR spectra revealed the structure of **2a** as (20R)-7-oxo-24-methylcholesta-5,24(28)-diene-3β,21-diol. The molecular formula of desulfated steroid **3a** was established to be $C_{28}H_{46}O_3$ from the $[M - H]^-$ ion peak at m/z 429.3376 in the (−)HRESIMS and from the $[M + Na]^+$ sodium adduct ion peak at m/z 453.3333 in the (+)HRESIMS, respectively (Figure S16). The ^{1}H- and ^{13}C-NMR spectra of **3a** contained signals for two angular methyl groups CH_3-18 (δ_H 0.70 s, δ_C 12.8) and CH_3-19 (δ_H 1.11 s, δ_C 12.1), an oxygenated methine CH-3 (δ_H 3.52 m, δ_C 71.3), a 7-oxo group (δ_C 214.4), an oxygenated methylene CH_2-21 [δ_H 3.68 dd (J = 10.9, 3.8), 3.53 dd (J = 10.9, 5.6); δ_C 63.2], and a 24(28) double bond [δ_H 4.72 br s, 4.68 br d (J = 1.4); δ_C 157.5, 106.9], two secondary methyls CH_3-26 [δ_H 1.03 d (J = 6.7); δ_C 22.5] and CH_3-27 [δ_H 1.03 d (J = 6.7); δ_C 22.3] that matched structure **3a** as (20R)-7-oxo-24-methyl-5α-cholest-24(28)-ene-3β,21-diol. All the proton and carbon signals belonging to **2a** and **3a** were derived from COSY, HSQC, HMBC, and ROESY experiments (Table 3, Figures S17–S29). The isolation of individual desulfated derivatives **2a** and **3a** additionally confirmed the structures of steroids **2** and **3**.

The molecular formula of steroid **4** was established to be $C_{28}H_{46}Na_2O_9S_2$ from the $[M - Na]^-$ and $[M - 2Na]^{2-}$ ion peaks at m/z 613.2483 and m/z 295.1304 in the (−)HRESIMS, respectively, and from the $[M + Na]^+$ sodium adduct ion peak at m/z 659.2243 in the (+)HRESIMS (Figure S30). The presence of sulfate groups in **4** is confirmed by HRESIMS as well as by the presence in the (−)HRESIMS/MS spectrum of $[M - 2Na]^{2-}$ of fragment ions at m/z 96.9604 $[HSO_4]^-$, 136.9909 $[C_3H_5O_4S]^-$, 191.0380 $[C_7H_{11}O_4S]^-$, 409.2047 $[M - Na - NaHSO_4 - C_6H_{12}]$, and 493.2987 $[M - Na - NaHSO_4]^-$. The detailed comparison of the ^{1}H- and ^{13}C-NMR spectroscopic data of compounds **4** and **3** revealed that the proton and carbon resonances belonging to the steroidal A, C, and D rings and side chains of **4** are close to those of **3**, indicating the 3β-hydroxy substitution in tetracyclic nucleus and $\Delta^{24(28)}$-21-sulfoxy-24-methyl-cholestane side chain in **4**, while the proton and carbon signals of the steroid B ring of **4** substantially differed from those of **3** (Tables 1 and 2, Figures S31 and S32). The absence of a carbon signal of the oxo group in the ^{13}C-NMR spectrum of **4** in comparison with the ^{13}C-NMR spectrum of **3** and the appearance of a triplet of doublets at δ_H 3.25 (J = 10.6, 5.2) in the ^{1}H-NMR spectrum of **4** in comparison with the ^{1}H-NMR spectrum of **3** indicated the presence of a hydroxyl function in the ring B. The attachment of the hydroxyl group at C-7 was deduced from proton and carbon correlations in the COSY, HSQC, and HMBC spectra (Figure 2 and Figures S33–S35). The key ROESY cross-peaks Hα-1/H-3, H-5, H-9; H-7/H-9; Hβ-12/H$_2$-21; Hα-16/H-17; H$_3$-18/H-8, Hβ-11, Hβ-15, H-20, H$_2$-21; and H$_3$-19/Hβ-1, Hβ-2, Hβ-4, Hβ-6; broad signal of H-3 and coupling constant J = 10.6 Hz of the triplet of doublets of axial proton H-7 confirmed the 3β,7β relative configurations of the oxygenated carbons in the $\Delta^{24(28)}$-24-methyl-5α-cholestane skeleton in **4** (Figure 3 and Figure S36). As a result, the structure of **4** was established as (20R)-24-methyl-7β-hydroxy-5α-cholest-24(28)-ene-3β,21-diyl disulfate disodium salt.

Table 3. ^{1}H-(700.13 MHz) and ^{13}C-(176.04 MHz) NMR chemical shifts of compounds **2a** and **3a** in CD$_3$OD, with δ in ppm and J values in Hz ^{a}.

Position	2a		3a	
	δ_H	δ_C	δ_H	δ_C
1β / α	1.98 m / 1.22 m	37.6	1.77 m / 1.03 m	37.3
2α / β	1.89 m / 1.61 m	31.9	1.80 m / 1.46 m	31.8
3	3.54 m	71.2	3.52 m	71.3
4α / β	2.48 ddd (13.5, 4.6, 2.1) / 2.39 ddd (13.5, 11.5, 2.0)	42.8	1.56 m / 1.44 m	48.4
5	–	169.1	1.48 m	169.1
6	5.65 m	126.3	2.45 t (13.0) / 1.92 dd (13.0, 3.2)	47.0
7	–	204.6	–	214.4
8	2.31 dd (12.8, 10.8)	46.6	2.47 t (12.1)	51.1
9	1.51 m	51.6	1.08 m	57.0
10	–	39.7	–	37.2
11	1.64 m	22.3	1.62 m / 1.56 m	22.9
12β / α	1.97 m / 1.19 m	39.3	1.92 m / 1.14 m	39.4
13	–	44.2	–	43.6
14	1.32 m	51.3	1.40 m	50.4
15α / β	2.39 m / 1.28 m	27.3	2.19 m / 1.01 m	25.9
16α / β	1.87 m / 1.39 m	28.4	1.86 m / 1.37 m	28.4
17	1.45 m	50.6	1.45 m	50.9
18	0.73 s	12.7	0.70 s	12.8
19	1.23 s	17.8	1.11 s	12.1
20	1.51 m	43.2	1.50 m	43.2
21	3.69 dd (10.7, 4.2) / 3.54 dd (10.7, 5.5)	63.2	3.68 dd (10.9, 3.8) / 3.53 dd (10.9, 5.6)	63.2
22	1.63 m / 1.44 m	29.4	1.61 m / 1.43 m	29.3
23	2.15 m / 1.98 m	32.3	2.13 m / 1.97 m	32.3
24	–	157.8	–	157.5
25	2.25 quin	34.9	2.25 quin	34.9
26	1.03 d (6.8)	22.5	1.03 d (6.7)	22.5
27	1.03 d (6.8)	22.3	1.03 d (6.7)	22.3
28	4.73 br s / 4.69 br d (1.4)	106.9	4.72 br s / 4.68 br d (1.4)	106.9

^{a} Assignments from 700.13 MHz COSY, HSQC, HMBC (8 Hz), and ROESY (250 msec) data.

The molecular formula of steroid **5** was established to be C$_{27}$H$_{42}$Na$_2$O$_8$S$_2$ from the [M − Na]$^-$ and [M − 2Na]$^{2-}$ ion peaks at *m/z* 581.2216 and *m/z* 279.1171 in the

(−)HRESIMS, respectively, and from the [M + Na]$^+$ sodium adduct ion peak at m/z 627.1993 in the (+)HRESIMS (Figure S37). The presence of sulfate groups in **5** is confirmed by HRESIMS as well as by the presence in the (−)HRESIMS/MS spectrum of [M − 2Na]$^{2-}$ of fragment ions at m/z 96.9601 [HSO$_4$]$^-$, 409.2041 [M − Na − NaHSO$_4$ − C$_5$H$_8$]$^-$, and 461.2722 [M − Na − NaHSO$_4$]$^-$. The examination of the ^{1}H-, ^{13}C-, and 2D NMR spectra of **5** and **1** revealed that both compounds have the identical $\Delta^{5(6)}$-3β-sulfoxy tetracyclic moiety, but the proton and carbon resonances of the steroid side chain of **5** differed from those of **1** (Tables 1 and 2, Figures S38–S43). The proton and carbon signals in the ^{1}H- and ^{13}C-NMR spectra belonging to the side chain of **1** showed the presence of three methyls CH$_3$-21 [δ_H 0.96 d (J = 6.7); δ_C 12.8], CH$_3$-26 (δ_H 1.69 s; δ_C 26.0), and CH$_3$-27 (δ_H 1.65 s; δ_C 18.1), an oxygenated methine CH-22 [δ_H 4.36 dd (J = 10.6, 4.5); δ_C 82.6], and the 24-double bond [δ_H 5.05 t (J = 7.7); δ_C 121.2, 134.8]. The proton connectivities from C-21 through C-20 to C-24 in the side chain were ascertained using the COSY and HSQC experiments. The attachment of the sulfoxy group at C-22 and a 24-double bond were supported from the HMBC cross-peaks H$_3$-21/C-17, C-20, C-22; H-22/C-17, C-20, C-24; H-23/C-24, C-25; H$_3$-26/C-24, C-25; and H$_3$-27/C-24, C-25 (Figure 2). The 20S configuration was elucidated by the ROESY correlations of Hβ-12/H-20, H-17/H$_3$-21, and H$_3$-18/H-20, H$_3$-21, and the downfield chemical shift of H$_3$-21 at δ_H 0.96 [21,23–25]. Based on the 20S configuration, we suggested the 22R configuration because the ROESY correlations of H-22/H$_2$-16 were observed (Figure 3). Similar correlations were observed in the NOEs spectrum of a natural steroid with a (20S,22R)-22-hydroxycholestane side chain [23]. Accordingly, the structure of **5** was elucidated as (20S)-cholesta-5,24-diene-3β,22-diyl disulfate disodium salt. The Δ^{24}-22-sulfoxycholestane side chain of the compound **5** has not been known earlier in other starfish or ophiuroid steroids. It's interesting that the desulfated derivative (20S,22R)-cholesta-5,24-diene-3β,22-diol or 22R-hydroxydesmosterol, related to compound **5**, is a derivative of desmosterol, a biosynthetic precursor of cholesterol. 22R-Hydroxydesmosterol was earlier obtained by stereospecific synthesis and shown to have a cytotoxic effect on tumor and hepatoma cells [26,27].

Previously reported feeding experiments labeled with deuterium precursors have shown that polyhydroxysteroids and related steroidal glycosides of starfish are biosynthesized from dietary cholesterol and cholesterol sulfate [28]. Obviously, the precursors of the biosynthesis of steroidal disulfates **1–5** are presumably cholesterol or cholesterol sulfate. The biosynthesis of these compounds takes place with the participation of enzymatic systems such as oxygenases, NAD and NADP-dependent dehydrogenases, SAM-methyltransferase, etc. The following hypothetical pathways for the biosynthesis of compounds **2–4** are proposed. Compound **1** undergoes changes only in the steroidal side chain in comparison with cholesterol sulfate by oxidation at CH$_3$-21 followed by sulfation and introduction of a methylene group by SAM-methyltransferase at C-24 with loss of a proton. The introduction of a hydroxyl group at C-7 of ring B of the steroidal nucleus of **1** gives an intermediate. Oxidation of the hydroxyl group at C-7 in the intermediate leads to the formation of steroid disulfate **2**, and reduction of the 5(6)-double bond leads to the formation of **4**. The end product, obviously, is the steroid disulfate **3**, which can be obtained from both compounds **2** and **4** (by oxidation or reduction). In compound **5**, as well as in **1**, there are no changes in the steroid nucleus, and only the side chain is modified by oxidation with the following sulfation at the C-22 position.

2.2. In Vitro Anticancer Activity of Compounds **1–5**

Currently, the main cellular model of cell biology is a two-dimensional (2D) monolayer. However, the cell growth in a monolayer does not reflect the true picture of tumor growth in a living organism by many parameters, where interactions not only between the cells of the tumor but also with the surrounding extracellular matrix are of great importance in its progression. The three-dimensional (3D cell culture) model is represented by spheroids, and proved to be the most effective system that is as close as possible in properties and organization to a natural tumor, which is used for screening the potential anticancer drugs [29]. So, the cytotoxic activity of **1**, **4**, and **5** and the mixture of **2** and **3** was determined on the models of 2D and 3D cultures of human epithelial kidney cells (HEK293), melanoma cells (SK-MEL-28), small intestine carcinoma cells (HuTu80), and breast carcinoma cells (ZR-75-1) using the MTS method.

The investigated compounds **1–5** were determined to possess moderate cytotoxic activity against normal and cancer cells with the greater impact of the mixture of **2** and **3**. It was found that this mixture inhibited the cell viability of 2D HEK293, SK-MEL-28, HuTu80, and ZR-75-1 by 28, 33, 34, and 55%, respectively, at a concentration of 100 µM after 24 h of treatment (Figure 4A–D). The concentration of the mixture of **2** and **3**, which caused inhibition of 50% cell viability (IC_{50}) was established against more sensitive breast carcinoma cells ZR-75-1 as 90.4 µM (Figure 4D). The IC_{50} of doxorubicin (Doxo), used as a positive control, was 35.7, 40.0, 11.2, and 19.2 µM against 2D HEK293, SK-MEL-28, HuTu80, and ZR-75-1, respectively (Figure 4A–D).

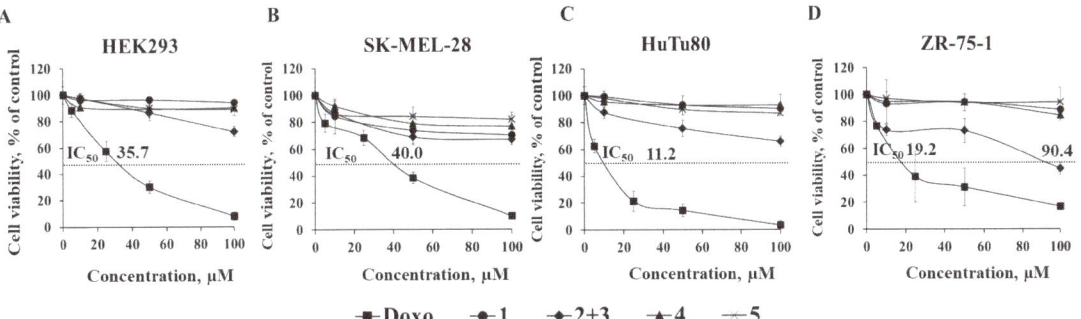

Figure 4. The cytotoxic effect of compounds **1–5** on the model of 2D (**A**) HEK293, (**B**) SK-MEL-28, (**C**) HuTu80, and (**D**) ZR-75-1 cells. Cells monolayer was treated with Doxo at concentrations of 5, 25, 50, and 100 µM or **1**, **4**, and **5** and the mixture of **2** and **3** at concentrations of 10, 50, and 100 µM and incubated for 24 h. Cell viability was assessed using the MTS test. Data are presented as means ± standard deviation, as determined in three experiments.

The investigated compounds insignificantly affect the size of the spheroids but inhibit their viability to varying degrees (Figure 5A–C). It was determined that the mixture of **2** and **3** inhibited viability of SK-MEL-28, HuTu80, and ZR-75-1 spheroids by 16, 36, and 51%, respectively, at 100 µM after 24 h of treatment. As in the case of 2D culture cells, ZR-75-1 spheroids were the most sensitive to the cytotoxic action of the mixture of **2** and **3**. IC_{50} of Doxo was 30.9 µM and 21.9 µM against HuTu80 and ZR-75-1, respectively.

It should be noted that 3D cell cultures were more resistant to the action of compounds than 2D cultures, which can be explained by dynamic cellular interactions between neighboring cells in spheroids. Moreover, the increased resistance of 3D spheroids may be associated with limited diffusion of the tested substances into the spheroid and hypoxia of cells within the spheroid, which leads to the activation of genes involved in cell survival and the formation of drug resistance [30].

In summary, the results of the present study described the significant inhibiting effect of the mixture of compounds **2** and **3** on the cell viability of human breast carcinoma cells ZR-75-1 in 2D and 3D cell culture models and may contribute to the development of effective chemotherapeutic methods for cancer treatment.

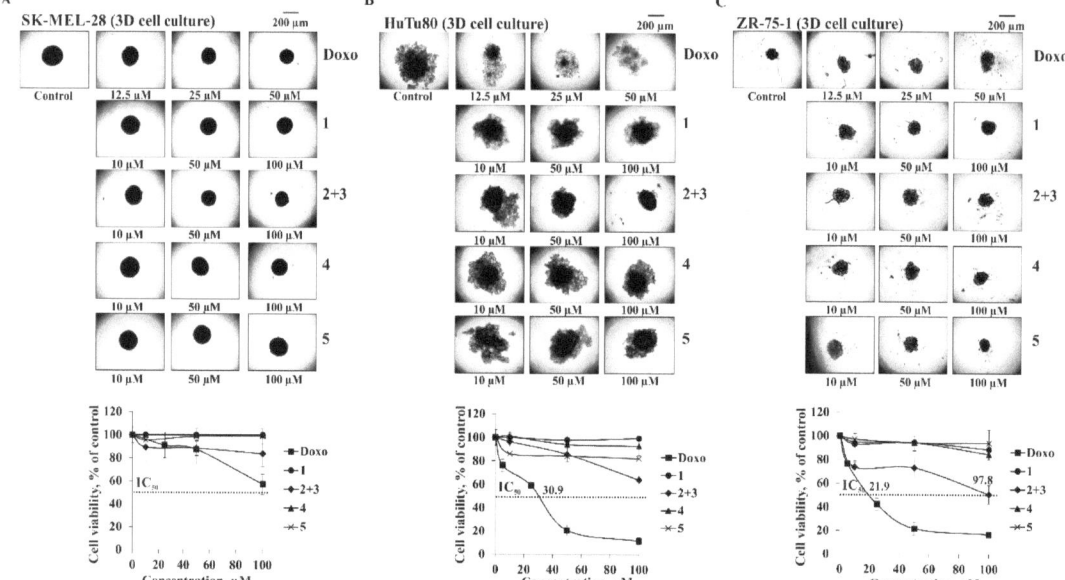

Figure 5. The cytotoxic effect of compounds **1–5** on the model of 3D (**A**) SK-MEL-28, (**B**) HuTu80, and (**C**) ZR-75-1 cells. Spheroids were treated with Doxo at concentrations of 5, 25, 50, and 100 µM or **1**, **4**, and **5** and the mixture of **2** and **3** at concentrations of 10, 50, and 100 µM and incubated for 24 h. Cell viability was assessed using the MTS test. Data are presented as means ± standard deviation, as determined in three experiments. Photographs (n = 6 for controls or cells treated with polysaccharides or derivatives, where n = number of photographs) of each spheroid were taken with the ZOE ™ Fluorescent Cell Imager. Spheroids were analyzed using ImageJ software.

3. Materials and Methods

3.1. General Procedures

Optical rotations were determined on a Perkin-Elmer 343 polarimeter (PerkinElmer, Waltham, MA, USA). The ^{1}H- and ^{13}C-NMR spectra were recorded on a Bruker Avance III 700 spectrometer (Bruker BioSpin, Bremen, Germany) at 700.13 and 176.04 MHz, respectively. Chemical shifts (ppm) were internally referenced to the corresponding residual solvent signals at δ_H 3.30/δ_C 49.0 for CD$_3$OD. HRESIMS mass spectra were recorded on a Bruker Impact II Q-TOF mass spectrometer (Bruker, Bremen, Germany); the samples were dissolved in MeOH (c 0.001 mg/mL). HPLC separations were carried out on an Agilent 1100 Series chromatograph (Agilent Technologies, Santa Clara, CA, USA), equipped with a differential refractometer; Discovery C18 (5 µm, 250 × 10 mm, Supelco, Bellefonte, PA, USA) and YMC-Pack Pro C18 (5 µm, 250 × 4.6 mm, YMC CO., LTD., Kyoto, Japan) columns were used. Low-pressure column liquid chromatography was performed using Polychrom 1 (powdered Teflon, 0.25–0.50 mm; Biolar, Olaine, Latvia) and silica gel KSK (50–160 µm, Sorbpolimer, Krasnodar, Russia). Sorbfil silica gel plates (4.5 × 6.0 cm, 5–17 µm, Sorbpolimer, Krasnodar, Russia) were used for thin-layer chromatography.

3.2. Animal Material

Specimens of *Pteraster marsippus* Fisher, 1910 (order Velatida, family Pterasteridae) were collected at a depth of 84–88 m using a small trawl off Urup Island in the Sea of Okhotsk (45.5280 N, 149.4230 E) during the research vessel *Akademik Oparin* 51th scientific cruise in May 2017. Species identification was carried out by Mr. B.B. Grebnev (G.B. Elyakov Pacific Institute of Bioorganic Chemistry of the FEB RAS, Vladivostok, Russia). A voucher specimen [no. 051-039] is on deposit at the marine specimen collection of the G.B. Elyakov Pacific Institute of Bioorganic Chemistry of the FEB RAS, Vladivostok, Russia.

3.3. Extraction and Isolation

Freshly collected specimens of *P. marsippus* were frozen and stored at −21 °C until used. The frozen animals (2.1 kg) were cut into small pieces and extracted twice with EtOH at room temperature (2.0 L/kg). The extract was evaporated and the residue (150 g) was dissolved in H_2O (1.0 L). The H_2O-soluble fraction was passed through a Polychrom 1 column (8 × 62 cm) and eluted with distilled H_2O until a negative chloride ion reaction was obtained, followed by elution with 50% aq. EtOH. The combined aq. EtOH eluate was evaporated to give a brownish residue (6.0 g). This fraction was chromatographed over a Si gel column (6.5 × 15 cm) using $CHCl_3$/EtOH (stepwise gradient, 4:1 to 1:2, v/v), EtOH, and EtOH/H_2O (9:1, v/v) and rechromatographed over a Florisil column (7 × 15 cm) using $CHCl_3$/EtOH (stepwise gradient, 2:1 to 1:1, v/v) to yield eleven main fractions (1–11) that were analyzed by TLC on Si gel plates in the eluent systems toluene/EtOH (9:5, v/v) and n-BuOH/EtOH/H_2O (4:1:2, $v/v/v$). Fractions 5 and 7 contained the mixtures of disulfated steroids. HPLC separation of fraction 5 (194 mg) on a Discovery C18 column with 54% aq. EtOH (2.0 mL/min) as an eluent system followed by the further separation on the same column with 62% aq. MeOH (2.0 mL/min) as an eluent system yielded pure **1** (1.1 mg, t_R 18.8 min). HPLC separation of fraction 7 (297 mg) on a Discovery C18 column with 60% aq. MeOH (2.0 mL/min) as an eluent system followed by the further separation on a YMC-Pack Pro C18 column with 60% aq. MeOH (0.6 mL/min) as an eluent system gave the mixture of **2** and **3** (16.1 mg, t_R 12.8 min), pure **4** (2.3 mg, t_R 8.5 min) and **5** (1.5 mg, t_R 16.5 min).

3.4. Compound Characterization Data

(20*R*)-24-Methylcholesta-5,24(28)-diene-3β,21-diyl disulfate disodium salt (**1**): Colorless amorphous powder; $[\alpha]_D^{25}$: −14.5 (*c* 0.11, MeOH); (−)HRESIMS *m/z* 595.2388 [M − Na]⁻ (calcd for $C_{28}H_{44}NaO_8S_2$, 595.2381); (−)HRESIMS *m/z* 286.1253 [M − 2Na]⁻ (calcd for $C_{28}H_{44}O_8S_2$, 286.1244); (+)HRESIMS *m/z* 641.2154 [M + Na]⁺ (calcd for $C_{28}H_{44}Na_3O_8S_2$, 641.2165); HRESIMS/MS of the [M − 2Na]²⁻ ion at *m/z* 286.1253: 475.2898 [M − Na − $NaHSO_4$]⁻, 459.2584 [M − Na − $NaHSO_4$ − CH_4]⁻, 391.1958 [M − Na − $NaHSO_4$ − C_6H_{12}]⁻, 136.9917 [$C_3H_5O_4S$]⁻, 96.9610 [HSO_4]⁻; ¹H-NMR data (see Table 1); ¹³C-NMR data (see Table 2).

(20*R*)-7-Oxo-24-methylcholesta-5,24(28)-diene-3β,21-diyl disulfate disodium salt (**2**); Colorless amorphous powder; the mixture of **2** and **3** $[\alpha]_D^{25}$: −28.8 (*c* 0.82, MeOH); (−)HRESIMS *m/z* 609.2177 [M − Na]⁻ (calcd for $C_{28}H_{42}NaO_9S_2$, 609.2173); (−)HRESIMS *m/z* 293.1148 [M − 2Na]²⁻ (calcd for $C_{28}H_{42}O_9S_2$, 293.1141); (+)HRESIMS *m/z* 655.1943 [M + Na]⁺ (calcd for $C_{28}H_{42}Na_3O_9S_2$, 655.1958); HRESIMS/MS of the [M − 2Na]²⁻ ion at *m/z* 293.1148: 489.2682 [M − Na − $NaHSO_4$]⁻, 405.1745 [M − Na − $NaHSO_4$ − C_6H_{12}]⁻, 136.9917 [$C_3H_5O_4S$]⁻, 96.9612 [HSO_4]⁻; ¹H-NMR data (see Table 1); ¹³C-NMR data (see Table 2).

(20*R*)-7-Oxo-24-methyl-5α-cholest-24(28)-ene-3β,21-diyl disulfate disodium salt (**3**); Colorless amorphous powder; the mixture of **2** and **3** $[\alpha]_D^{25}$: −28.8 (*c* 0.82, MeOH); (−)HRESIMS *m/z* 611.2299 [M − Na]⁻ (calcd for $C_{28}H_{44}NaO_9S_2$, 611.2330); (−)HRESIMS *m/z* 294.1222 [M − 2Na]²⁻ (calcd for $C_{28}H_{44}O_9S_2$, 294.1219); (+)HRESIMS *m/z* 657.2077 [M + Na]⁺ (calcd for $C_{28}H_{44}Na_3O_9S_2$, 657.2114); HRESIMS/MS of the [M − 2Na]²⁻ ion at *m/z* 294.1222: 491.2825 [M − Na − $NaHSO_4$]⁻, 407.1891 [M − Na − $NaHSO_4$ − C_6H_{12}]⁻, 136.9917 [$C_3H_5O_4S$]⁻, 96.9612 [HSO_4]⁻; ¹H-NMR data (see Table 1); ¹³C-NMR data (see Table 2).

(20*R*)-24-Methyl-7β-hydroxy-5α-cholest-24(28)-ene-3β,21-diyl disulfate disodium salt (**4**); Colorless amorphous powder; $[\alpha]_D^{25}$: +9.6 (*c* 0.23, MeOH); (−)HRESIMS *m/z* 613.2483 [M − Na]⁻ (calcd for $C_{28}H_{46}NaO_9S_2$, 613.2486); (−)HRESIMS *m/z* 295.1304 [M − 2Na]²⁻ (calcd for $C_{28}H_{46}O_9S_2$, 295.1297); (+)HRESIMS *m/z* 659.2243 [M + Na]⁺ (calcd for

$C_{28}H_{46}Na_3O_9S_2$, 659.2271); HRESIMS/MS of the $[M - 2Na]^{2-}$ ion at m/z 295.1304: 493.2987 $[M - Na - NaHSO_4]^-$, 409.2047 $[M - Na - NaHSO_4 - C_6H_{12}]^-$, 191.0380 $[C_7H_{11}O_4S]^-$, 136.9909 $[C_3H_5O_4S]^-$, 96.9604 $[HSO_4]^-$; ^{1}H-NMR data (see Table 1); ^{13}C-NMR data (see Table 2).

(20S)-Cholesta-5,24-diene-3β,22-diyl disulfate disodium salt (**5**); Colorless amorphous powder; $[\alpha]_D^{25}$: −14.0 (c 0.15, MeOH); (−)HRESIMS m/z 581.2216 $[M - Na]^-$ (calcd for $C_{27}H_{42}NaO_8S_2$, 581.2224); (−)HRESIMS m/z 279.1171 $[M - 2Na]^{2-}$ (calcd for $C_{27}H_{42}O_8S_2$, 279.1166); (+)HRESIMS m/z 627.1993 $[M + Na]^+$ (calcd for $C_{27}H_{42}Na_3O_8S_2$, 627.2009); HRESIMS/MS of the $[M - 2Na]^{2-}$ ion at m/z 279.1171: 461.2722 $[M - Na - NaHSO_4]^-$, 409.2041 $[M - Na - NaHSO_4 - C_5H_8]^-$, 96.9601 $[HSO_4]^-$. ^{1}H-NMR data (see Table 1); ^{13}C-NMR data (see Table 2).

*3.5. Solvolysis of the Mixture of **2** and **3***

A solution of the mixture of **2** and **3** (5.0 mg) in 2 mL of dioxane/pyridine (1:1) was heated at 100 °C for 4 h. The reaction mixture was evaporated under reduced pressure and separated by HPLC on a YMC-Pack Pro C18 column with 80% aq. MeOH (0.7 mL/min) as an eluent system to give pure desulfated derivatives **2a** (0.5 mg, t_R 40.6 min) and **3a** (0.4 mg, t_R 39.6 min).

(20R)-7-Oxo-24-methylcholesta-5,24(28)-diene-3β,21-diol (**2a**); Colorless amorphous powder; $[\alpha]_D^{25}$: −38.0 (c 0.05, MeOH); (−)HRESIMS m/z 427.3215 $[M - H]^-$ (calcd for $C_{28}H_{43}O_3$, 427.3218); (+)HRESIMS m/z 451.3175 $[M + Na]^+$ (calcd for $C_{28}H_{44}NaO_3$, 451.3183); ^{1}H- and ^{13}C-NMR data (see Table 3).

(20R)-7-Oxo-24-methyl-5α-cholest-24(28)-ene-3β,21-diol (**3a**); Colorless amorphous powder; $[\alpha]_D^{25}$: −5.0 (c 0.04, MeOH); (−)HRESIMS m/z 429.3376 $[M - H]^-$ (calcd for $C_{28}H_{45}O_3$, 429.3374); (+)HRESIMS m/z 453.3333 $[M + Na]^+$ (calcd for $C_{28}H_{46}NaO_3$, 453.3339); ^{1}H- and ^{13}C-NMR data (see Table 3).

3.6. Bioactivity Assay

3.6.1. Cell Lines

American Type Culture Collection (Manassas, VA, USA) provided human epithelial kidney cells HEK293 (ATCC® no. CRL-1573™) and melanoma cells SK-MEL-28 (ATCC® no. HTB-72™). Human small intestine carcinoma cells HuTu80 and breast carcinoma cells ZR-75-1 were obtained from the Shared Research Facility's Vertebrate cell culture collection (Saint-Petersburg, Russia).

3.6.2. Cell Culture Conditions

HEK293 and SK-MEL-28 cells were cultured in Dulbecco's Modified Eagle Medium (DMEM), HuTu80 cells were maintained in Minimum Essential Medium (MEM), and ZR-75-1 cells were cultured in Roswell Park Memorial Institute Medium (RPMI-1640) in a humidified 5% CO_2 incubator. The culture medium was supplemented with 10% of fetal bovine albumin (FBS), 100 mg/mL streptomycin, and 100 U/mL penicillin. At 90% confluence, cells were rinsed with PBS, detached from the tissue culture flask by 0.25% trypsin/0.5 mM EDTA, and 10–20% of the harvested cells were transferred to a new flask containing fresh complete appropriate medium. The passage number was carefully controlled and the mycoplasma contamination was monitored on a regular basis.

3.6.3. Preparation of Compounds for the Determination of Cytotoxic Activity

Compounds **1**, **4**, and **5** and the mixture of **2** and **3** were dissolved in sterile dimethyl sulfoxide (DMSO) to prepare stock concentrations of 20 mM. Cells were treated with serially diluted **1**–**5** (10, 50, 100 μM) (culture medium used as diluent) (final concentration of DMSO was less than 0.5%).

Doxorubicin (Doxo) (Teva Pharmaceutical Industries, Ltd., Petah Tikva, Israel) was dissolved in sterile PBS to prepare stock concentrations of 10 mM. Cells were treated with serially diluted Doxo (5, 25, 50, 100 μM) (culture medium used as diluent).

The vehicle control is the cells treated with the equivalent volume of DMSO (final concentration was less than 0.5%) for all of the presented experiments.

3.6.4. Formation of 3D Spheroids by Liquid Overlay Technique (LOT)

SK-ME-28, HuTu80, and ZR-75-1 spheroids were formed by the liquid overlay technique (LOT) method with slight modifications. Briefly, to create non-adherent surfaces for the efficient spheroids' formation, 50 µL of preheated (60 °C) agarose (1.5%) was overlaid the bottom of 96-well plates and left to solidify for 1 h at room temperature under sterile conditions.

SK-MEL-28 cells (5.0×10^3), HuTu80 (3.0×10^3), and ZR-75-1 (3.0×10^3) were inoculated in an agarose layer and cultured in 200 µL of a complete appropriate culture medium for 96 h at 37 °C in a 5% CO_2 incubator. An image of each spheroid was made with a ZOE™ Fluorescent Cell Imager (Bio Rad, Hercules, CA, USA). ImageJ software bundled with 64-bit Java 1.8.0_112 (NIH, Bethesda, MD, USA) was used to measure the spheroid integrity, diameter, and volume.

3.6.5. Cytotoxic Activity Assay (MTS)

2D Cell Culture (Monolayer)

HEK293 (0.8×10^3/200 µL), SK-MEL-28 (0.8×10^3/200 µL), HuTu80 (1.0×10^3/200 µL), and ZR-75-1 (1.2×10^3/200 µL) cells were seeded into 96-well plates (Jet Biofil, Guangzhou, China) for 24 h at 37 °C in a 5% CO_2 incubator. Then cell monolayer was treated either with DMSO (control), Doxo (positive control) (5, 25, 50, 100 µM) or various concentrations of compounds **1**, **4**, and **5** and the mixture of **2** and **3** (10, 50, 100 µM) in fresh appropriate culture medium for 24 h. Subsequently, the cells were incubated with 15 µL of 3-(4,5-dimethylthiazol-2-yl)-5-(3-carboxymethoxyphenyl)-2-(4-sulfophenyl)-2H-tetrazolium (MTS reagent) (Promega, Madison, WI, USA) for 3 h, and the absorbance of each well was measured at 490/630 nm using Power Wave XS microplate reader (BioTek, Wynusky, VT, USA). The concentration at which the compounds exert half of its maximal inhibitory effect on cell viability (IC_{50}) was calculated by the AAT-Bioquest® online calculator [31].

3D Cell Culture (Spheroids)

The spheroids were treated by replacing 100 µL of supernatant with a complete medium containing DMSO (control), Doxo (positive control) at 5, 25, 50, 100 µM or compounds **1**, **4**, and **5** and the mixture of **2** and **3** at 10, 50, 100 µM for 24 h. Then, 15 µL of 3-(4,5-dimethylthiazol-2-yl)-5-(3-carboxymethoxyphenyl)-2-(4-sulfophenyl)-2H-tetrazolium (MTS) reagent (Promega, Madison, WI, USA) was added to each well with spheroids and incubated for 3 h at 37 °C in a 5% CO_2 incubator. The absorbance of each well was measured at 490/630 nm using Power Wave XS microplate reader. A photo of the 3D spheroids (40×200 µm scale) was made with the aid of a microscope Motic AE 20 (XiangAn, Xiamen 361101, China) and the ImageJ software.

3.6.6. Statistical Analysis

All of the assays were performed in at least three independent experiments. Results are expressed as the mean ± standard deviation (SD). The Student's t-test was used to evaluate the data with the following significance levels: * $p < 0.05$, ** $p < 0.01$, *** $p < 0.001$.

4. Conclusions

Three new 3β,21-disulfated steroids and one new 3β,22-disulfated steroid, along with a previously known related compound, were isolated from the Far Eastern starfish *P. marsippus*, and their chemical structures were established. Two steroids have an oxo-group at position C-7 in steroid nucleus; moreover, one of them additionally includes the conjugated 5,6-double bond. The Δ^{24}-22-sulfoxycholestane side chain, indicated in another new steroid, has not been earlier found in starfish and ophiuroid steroidal compounds.

Thus, in one more species of starfish, *P. marsippus*, belonging to the Pterasteridae family, like the previously studied six species of starfish of the same family, disulfated steroids of «the ophiuroid type» were found. It should be noted that the polyhydroxylated compounds and asterosaponins common in starfish were absent in the *P. marsippus* as well as in the previously studied species of this family. This fact once again confirms the assumption about a closer phylogenetic relationship between Asteroidea and Ophiuroidea classes compared to other classes of Echinodermata. The mixture of two steroids, having an oxo-group at position C-7 in steroid nucleus, was found to possess the highest cytotoxic activity against 2D and 3D human breast carcinoma cells ZR-75-1 among other investigated by us compounds and can be a candidate for further examination of the molecular mechanism of its anticancer action.

Supplementary Materials: The following are available online at https://www.mdpi.com/article/10.3390/md20030164/s1, Copies HRESIMS (Figures S1, S14–S18, S31 and S38), 1H-NMR (Figures S2, S8, S19, S25, S32, and S39), 13C-NMR (Figures S3, S9, S20, S26, S33, and S40), COSY (Figures S4, S10, S21, S27, S34, and S41), HSQC (Figures S5, S11, S22, S28, S20, S35, and S42), HMBC (Figures S6, S12, S23, S29, S36, and S43), and ROESY (Figures S7, S13, S24, S30, S37, and S44) spectra of compounds 1, the mixture of 2 and 3, 2a, 3a, 4, and 5, respectively. COSY, key HMBC, and key ROESY correlations of compounds 2a and 3a (Figure S18).

Author Contributions: Conceptualization, A.A.K. and O.S.M.; data curation, A.I.K. and R.S.P.; funding acquisition, V.A.S.; investigation, A.A.K., A.I.K., O.S.M. and R.S.P.; methodology, A.A.K., A.I.K., T.V.M., O.S.M., R.S.P. and N.V.I.; writing—original draft, A.A.K. and O.S.M.; writing—review and editing, T.V.M., S.P.E., V.A.S. and N.V.I. All authors have read and agreed to the published version of the manuscript.

Funding: This research was funded by RFBR (Russian Foundation for Basic Research), grant number 20-03-00014.

Institutional Review Board Statement: Not applicable.

Informed Consent Statement: Not applicable.

Data Availability Statement: Not applicable.

Acknowledgments: The study was carried out on the equipment of the Collective Facilities Center —The Far Eastern Center for Structural Molecular Research (NMR/MS) of PIBOC FEB RAS. We are grateful to B.B. Grebnev (G.B. Elyakov Pacific Institute of Bioorganic Chemistry FEB RAS, Vladivostok, Russia) for species identification of the starfish.

Conflicts of Interest: The authors declare no conflict of interest.

References

1. Kornprobst, J.M.; Sallenave, C.; Barnathan, G. Sulfated compounds from marine organisms. *Comp. Biochem. Physiol.* **1998**, *119B*, 1–51. [CrossRef]
2. Stonik, V.A. Marine polar steroids. *Russ. Chem. Rev.* **2001**, *70*, 673–715. [CrossRef]
3. Carvalhal, F.; Correia-da-Silva, M.; Sousa, E.; Pinto, M.; Kijjoa, A. SULFATION PATHWAYS: Sources and biological activities of marine sulfated steroids. *J. Mol. Endocrinol.* **2018**, *61*, T211–T231. [CrossRef] [PubMed]
4. Minale, L.; Riccio, R.; Zollo, F. Steroidal oligoglycosides and polyhydroxysteroids from Echinoderms. *Fortschr. Chem. Org. Naturst.* **1993**, *62*, 75–308. [CrossRef]
5. Stonik, V.A.; Ivanchina, N.V.; Kicha, A.A. New polar steroids from starfish. *Nat. Prod. Commun.* **2008**, *3*, 1587–1610. [CrossRef]
6. Ivanchina, N.V.; Kicha, A.A.; Stonik, V.A. Steroid glycosides from marine organisms. *Steroids* **2011**, *76*, 425–454. [CrossRef] [PubMed]
7. Dong, G.; Xu, T.H.; Yang, B.; Lin, X.P.; Zhou, X.F.; Yang, X.W.; Liu, Y.H. Chemical constituents and bioactivities of starfish. *Chem. Biodivers.* **2011**, *8*, 740–791. [CrossRef]
8. Ivanchina, N.V.; Kicha, A.A.; Malyarenko, T.V.; Stonik, V.A. *Advances in Natural Products Discovery*; Gomes, A.R., Rocha-Santos, T., Duarte, A., Eds.; Nova Science Publishers: Hauppauge, NY, USA, 2017; Volume 6, pp. 191–224.
9. Xia, J.M.; Miao, Z.; Xie, C.L.; Zhang, J.W.; Yang, X.W. Chemical constituents and bioactivities of starfishes: An update. *Chem. Biodivers.* **2020**, *17*, e1900638. [CrossRef]
10. Stonik, V.A.; Kicha, A.A.; Malyarenko, T.V.; Ivanchina, N.V. Asterosaponins: Structures, taxonomic distribution, biogenesis and biological activities. *Mar. Drugs* **2020**, *18*, 584. [CrossRef]

11. D'Auria, M.V.; Finamore, E.; Minale, L.; Pizza, C.; Riccio, R.; Zollo, F.; Pusset, M.; Tirard, P. Steroids from the starfish *Euretaster insignis*: A novel group of sulphated 3β,21-dihydroxysteroids. *J. Chem. Soc. Perkin Trans.* **1984**, *1*, 2277–2282. [CrossRef]
12. Levina, E.V.; Andriyaschenko, P.V.; Stonik, V.A.; Kalinovsky, A.I. Ophiuroid-type steroids in starfish of the genus *Pteraster*. *Comp. Biochem. Physiol. B Biochem. Mol. Biol.* **1996**, *114B*, 49–52. [CrossRef]
13. Levina, E.V.; Andriyaschenko, P.V.; Kalinovsky, A.I.; Stonik, V.A. New ophiuroid-type steroids from the starfish *Pteraster tesselatus*. *J. Nat. Prod.* **1998**, *61*, 1423–1426. [CrossRef] [PubMed]
14. Levina, E.V.; Andriyashchenko, P.V.; Kalinovsky, A.I.; Dmitrenok, P.S.; Stonik, V.A. Steroid compounds from the Far Eastern starfish *Diplopteraster multipes*. *Russ. J. Bioorgan. Chem.* **2002**, *28*, 189–193. [CrossRef] [PubMed]
15. Ivanchina, N.V.; Kicha, A.A.; Kalinovsky, A.I.; Dmitrenok, P.S.; Stonik, V.A. Hemolytic steroid disulfates from the Far Eastern starfish *Pteraster pulvillus*. *J. Nat. Prod.* **2003**, *66*, 298–301. [CrossRef] [PubMed]
16. Levina, E.V.; Kalinovsky, A.I.; Dmitrenok, P.S. Steroid compounds from the Far East starfish *Pteraster obscurus* and the ophiura *Asteronyx loveni*. *Russ. J. Bioorg. Chem.* **2007**, *33*, 341–346. [CrossRef]
17. Fu, X.; Schmitz, F.J.; Lee, R.H.; Papkoff, J.S.; Slate, D.L. Inhibitors of protein tyrosine kinase pp60^{v-src}: Sterol sulfates from the brittle star *Ophiarachna incrassata*. *J. Nat. Prod.* **1994**, *57*, 1591–1594. [CrossRef]
18. McKee, T.C.; Cardellina, J.H.; Riccio, R.; D'Auria, M.V.; Iorizzi, M.; Minale, L.; Moran, R.A.; Gulakowski, R.J.; McMahon, J.B.; Buckheit, R.W.; et al. HIV-inhibitory natural products. 11. Comparative studies of sulfated sterols from marine invertebrate. *J. Med. Chem.* **1994**, *37*, 793–797. [CrossRef]
19. Sepe, V.; Bifulco, G.; Renga, B.; D'Amore, C.; Fiorucci, S.; Zampella, A. Discovery of sulfated sterols from marine invertebrates as a new class of marine natural antagonists of farnesoid-X-receptor. *J. Med. Chem.* **2011**, *54*, 1314–1320. [CrossRef]
20. Gazha, A.K.; Ivanushko, L.A.; Levina, E.V.; Fedorov, S.N.; Zaporozets, T.S.; Stonik, V.A.; Besednova, N.N. Steroid sulfates from ophiuroids (brittle stars): Action on some factors of innate and adaptive immunity. *Nat. Prod. Commun.* **2016**, *11*, 749–752. [CrossRef]
21. Kicha, A.A.; Kalinovsky, A.I.; Antonov, A.S.; Radchenko, O.S.; Ivanchina, N.V.; Malyarenko, T.V.; Savchenko, A.M.; Stonik, V.A. Determination of C-23 configuration in (20R)-23-hydroxycholestane side chain of steroid compounds by ^{1}H and ^{13}C NMR spectroscopy. *Nat. Prod. Commun.* **2013**, *8*, 1219–1222. [CrossRef]
22. D'Auria, M.V.; Riccio, R.; Minale, L.; La Barre, S.; Pusset, J. Novel marine steroid sulfates from Pacific ophiuroids. *J. Org. Chem.* **1987**, *52*, 3947–3952. [CrossRef]
23. Hamdy, A.-H.A.; Aboutabl, E.A.; Sameer, S.; Hussein, A.A.; Díaz-Marrero, A.R.; Darias, J.; Cueto, M. 3-Keto-22-*epi*-28-nor-cathasterone, a brassinosteroid-related metabolite from *Cystoseira myrica*. *Steroids* **2009**, *74*, 927–930. [CrossRef] [PubMed]
24. Nes, W.R.; Varkey, T.E.; Krevitz, K. The stereochemistry of sterols at C-20 and its biosynthetic implications. *J. Am. Chem. Soc.* **1977**, *99*, 260–262. [CrossRef] [PubMed]
25. Vanderach, D.J.; Djerassi, C. Marine natural products. Synthesis of four naturally occurring 20.beta.-H cholanic acid derivatives. *J. Org. Chem.* **1978**, *43*, 1442–1448. [CrossRef]
26. Amann, A.; Ourisson, G.; Luu, B. A novel stereospecific synthesis of 22-hydroxylated triterpenes and steroids: Syntheses of 22R-hydroxylanosterol and 22R-hydroxydesmosterol. *Synthesis* **1987**, *1987*, 696–700. [CrossRef]
27. Hietter, H.; Trifilieff, E.; Richert, L.; Beck, J.-P.; Luu, B.; Ourisson, G. Antagonistic action of cholesterol towards the toxicity of hydroxysterols on cultured hepatoma cells. *Biochem. Biophys. Res. Commun.* **1984**, *120*, 657–664. [CrossRef]
28. Ivanchina, N.V.; Kicha, A.A.; Malyarenko, T.V.; Kalinovsky, A.I.; Dmitrenok, P.S.; Stonik, V.A. Biosynthesis of polar steroids from the Far Eastern starfish *Patiria (=Asterina) pectinifera*. Cholesterol and cholesterol sulfate are converted into polyhydroxylated sterols and monoglycoside asterosaponin P$_1$ in feeding experiments. *Steroids* **2013**, *78*, 1183–1191. [CrossRef]
29. Amelian, A.; Wasilewska, K.; Megias, D.; Winnicka, K. Application of standard cell cultures and 3D in vitro tissue models as an effective tool in drug design and development. *Pharmacol. Rep.* **2017**, *69*, 861–870. [CrossRef]
30. Edmondson, R.; Broglie, J.J.; Adcock, A.F.; Yang, L. Three-dimensional cell culture systems and their applications in drug discovery and cell-based biosensors. *Assay Drug Dev. Technol.* **2014**, *12*, 207–218. [CrossRef]
31. AAT Bioquest. Available online: https://www.aatbio.com/tools/ic50-calculator (accessed on 10 November 2020).

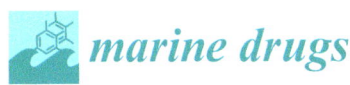

Article

Triterpene Glycosides from the Far Eastern Sea Cucumber *Psolus chitonoides*: Chemical Structures and Cytotoxicities of Chitonoidosides E_1, F, G, and H

Alexandra S. Silchenko, Anatoly I. Kalinovsky, Sergey A. Avilov, Pelageya V. Andrijaschenko, Roman S. Popov, Ekaterina A. Chingizova, Vladimir I. Kalinin * and Pavel S. Dmitrenok *

G.B. Elyakov Pacific Institute of Bioorganic Chemistry, Far Eastern Branch of the Russian Academy of Sciences, Pr. 100-letya Vladivostoka 159, 690022 Vladivostok, Russia; silchenko_als@piboc.dvo.ru (A.S.S.); kaaniv@piboc.dvo.ru (A.I.K.); avilov_sa@piboc.dvo.ru (S.A.A.); andrijashchenko_pv@piboc.dvo.ru (P.V.A.); popov_rs@piboc.dvo.ru (R.S.P.); chingizova_ea@piboc.dvo.ru (E.A.C.)
* Correspondence: kalininv@piboc.dvo.ru (V.I.K.); paveldmt@piboc.dvo.ru (P.S.D.);
  Tel./Fax: +7-(423)2-31-40-50 (V.I.K.)

Citation: Silchenko, A.S.; Kalinovsky, A.I.; Avilov, S.A.; Andrijaschenko, P.V.; Popov, R.S.; Chingizova, E.A.; Kalinin, V.I.; Dmitrenok, P.S. Triterpene Glycosides from the Far Eastern Sea Cucumber *Psolus chitonoides*: Chemical Structures and Cytotoxicities of Chitonoidosides E_1, F, G, and H. *Mar. Drugs* **2021**, *19*, 696. https://doi.org/10.3390/md19120696

Academic Editor: Hitoshi Sashiwa

Received: 16 November 2021
Accepted: 6 December 2021
Published: 7 December 2021

Publisher's Note: MDPI stays neutral with regard to jurisdictional claims in published maps and institutional affiliations.

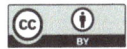

Copyright: © 2021 by the authors. Licensee MDPI, Basel, Switzerland. This article is an open access article distributed under the terms and conditions of the Creative Commons Attribution (CC BY) license (https://creativecommons.org/licenses/by/4.0/).

Abstract: Four new triterpene disulfated glycosides, chitonoidosides E_1 (**1**), F (**2**), G (**3**), and H (**4**), were isolated from the Far-Eastern sea cucumber *Psolus chitonoides* and collected near Bering Island (Commander Islands) at depths of 100–150 m. Among them there are two hexaosides (**1** and **3**), differing from each other by the terminal (sixth) sugar residue, one pentaoside (**4**) and one tetraoside (**2**), characterized by a glycoside architecture of oligosaccharide chains with shortened bottom semi-chains, which is uncommon for sea cucumbers. Some additional distinctive structural features inherent in **1**–**4** were also found: the aglycone of a recently discovered new type, with 18(20)-ether bond and lacking a lactone in chitonoidoside G (**3**), glycoside 3-*O*-methylxylose residue in chitonoidoside E_1 (**1**), which is rarely detected in sea cucumbers, and sulfated by uncommon position 4 terminal 3-*O*-methylglucose in chitonoidosides F (**2**) and H (**4**). The hemolytic activities of compounds **1**–**4** and chitonoidoside E against human erythrocytes and their cytotoxic action against the human cancer cell lines, adenocarcinoma HeLa, colorectal adenocarcinoma DLD-1, and monocytes THP-1, were studied. The glycoside with hexasaccharide chains (**1**, **3** and chitonoidoside E) were the most active against erythrocytes. A similar tendency was observed for the cytotoxicity against adenocarcinoma HeLa cells, but the demonstrated effects were moderate. The monocyte THP-1 cell line and erythrocytes were comparably sensitive to the action of the glycosides, but the activity of chitonoidosides E and E_1 (**1**) significantly differed from that of **3** in relation to THP-1 cells. A tetraoside with a shortened bottom semi-chain, chitonoidoside F (**2**), displayed the weakest membranolytic effect in the series.

Keywords: *Psolus chitonoides*; triterpene glycosides; chitonoidosides; sea cucumber; cytotoxic activity

1. Introduction

Triterpene glycosides are characteristic secondary metabolites of the sea cucumbers. Extensive studies on glycosides provide significant information on the exploration of chemical diversity, properties and biological activity of a huge collection of natural products, which are a valuable and promising resource of new drugs and medicines [1–8]. The interest in these compounds is also driven by their taxonomic specificity [9–11] as well as the possibility of reconstructing the sequences of the biosynthetic transformations of aglycones and carbohydrate chains during biosynthesis [12,13] and of defining the peculiarities of «structure-activity relationships» based on knowledge about their structural diversity [14]. All this indicates the relevance of searching for new glycosides. The Far Eastern sea cucumber *Psolus chitonoides* is the fourth chemically studied representative of the genus *Psolus*. The animals of this species contain a complicated multicomponent mixture of triterpene glycosides. Therefore, their separation and purification are difficult and time-consuming. Recently, we published a paper concerning the isolation, structural elucidation, and biologic activity of a series of the glycosides, named chitonoidosides A–E, isolated from *P. chitonoides* [15]. These compounds feature some interesting structural features, such as a new, non-holostane aglycone lacking a lactone and featuring an 18(20)-epoxy cycle, 3-*O*-methylxylose residue in the carbohydrate chains of three of them, the sulfation of 3-*O*-methylxylose by C-4, and, finally, a rather rare architecture of tetrasaccharide carbohydrate chain branched by C-4 Xyl1. As a continuation of our research on the glycosides from this species, four new chitonoidosides, E_1 (**1**), F (**2**), G (**3**), and H (**4**), are reported. The chemical structures of **1**–**4** were established through the analyses of the ^{1}H, ^{13}C NMR, 1D TOCSY, and 2D NMR (^{1}H, ^{1}H-COSY, HMBC, HSQC, and ROESY) spectra as well as HR-ESI mass spectra. All the original spectra are presented in Figures S1–S33 in the Supplementary Data section. The hemolytic activity against human erythrocytes and cytotoxic activities against human adenocarcinoma HeLa, colorectal adenocarcinoma DLD-1, and monocyte THP-1 cells were examined.

2. Results and Discussion

2.1. Structural Elucidation of the Glycosides

The concentrated ethanolic extract of the sea cucumber *Psolus chitonoides* was submitted to hydrophobic chromatography on a Polychrom-1 column (powdered Teflon, Biolar, Latvia). The glycosides were eluted after washing with water as a mobile phase to eliminate salts and inorganic impurities with 50% EtOH. The obtained glycoside fraction was separated by the chromatography on Si gel columns with the stepped gradient of eluents CHCl3/EtOH/H2O (100:75:10), (100:100:17), and (100:125:25) to give the fractions (I–IV). The individual compounds **1**–**4** (Figure 1) were isolated by HPLC of the fractions III and IV on a silica-based column, Supelcosil LC-Si (4.6 × 150 mm) and reversed-phase semipreparative column Supelco Ascentis RP-Amide (10 × 250 mm).

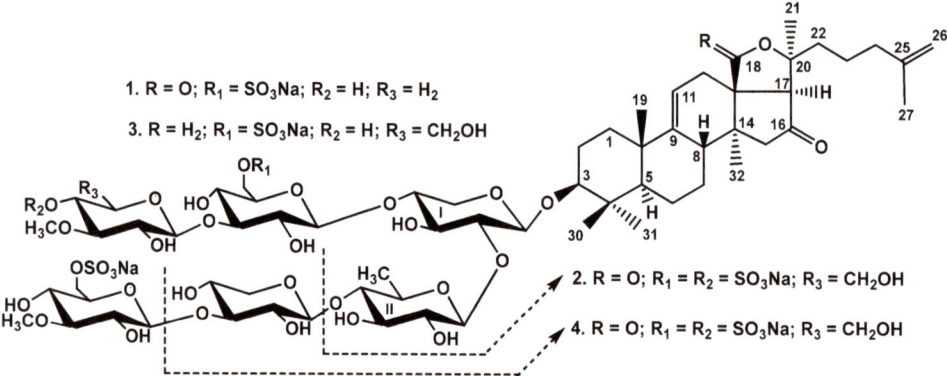

Figure 1. Chemical structures of glycosides isolated from *Psolus chitonoides*: **1**—chitonoidoside E_1; **2**—chitonoidoside F; **3**—chitonoidoside G; **4**—chitonoidoside H.

The configurations of the monosaccharide residues in glycosides **1**–**4** were assigned as *D* based on their biogenetic analogies with all other known sea cucumber triterpene glycosides.

It was found that chitonoidosides E_1 (**1**), F (**2**) and H (**4**) are characterized by holotoxinogenin as aglycone, which was first found in *Apostichopus japonicus* and is broadly distributed in sea cucumber glycosides [16]. This was deduced from the analyses of their ^{1}H and ^{13}C NMR spectra (Tables S1–S3, Figures S1–S6, S9–S14 and S25–S31), which coincided with each other as well as with those of the aglycones of chitonoidosides A_1, C, and D isolated earlier from the same species—*P. chitonoides* [9].

The molecular formula of chitonoidoside E$_1$ (**1**) was determined to be C$_{65}$H$_{100}$O$_{36}$S$_2$Na$_2$ from the [M$_{2Na}$–Na]$^-$ ion peak at *m/z* 1543.5315 (calc. 1543.5339) and [M$_{2Na}$–2Na]$^{2-}$ at *m/z* 760.2734 (calc. 760.2723) in the (−)HR-ESI-MS (Figure S8). The ^{1}H and ^{13}C NMR spectra of the carbohydrate chain of chitonoidoside E$_1$ (**1**) (Table 1, Figures S1–S7) were coincident with those for chitonoidoside E, isolated recently [15] and demonstrated six characteristic doublets of anomeric protons at δ$_H$ 4.67–5.11 (*J* = 7.1–8.0 Hz) and six signals of anomeric carbons at δ$_C$ 102.3–105.2. The analysis of the ^{1}H,^{1}H-COSY, 1D TOCSY, HSQC and ROESY spectra of **1** resulted in the assignment of the signals of two xylose residues, one quinovose, one glucose and 3-*O*-methylglucose, as well as 3-*O*-methylxylose residues. The positions of the sulfate groups were determined based on the deshielding, due to α-shifting effect, of the sulfate group's doubled signal at δ$_C$ 67.1, which is characteristic of glucopyranose units sulfated by C-6 (C-6 signals of non-sulfated glucopyranose residues are usually observed at ~δ$_C$ 61.2). The signals of C-5 MeGlc4 and C-5 Glc5 were shielded due to the β-effect of the sulfate groups to δ$_C$ 75.3 and 75.5, respectively. These data indicate the presence of a hexasaccharide chain with two sulfate groups attached to C-6 MeGlc4 and to C-6 Glc5, and 3-*O*-methylxylose residue as the sixth sugar unit in chitonoidoside E$_1$ (**1**). The sequence of monosaccharides and the positions of the glycosidic bonds were confirmed by the correlations H-1 Xyl1/H-3 (C-3) of the aglycone, H-1 Qui2/H-2 (C-2) Xyl1, H-1 Xyl3/H-4 (C-4) Qui2, H-1 MeGlc4/H-3 (C-3) Xyl3, H-1 Glc5/H-4 (C-4) Xyl1, and H-1 MeXyl6/H-3 (C-3) Glc5 in the ROESY and HMBC spectra of **1**, respectively (Table 1, Figures S5–S7).

Table 1. ^{13}C and ^{1}H NMR chemical shifts, HMBC and ROESY correlations of carbohydrate moiety of chitonoidoside E$_1$ (**1**).

Atom	δ$_C$ Mult. $^{a-c}$	δ$_H$ Mult. (*J* in Hz) ^{d}	HMBC	ROESY
Xyl1 (1→C-3)				
1	104.8 CH	4.67 d (7.1)	C: 3	H-3; H-3, 5 Xyl1
2	**82.2** CH	3.96 m	C: 1 Qui2	H-1 Qui2
3	75.1 CH	4.16 m		H-1, 5 Xyl1
4	**77.9** CH	4.16 m		H-1 Glc5
5	63.5 CH$_2$	4.38 dd (4.3; 12.2)	C: 3 Xyl1	
		3.64 m		H-1 Xyl1
Qui2 (1→2Xyl1)				
1	104.6 CH	5.03 d (8.0)	C: 2 Xyl1	H-2 Xyl1; H-3, 5 Qui2
2	75.7 CH	3.87 t (8.0)	C: 1, 3 Qui2	H-1 Qui2
3	74.8 CH	3.98 t (9.3)	C: 2 Qui2	H-1 Qui2
4	**85.6** CH	3.49 t (9.3)	C: 1 Xyl3; 3, 5 Qui2	H-1 Xyl3
5	71.4 CH	3.67 dd (6.2; 9.3)		H-1 Qui2
6	17.8 CH$_3$	1.61 d (6.2)	C: 4, 5 Qui2	H-4 Qui2
Xyl3 (1→4Qui2)				
1	104.5 CH	4.75 d (7.7)	C: 4 Qui2	H-4 Qui2; H-3, 5 Xyl3
2	73.2 CH	3.84 t (8.5)	C: 1 Xyl3	
3	**87.1** CH	4.04 t (8.5)	C: 1 MeGlc4; 2, 4 Xyl3	H-1 MeGlc4
4	68.7 CH	3.90 m		
5	65.7 CH$_2$	4.13 dd (4.3; 11.1)	C: 4 Xyl3	
		3.60 t (11.1)	C: 1, 3 Xyl3	H-1 Xyl3
MeGlc4 (1→3Xyl3)				
1	104.4 CH	5.11 d (7.9)	C: 3 Xyl3	H-3 Xyl3; H-3, 5 MeGlc4
2	74.3 CH	3.80 t (7.9)	C: 1 MeGlc4	
3	86.4 CH	3.64 t (9.1)	C: 2, 4 MeGlc4, OMe	H-1, 5 MeGlc4
4	69.7 CH	3.96 t (9.1)		
5	75.3 CH	4.03 m		H-1, 3 MeGlc4
6	67.1 CH$_2$	4.97 dd (3.0; 11.5)	C: 5 MeGlc4	
		4.71 dd (6.1; 11.5)	C: 5 MeGlc4	
OMe	60.5 CH$_3$	3.76 s	C: 3 MeGlc4	

Table 1. Cont.

Atom	δ_C Mult. [a–c]	δ_H Mult. (J in Hz) [d]	HMBC	ROESY
Glc5 (1→4Xyl1)				
1	102.3 CH	4.90 d (7.9)	C: 4 Xyl1	H-4 Xyl1; H-3, 5 Glc5
2	73.2 CH	3.84 t (9.1)	C: 1, 3 Glc5	
3	**86.0** CH	4.07 t (9.1)	C: 1 MeXyl6; 2 Glc5	H-1 MeXyl6; H-1 Glc5
4	68.9 CH	3.88 t (9.1)		
5	75.5 CH	4.05 m		H-1 Glc5
6	*67.1* CH$_2$	4.97 dd (1.9; 11.5)	C: 4, 5 Glc5	
		4.70 dd (5.5; 11.5)		
MeXyl6 (1→3Glc5)				
1	105.2 CH	5.07 d (7.9)	C: 3 Glc5	H-3 Glc5; H-3,5 MeXyl6
2	74.2 CH	3.79 t (8.5)	C: 1 MeXyl6	
3	86.6 CH	3.57 t (9.1)	C: 2, 4 MeXyl6; OMe	H-1 MeXyl6; OMe
4	69.9 CH	3.98 t (9.1)	C: 3, 5 MeXyl6	
5	66.4 CH$_2$	4.14 dd (5.5; 12.1)	C: 1, 3, 4 MeXyl6	
		3.61 t (11.5)		H-1 MeXyl6
OMe	60.5 CH$_3$	3.79 s	C: 3 MeXyl6	H-3 MeXyl6

[a] Recorded at 125.67 MHz in C$_5$D$_5$N/D$_2$O (4/1). [b] Bold = interglycosidic positions. [c] Italic = sulfate position. [d] Recorded at 500.12 MHz in C$_5$D$_5$N/D$_2$O (4/1). Multiplicity by 1D TOCSY. The original spectra of **1** are provided in Figures S1–S7.

The (−)ESI-MS/MS of **1** (Figure S8) demonstrated the fragmentation of [M$_{2Na}$–Na]$^-$ ion at m/z 1543.5 with the ion-peaks observed at m/z 1423.6 [M$_{2Na}$–Na–NaHSO$_4$]$^-$, 1266.5 [M$_{2Na}$–Na–MeGlcOSO$_3$Na+H]$^-$, 1133.5 [M$_{2Na}$–Na–MeGlcOSO$_3$Na–Xyl+H]$^-$, 987.4 [M$_{2Na}$–Na–MeGlcOSO$_3$Na–Xyl–Qui+H]$^-$, 841.4 [M$_{2Na}$–Na–MeGlcOSO$_3$Na–Xyl––Qui–MeXyl+2H]$^-$, 665.1 [M$_{2Na}$–Na–Agl–MeXyl–GlcOSO$_3$Na+H]$^-$, 533.1 [M$_{2Na}$–Na–Agl–MeXyl–GlcOSO$_3$Na–Xyl+H]$^-$, 387.0 [M$_{2Na}$–Na–Agl–MeXyl–GlcOSO$_3$Na–Xyl–Qui+H]$^-$, 255.0 [M$_{2Na}$–Na–Agl–MeXyl–GlcOSO$_3$Na–Xyl–Qui–Xyl+H]$^-$. All these ion peaks corroborated the sequence of monosaccharides and the aglycone structure of **1**.

Therefore, chitonoidosides E [15] and E$_1$ (**1**) share the identical oligosaccharide moiety (they belong to the same group of glycosides) and differ from each other through the presence/absence of a carbonyl group at C-18 in the aglycones (the difference of their exact masses by 14 *amu* in (−) HR-ESI-MS confirmed this). These data indicate that chitonoidoside E$_1$ (**1**) is 3β-O-{6-O-sodium sulfate-3-O-methyl-β-D-glucopyranosyl-(1→3)-β-D-xylopyranosyl-(1→4)-β-D-quinovopyranosyl-(1→2)-[3-O-methyl-β-D-xylopyranosyl-(1→3)-6-O-sodium sulfate-β-D-glucopyranosyl-(1→4)]-β-D-xylopyranosyl}-16-oxo-holosta-9(11), 25(26)-diene.

The molecular formula of chitonoidoside F (**2**) was determined to be C$_{54}$H$_{82}$O$_{28}$S$_2$Na$_2$ from the [M$_{2Na}$–Na]$^-$ ion peak at m/z 1265.4337 (calc. 1265.4337) and [M$_{2Na}$–2Na]$^{2-}$ ion peak at m/z 621.2244 (calc. 621.2269) in the (−)HR-ESI-MS (Figure S16). The 1H NMR spectrum of the carbohydrate part of chitonoidoside F (**2**) exhibited four characteristic doublets at δ_H 4.67–5.18 (J = 7.6–8.1 Hz), correlated by the HSQC spectrum with corresponding anomeric carbon signals at δ_C 102.2–104.9. These signals were indicative of a tetrasaccharide chain with β-configurations of glycosidic bonds (Table 2, Figures S9–S15).

An isolated spin system from each monosaccharide residue was analyzed using the ^{1}H,^{1}H-COSY and 1D TOCSY spectra. Further analysis of the HSQC, ROESY and HMBC spectra resulted in the assignment of all monosaccharide NMR signals. Using this algorithm, the monosaccharides composing the carbohydrate moiety of chitonoidoside F (**2**) were found to be xylose (Xyl1), quinovose (Qui2), glucose (Glc3), and 3-O-methylglucose (MeGlc4). The monosaccharide compositions of the other glycosides, reported herein, were established in the same manner.

Table 2. ^{13}C and ^{1}H NMR chemical shifts, HMBC and ROESY correlations of carbohydrate moiety of chitonoidoside F (**2**).

Atom	δ_C Mult. $^{a-c}$	δ_H Mult. (J in Hz) ^{d}	HMBC	ROESY
Xyl1 (1→C-3)				
1	104.8 CH	4.67 d (7.6)	C: 3	H-3; H-3, 5 Xyl1
2	**82.1** CH	3.98 t (8.3)	C: 1 Qui2; 3 Xyl1	H-1 Qui2
3	75.1 CH	4.17 t (8.3)	C: 4 Xyl1	
4	**78.0** CH	4.16 m		H-1 Xyl1; H-1 Glc3
5	63.5 CH$_2$	4.38 d (10.2)		
		3.63 m		H-1, 3 Xyl1
Qui2 (1→2Xyl1)				
1	104.9 CH	5.06 d (8.1)	C: 2 Xyl1	H-2 Xyl1; H-3, 5 Qui2
2	76.2 CH	3.88 t (9.1)	C: 1 Qui2	H-4 Qui2
3	76.8 CH	4.06 t (9.1)	C: 2, 4 Qui2	H-1, 5 Qui2
4	76.2 CH	3.58 t (9.1)	C: 3, 5 Qui2	H-2 Qui2
5	72.8 CH	3.70 dd (6.3; 9.9)	C: 4 Qui2	H-1, 3 Qui2
6	18.2 CH$_3$	1.53 d (6.3)	C: 4, 5 Qui2	
Glc3 (1→4Xyl1)				
1	102.2 CH	4.90 d (8.0)	C: 4 Xyl1	H-4 Xyl1; H-3, 5 Glc3
2	73.3 CH	3.83 t (9.2)	C: 1 Glc3	
3	**86.0** CH	4.17 t (9.2)	C: 2, 4 Glc3; 1 MeGlc4	H-1 MeGlc4; H-1 Glc3
4	68.9 CH	3.87 t (9.2)	C: 5 Glc3	
5	75.1 CH	4.04 m		H-1 Glc3
6	67.2 CH$_2$	4.94 d (10.3)		
		4.68 m		
MeGlc4 (1→3Glc3)				
1	104.3 CH	5.18 d (8.0)	C: 3 Glc3	H-3 Glc3; H-3, 5 MeGlc4
2	74.0 CH	3.86 t (8.7)	C: 1, 3 MeGlc4	H-4 MeGlc4
3	85.3 CH	3.71 t (8.7)	C: 4, 5 MeGlc4, OMe	H-1, 5 MeGlc4; Ome
4	*76.3* CH	4.88 t (9.6)	C: 3, 5 MeGlc4	H-2 MeGlc4
5	76.4 CH	3.86 t (8.7)		H-1 MeGlc4
6	61.2 CH$_2$	4.51 d (11.4)		
		4.33 dd (4.4; 11.4)		
OMe	60.7 CH$_3$	3.93 s	C: 3 MeGlc4	

^{a} Recorded at 125.67 MHz in C$_5$D$_5$N/D$_2$O (4/1). ^{b} Bold = interglycosidic positions. ^{c} Italic = sulfate position. ^{d} Recorded at 500.12 MHz in C$_5$D$_5$N/D$_2$O (4/1). Multiplicity by 1D TOCSY. The original spectra of **2** are provided in Figures S9–S15.

The signal of C-6 Glc3 in the ^{13}C NMR spectrum of **2** was deshielded to δ_C 67.2, which is characteristic of sulfation at this position. The signal of C-6 MeGlc4 was observed at δ_C 61.2, indicating the absence of a sulfate group at this position, although the MS data indicated the presence of two sulfate groups in **2**. The signal of C-4 MeGlc4 was deshielded to δ_C 76.3 when compared to the same signal of terminal 3-O-methylglucose residues of the glycosides lacking a sulfate group (δ_C ~70.0) [12]. Moreover, the signals of C-3 and C-5 MeGlc4 in the spectrum of **2** were shielded to δ_C 85.3 and 76.4, respectively, due to the β-shifting effect of a sulfate group. Therefore, the 3-O-methylglucose residue in the sugar part of **2** was sulfated by C-4. This structural feature was only found once in previous research—in the glycosides of *Colochirus quadrangularis* [17]. The observation of 3-O-methylxylose residue sulfated by C-4 in the glycosides of *P. chitonoides* [15] clearly demonstrates the presence of a specific sulfatase capable of attaching a sulfate group to C-4 of monosaccharides in pyranose form.

The positions of glycosidic linkages, established by the ROESY and HMBC spectra of **2** revealed the uncommon architecture of the sugar chain with disaccharide fragment 4-O-sodium sulfate-3-O-methyl-β-D-glucopyranosyl-(1→3)-6-O-sodium sulfate-β-D-glucopyranosyl-(1→4) attached to the first (Xyl1) residue, while quinovose was a terminal unit in the reduced bottom semi-chain (Table 2). Two tetraosides whose carbohydrate part featured the same architecture were found only in the sea cucumber *Thyonidium kurilensis* [18].

The (−)ESI-MS/MS of **2** (Figure S16) demonstrated the fragmentation of [M$_{2Na}$−Na]$^-$ ion at m/z 1265.4 resulting in the ion-peaks appearance at m/z 1146.5 [M$_{2Na}$−Na−NaSO$_4$]$^-$, 987.4 [M$_{2Na}$−Na−MeGlcOSO$_3$Na+H]$^-$, 841.4, [M$_{2Na}$−Na−MeGlcOSO$_3$Na−Qui)+H]$^-$, corroborating the notion that sulfated 3-O-methylglucose and quinovose are terminal monosaccharides. All these data indicate that chitonoidoside F (**2**) is 3β-O-{β-D-quinovopyranosyl-(1→2)-(4-O-sodium sulfate-3-O-methyl-β-D-glucopyranosyl-(1→3)-6-O-sodium sulfate-β-D-glucopyranosyl-(1→4))-β-D-xylopyranosyl}-16-oxo-holosta-9(11),25(26)-diene.

The molecular formula of chitonoidoside G (**3**) was determined to be C$_{66}$H$_{104}$O$_{36}$S$_2$Na$_2$ from the [M$_{2Na}$−Na]$^-$ ion peak at m/z 1559.5646 (calc. 1559.5652) and [M$_{2Na}$−2Na]$^{2-}$ ion peak at m/z 768.2895 (calc. 768.2880) in the (−)HR-ESI-MS (Figure S24).

Based on the absence of the signals of 18(20)-lactone at δ$_C$ ~178 (C-18) and ~83 (C-20) in the ^{13}C NMR spectrum of **3**, the aglycone with 18(20)-ether bond instead of the lactone was supposed to be present. The NMR spectra of the aglycone part of chitonoidosides G (**3**) and A [15], where this aglycone was first found, were almost coincident with each other (Table 3, Figures S17–S22).

Table 3. ^{13}C and ^{1}H NMR chemical shifts, HMBC and ROESY correlations of the aglycone moiety of chitonoidoside G (**3**).

Position	δ$_C$ Mult. ^{a}	δ$_H$ Mult. (J in Hz) ^{b}	HMBC	ROESY
1	35.9 CH$_2$	1.60 m 1.28 m		H-11
2	26.7 CH$_2$	2.08 m 1.83 m		H-19, H-30
3	88.7 CH	3.12 dd (4.2; 11.8)	C: 1 Xyl1	H-5, H-31, H1-Xyl1
4	39.6 C			
5	52.7 CH	0.75 brd (12.0)	C: 10, 19	H-3, H-31
6	20.9 CH$_2$	1.57 m 1.35 m		H-31 H-19, H-30
7	28.7 CH$_2$	1.57 m 1.17 m		
8	40.9 CH	2.31 m		H-18, H-19
9	150.9 C			
10	39.5 C			
11	114.7 CH	5.30 m		H-1
12	33.8 CH$_2$	2.38 m 2.25 m		H-32 H-21
13	56.3 C			
14	40.3 C			
15	50.5 CH$_2$	2.47 d (15.9) 2.19 d (15.9)	C: 14, 16, 32 C: 13, 16	H-18 H-32
16	218.1 C			
17	63.8 CH	2.35 s	C: 12, 13, 16, 18, 20, 21	H-12, H-21, H-22, H-32
18	73.8 CH$_2$	4.02 m 3.65 d (9.1)	C: 12, 20	
19	22.2 CH$_3$	0.97 s	C: 1, 5, 9, 10	H-1, H-2, H-6, H-8, H-18
20	86.6 C			
21	26.1 CH$_3$	1.32 s	C: 17, 20, 22	H-12, H-17, H-18, H-22
22	37.8 CH$_2$	1.70 m 1.57 m		H-21, H-24
23	22.7 CH$_2$	1.69 m 1.56 m		
24	38.2 CH$_2$	1.95 m	C: 23	H-21
25	146.0 C			
26	110.2 CH$_2$	4.72 brs 4.71 brs	C: 24, 27 C: 24, 27	
27	22.2 CH$_3$	1.65 s	C: 24, 25, 26	H-24
30	16.5 CH$_3$	0.97 s	C: 3, 4, 5, 31	H-31
31	27.9 CH$_3$	1.13 s	C: 3, 4, 5, 30	H-1, H-3, H-5, H-30
32	21.4 CH$_3$	0.78 s	C: 13, 14, 15	H-15, H-17

^{a} Recorded at 125.67 MHz in C$_5$D$_5$N/D$_2$O (4/1). ^{b} Recorded at 500.12 MHz in C$_5$D$_5$N/D$_2$O (4/1). The original spectra of **3** are provided in Figures S17–S23.

The ^{1}H and ^{13}C NMR spectra of the carbohydrate chain of chitonoidoside G (**3**) (Table 4, Figures S17–S23) demonstrated six signals of anomeric protons at δ$_H$ 4.66–5.18 (d, J = 6.9–7.9 Hz), corresponding to the signals of the anomeric carbons at δ$_C$ 102.2–104.8.

These signals indicated the presence of a hexasaccharide moiety with β-glycosidic bonds. The monosaccharide composition of **3** was determined as two xyloses (Xyl1 and Xyl3), quinovose (Qui2), glucose (Glc5), and two 3-*O*-methylglucoses (MeGlc4 and MeGlc6). The doubled signal at δ_C 67.1 indicated the presence of two sulfate groups. Using the 1H,1H-COSY and 1D TOCSY spectra their positions were deduced as C-6 MeGlc4 and C-6 Glc5. The comparison of the ^{13}C NMR spectra of the carbohydrate parts of the chitonoidosides G (**3**) and E$_1$ (**1**) demonstrated the closeness of the signals of the monosaccharide units from first to fifth. The signals of the terminal sixth monosaccharide residue in **3** were assigned as 3-*O*-methylglucose instead of 3-*O*-methylxylose in **1**. The sequence of monosaccharides and the positions of the glycosidic bonds were confirmed by the correlations in the ROESY and HMBC spectra of **3** (Table 4, Figures S17–S23). Therefore, chitonoidoside G (**3**) is the first compound in the combinatorial library of the glycosides from *P. chitonoides* to feature non-sulfated 3-*O*-methylglucose as terminal residue in the upper semi-chain.

Table 4. ^{13}C and ^{1}H NMR chemical shifts, HMBC and ROESY correlations of carbohydrate moiety of chitonoidoside G (**3**).

Atom	δ_C Mult. $^{a-c}$	δ_H Mult. (*J* in Hz) ^{d}	HMBC	ROESY
Xyl1 (1→C-3)				
1	104.8 CH	4.66 d (6.9)	C: 3	H-3; H-3, 5 Xyl1
2	**82.1** CH	3.97 t (8.8)	C: 1 Qui2; 1, 3 Xyl1	H-1 Qui2
3	75.1 CH	4.16 t (8.8)	C: 4 Xyl1	
4	**77.8** CH	4.16 m		
5	63.5 CH$_2$	4.37 dd (4.1; 11.8)		
		3.62 m		H-1 Xyl1
Qui2 (1→2Xyl1)				
1	104.5 CH	5.04 d (7.3)	C: 2 Xyl1	H-2 Xyl1; H-3, 5 Qui2
2	75.7 CH	3.87 t (9.0)	C: 1, 3 Qui2	H-4 Qui2
3	74.8 CH	3.98 t (9.0)	C: 2, 4 Qui2	H-5 Qui2
4	**85.6** CH	3.49 t (9.0)	C: 1 Xyl3; 3, 5 Qui2	H-1 Xyl3; H-2 Qui2
5	71.4 CH	3.68 dd (6.2; 9.0)		H-1 Qui2
6	17.8 CH$_3$	1.62 d (6.2)	C: 4, 5 Qui2	H-4, 5 Qui2
Xyl3 (1→4Qui2)				
1	104.4 CH	4.75 d (7.7)	C: 4 Qui2	H-4 Qui2; H-3, 5 Xyl3
2	73.2 CH	3.84 t (8.3)	C: 1, 3 Xyl3	
3	**87.0** CH	4.04 t (8.3)	C: 1 MeGlc4; 2, 4 Xyl3	H-1 MeGlc4; H-1 Xyl3
4	68.8 CH	3.89 m	C: 5 Xyl3	
5	65.7 CH$_2$	4.12 dd (5.3; 11.2)		
		3.59 d (11.2)	C: 1 Xyl3	H-1 Xyl3
MeGlc4 (1→3Xyl3)				
1	104.6 CH	5.12 d (7.9)	C: 3 Xyl3	H-3 Xyl3; H-3, 5 MeGlc4
2	74.3 CH	3.80 t (8.5)	C: 1 MeGlc4	
3	86.4 CH	3.64 t (8.5)	C: 4 MeGlc4, OMe	H-1 MeGlc4; OMe
4	69.9 CH	3.96 t (8.5)	C: 3, 5, 6 MeGlc4	H-2, 6 MeGlc4
5	75.5 CH	4.03 m		H-1, 3 MeGlc4
6	67.1 CH$_2$	4.97 d (10.7)		
		4.71 dd (5.6; 11.3)	C: 5 MeGlc4	
OMe	60.5 CH$_3$	3.76 s	C: 3 MeGlc4	
Glc5 (1→4Xyl1)				
1	102.2 CH	4.88 d (7.9)	C: 4 Xyl1	H-4 Xyl1; H-3, 5 Glc5
2	73.2 CH	3.84 t (9.0)	C: 1, 3 Glc5	
3	**86.0** CH	4.16 t (9.0)	C: 1 MeGlc6; 2 Glc5	H-1 MeGlc6; H-1 Glc5
4	69.0 CH	3.89 t (9.0)	C: 3 Glc5	
5	75.5 CH	4.02 m		H-1 Glc5
6	67.1 CH$_2$	4.93 d (10.7)		
		4.68 dd (6.2; 11.3)		

Table 4. Cont.

Atom	δ$_C$ Mult. $^{a-c}$	δ$_H$ Mult. (J in Hz) ^{d}	HMBC	ROESY
MeGlc6 (1→3Glc5)				
1	104.4 CH	5.18 d (7.5)	C: 3 Glc5	H-3 Glc5; H-3, 5 MeGlc6
2	74.5 CH	3.84 t (8.8)	C: 1 MeGlc6	
3	86.8 CH	3.66 t (8.8)	C: 2, 4 MeGlc6, OMe	H-1 MeGlc6
4	70.3 CH	3.89 m	C: 5 MeGlc6	H-6 MeGlc6
5	77.5 CH	3.89 m		H-1 MeGlc6
6	61.7 CH$_2$	4.34 dd (2.2; 11.7)		
		4.05 dd (5.1; 11.7)	C: 4 MeGlc6	
OMe	60.6 CH$_3$	3.80 s	C: 3 MeGlc6	

^{a} Recorded at 125.67 MHz in C$_5$D$_5$N/D$_2$O (4/1). ^{b} Bold = interglycosidic positions. ^{c} Italic = sulfate position. ^{d} Recorded at 500.12 MHz in C$_5$D$_5$N/D$_2$O (4/1). Multiplicity by 1D TOCSY. The original spectra of **1** are provided in Figures S17–S23.

The (−)ESI-MS/MS of **3** (Figure S24) demonstrated the fragmentation of [M$_{2Na}$−Na]$^-$ ion at m/z 1559.6 leading to the ion-peaks appearance at m/z 1439.6 [M$_{2Na}$−Na−NaHSO$_4$]$^-$, 1383.6 [M$_{2Na}$−Na−MeGlc+H]$^-$, 1281.6 [M$_{2Na}$−Na−MeGlcOSO$_3$Na+H]$^-$, 1149.5 [M$_{2Na}$−Na−MeGlcOSO$_3$Na−Xyl+H]$^-$, 1003.5 [M$_{2Na}$−Na−MeGlcOSO$_3$Na−Xyl−Qui+H]$^-$, 533.1 [M$_{2Na}$−Na−Agl−MeGlc−MeGlcOSO$_3$Na−Xyl+H]$^-$, 387.0 [M$_{2Na}$−Na−Agl−MeGlc−MeGlcOSO$_3$Na−Xyl−Qui+H]$^-$, 255.0 [M$_{2Na}$−Na−Agl−MeGlc−MeGlcOSO$_3$Na−Xyl−Qui−Xyl+H]$^-$, confirming the sequence of monosaccharides and the aglycone structure of **3**.

These data indicate that chitonoidoside G (**3**) is 3β-O-{6-O-sodium sulfate-3-O-methyl-β-D-glucopyranosyl-(1→3)-β-D-xylopyranosyl-(1→4)-β-D-quinovopyranosyl-(1→2)-[3-O-methyl-β-D-glucopyranosyl-(1→3)-6-O-sodium sulfate-β-D-glucopyranosyl-(1→4)]-β-D-xylopyranosyl}-16-oxo-18(20)-epoxylanosta-9(11),25(26)-diene.

The molecular formula of chitonoidoside H (**4**) was determined to be C$_{59}$H$_{90}$O$_{32}$S$_2$Na$_2$ from the [M$_{2Na}$−Na]$^-$ ion peak at m/z 1397.4749 (calc. 1397.4760) and [M$_{2Na}$−2Na]$^{2-}$ ion peak at m/z 687.2442 (calc. 687.2434) in the (−)HR-ESI-MS (Figure S33).

The ^{1}H and ^{13}C NMR spectra of the carbohydrate chain of chitonoidoside H (**4**) (Table 5, Figures S25–S32) demonstrated five signals of anomeric protons at δ$_H$ 4.66–5.18 (d, J = 6.9–8.1 Hz), corresponding to the signals of the anomeric carbons at δ$_C$ 102.3–104.8, which indicated the presence of a pentasaccharide oligosaccharide chain with β-glycosidic bonds between the monosaccharides. The analysis of the 1H,1H-COSY, 1D, and 2D TOCSY and HSQC spectra resulted in the assignment of the signals of two xyloses (Xyl1 and Xyl3), quinovose (Qui2), glucose (Glc4), and 3-O-methylglucose (MeGlc5). One sulfate group in chitonoidoside H (**4**) was attached to C-6 Glc4 (in the upper semi-chain), which is a typical position for chitonoidosides that feature a branch point in the sugar chain at C-4 Xyl1, with the exception of chitonoidoside B [15], containing one sulfate group. The position of the second sulfate group was determined as C-4 MeGlc5, based on the deshielding of the signal of C-4 MeGlc5 to δ$_C$ 76.2 (α-shifting effect of sulfate group) and the shielding of the signals C-3 and C-5 MeGlc5 to δ$_C$ 85.2 and 76.4 (β-shifting effect of sulfate group), respectively, compared to the signals in the chitonoidoside G (**3**). The sequence of the monosaccharides and the positions of the glycosidic bonds deduced by the ROESY and HMBC spectra of **4** displayed the bottom semi-chain, composed of two monosaccharide units, and the upper semi-chain, composed of three monosaccharide units, forming a chain with an uncommon architecture (Table 5, Figures S25–S32).

Table 5. ^{13}C and ^{1}H NMR chemical shifts, HMBC and ROESY correlations of carbohydrate moiety of chitonoidoside H (**4**).

Atom	δ$_C$ Mult. $^{a-c}$	δ$_H$ Mult. (J in Hz) ^{d}	HMBC	ROESY
Xyl1 (1→C-3)				
1	104.6 CH	4.66 d (6.9)	C: 3	H-3; H-3, 5 Xyl1
2	**81.9** CH	3.97 m	C: 1 Qui2; 1 Xyl1	H-1 Qui2
3	75.1 CH	4.16 m	C: 4 Xyl1	H-1 Xyl1
4	**78.0** CH	4.15 m		H-1 Glc4
5	63.5 CH$_2$	4.38 m	C: 3 Xyl1	
		3.62 m		H-1 Xyl1
Qui2 (1→2Xyl1)				
1	104.4 CH	5.07 d (6.9)	C: 2 Xyl1	H-2 Xyl1; H-5 Qui2
2	75.7 CH	3.87 t (9.2)	C: 1, 3 Qui2	H-4 Qui2
3	74.8 CH	4.00 t (9.2)	C: 2, 4 Qui2	H-1 Qui2
4	**85.6** CH	3.47 t (9.2)	C: 1 Xyl3; 3, 5 Qui2	H-1 Xyl3; H-2 Qui2
5	71.4 CH	3.70 dd (6.2; 9.2)		H-1, 3 Qui2
6	17.8 CH$_3$	1.61 d (6.2)	C: 4, 5 Qui2	H-4, 5 Qui2
Xyl3 (1→4Qui2)				
1	104.8 CH	4.70 d (6.6)	C: 4 Qui2	H-4 Qui2; H-3, 5 Xyl3
2	73.3 CH	3.82 t (8.4)	C: 1, 3 Xyl3	
3	77.2 CH	4.05 t (8.4)	C: 2, 4 Xyl3	
4	70.1 CH	4.03 m	C: 3 Xyl3	
5	66.5 CH$_2$	4.14 brd (11.2)	C: 3 Xyl3	
		3.59 t (11.2)	C: 1, 3, 4 Xyl3	H-1 Xyl3
Glc4 (1→4Xyl1)				
1	102.3 CH	4.89 d (8.1)	C: 4 Xyl1	H-4 Xyl1; H-3, 5 Glc4
2	74.0 CH	3.82 t (9.1)	C: 1 Glc4	
3	86.0 CH	4.16 t (9.1)	C: 1 MeGlc5	H-1 MeGlc5; H-1 Glc4
4	69.0 CH	3.86 t (9.1)	C: 3 Glc4	
5	75.2 CH	4.03 m		H-1 Glc4
6	67.2 CH$_2$	4.96 d (12.2)		
		4.69 m		
MeGlc5 (1→3Glc4)				
1	104.3 CH	5.18 d (8.1)	C: 3 Glc4	H-3 Glc4; H-3, 5 MeGlc5
2	74.1 CH	3.86 t (9.1)	C: 1 MeGlc5	H-4 MeGlc5
3	85.2 CH	3.71 t (9.1)	C: 4 MeGlc5; OMe	H-1 MeGlc5
4	76.2 CH	4.88 t (9.1)	C: 3, 5 MeGlc5	H-6 MeGlc5
5	76.4 CH	3.84 t (9.1)		
6	61.7 CH$_2$	4.50 d (12.2)		
		4.33 dd (6.2; 12.2)		
OMe	60.7 CH$_3$	3.93 s	C: 3 MeGlc5	

^{a} Recorded at 125.67 MHz in C$_5$D$_5$N/D$_2$O (4/1). ^{b} Bold = interglycosidic positions. ^{c} Italic = sulfate position. ^{d} Recorded at 500.12 MHz in C$_5$D$_5$N/D$_2$O (4/1). Multiplicity by ^{1}H, and 1D TOCSY. The original spectra of **1** are provided in Figures S25–S32.

The comparison of the ^{13}C NMR spectra of the carbohydrate parts of **4** and **2** displayed their difference only in the presence of the signals of additional xylose residue (in the bottom semi-chain of **4**), as well as the glycosylation effect at C-4 Qui2, whose signal was observed at δ$_C$ 85.6, instead of δ$_C$ 76.2 (C-4 Qui2), observed in **2**. Therefore, the chitonoidosides F (**2**) and H (**4**) can be considered as sequential steps in the biosynthesis of the glycosides in *P. chitonoides*.

The (−)ESI-MS/MS of **4** (Figure S33) demonstrated the fragmentation of [M$_{2Na}$−Na]$^−$ ion at *m/z* 1397.5 resulted in the fragmentary ion-peaks at *m/z* 1277.5 [M$_{2Na}$−Na−NaHSO$_4$]$^−$, 1119.5 [M$_{2Na}$−Na−MeGlcOSO$_3$Na+H]$^−$, 1119.5 [M$_{2Na}$−Na−Xyl−Qui]$^−$, 987.4 [M$_{2Na}$−Na−MeGlcOSO$_3$Na−Xyl+H]$^−$, 841.4 [M$_{2Na}$−Na−MeGlcOSO$_3$Na−Xyl−Qui+H]$^−$, 519.0 [M$_{2Na}$−Na−Agl−MeGlcOSO$_3$Na−Xyl+H]$^−$, 399.0 [M$_{2Na}$−Na−Agl−MeGlcOSO$_3$Na−Xyl−NaHSO$_4$]$^−$, 373.0 [M$_{2Na}$−Na−Agl−Xyl−Qui−MeGlcOSO$_3$Na+H]$^−$, 255.0 [M$_{2Na}$−Na−Agl−MeGlcOSO$_3$Na−GlcOSO$_3$Na−Xyl+H]$^−$, confirming both the sequence of monosaccharides and the aglycone structure of **4**.

These data indicate that chitonoidoside H (**4**) is 3β-O-{β-D-xylopyranosyl-(1→4)-β-D-quinovopyranosyl-(1→2)-[4-O-sodium sulfate-3-O-methyl-β-D-glucopyranosyl-(1→3)-6-O-sodium sulfate-β-D-glucopyranosyl-(1→4)]-β-D-xylopyranosyl}-16-oxo-holosta-9(11), 25(26)-diene.

2.2. Bioactivity of the Glycosides

The cytotoxic activity of sea cucumber glycosides against different cell types and cell lines, including HeLa and THP-1, has been extensively studied [1,19]. This has led to deeper understanding of the mechanisms of the anticancer activities of glycosides [7,8,20]. Different tumor cell lines exhibit different sensitivities to the cytotoxic effects of sea cucumber glycosides, depending on their chemical structures. This can be of special interest for the development of therapy for certain types of cancer [21].

The cytotoxic activities of compounds **1–4** and chitonoidoside E against human erythrocytes and the human cancer cell lines, adenocarcinoma HeLa, colorectal adenocarcinoma DLD-1, monocytes THP-1, and leukemia promyeloblast HL-60 were investigated (Table 6). The previously tested chitonoidoside A [9] and cisplatin were used as the positive controls.

Table 6. The cytotoxic activities of glycosides **1–4**, chitonoidoside E, cisplatin and chitonoidoside A (positive controls) against human erythrocytes, HeLa, DLD-1, THP-1 human cell lines.

Glycosides	ED$_{50}$, μM, Erythrocytes	Cytotoxicity, ED$_{50}$ μM			
		HeLa	DLD-1	THP-1	HL-60
Chitonoidoside E	0.45 ± 0.01	5.73 ± 0.10	8.93 ± 1.28	0.58 ± 0.07	5.73 ± 0.37
Chitonoidoside E$_1$ (**1**)	0.64 ± 0.01	18.00 ± 0.59	34.12 ± 2.12	0.58 ± 0.04	9.97 ± 0.94
Chitonoidoside F (**2**)	1.17 ± 0.07	37.99 ± 1.36	71.11 ± 1.22	4.87 ± 0.47	41.23 ± 1.11
Chitonoidoside G (**3**)	0.65 ± 0.01	14.52 ± 1.08	12.44 ± 1.07	4.81 ± 0.46	8.23 ± 0.33
Chitonoidoside H (**4**)	0.89 ± 0.05	17.02 ± 1.18	36.62 ± 1.51	2.88 ± 0.23	8.13 ± 0.45
Chitonoidoside A	1.27 ± 0.03	39.48 ± 1.15	32.68 ± 2.56	2.93 ± 0.17	8.95 ± 0.35
Cisplatin	-	16.94 ± 0.25	> 80.00	56.12 ± 3.91	8.58 ± 0.54

All the tested compounds demonstrated strong hemolytic activity, with hexaosides **1**, **3** and chitonoidoside E proving to be the most active. The human erythrocytes were more sensitive to the membranolytic action of tested compounds (Table 6) compared to the cancer cells, which is similar to previous data concerning mouse erythrocytes [12,13,15,17]. The monocyte cell line THP-1 and the erythrocytes were comparably sensitive to the action of the glycosides.

A similar tendency for **1**, **3**, and chitonoidoside E was observed for the cytotoxicity against the adenocarcinoma HeLa and HL-60 cells, but the demonstrated effects were moderate. Chitonoidoside E possessing a hexasaccharide chain and the aglycone with a 18(20)-ether bond was the most active; the activity of hexaosides **1** and **3**, which differed through the sixth monosaccharide residue, and the activity of pentaoside **4**, were close to each other against erythrocytes and HeLa and HL-60 cells, but significantly differed in relation to DLD-1 and THP-1 cells. The tetraoside with a shortened bottom semi-chain, chitonoidoside F (**2**), exhibited the weakest membranolytic effect in the series. The most significant difference in the activity of **2** and the other compounds of the series was observed for the DLD-1 and HL-60 cell lines, confirming the diversity in the sensitivities of the cancer cell lines. The presence of the aglycone with an 18(20)-ether bond (in **3**) did not decrease the activity of the glycosides. The latter two peculiarities are in good accordance with the biologic activity of a previously analyzed series of chitonoidosides—the glycosides of *P. chitonoides* [15].

2.3. Metabolic Network of Carbohydrate Chains of Chitonoidosides of the Groups A–H

The aglycones and carbohydrate chains of triterpene glycosides are biosynthesized simultaneously and independently from each other [12,22,23], leading to the tremendous structural diversity in this class of natural products from sea cucumbers. Glycosides with identical to sugar moieties that differ in their aglycone structures are considered to belong to a group of glycosides named by particular letter (some groups may consist of one compound). Thus, eight groups of chitonoidosides, A–H, were discovered in *P. chitonoides*, including three types of tetraosides (groups A, C, and F), differing in their architecture and monosaccharide composition, two types of pentaosides (groups D and H) with analogical differences, and three types of hexaosides (groups B, E, and G), differing in their terminal monosaccharide residues and the positions of their sulfate groups. The biosynthesis of sugar moieties occurs through the sequential connection of monosaccharides to certain positions, forming carbohydrate chains. The first branchpoint in the biosynthesis of the chitonoidosides of diverse groups is the attachment of the third sugar residue to the bioside consisting of Xyl1 and Qui2. When the third sugar (xylose) attaches to C-4 Qui2, with the subsequent attachment of 3-OMeGlc and sulfation, the growth of the sugar chain ends with the formation of tetraosides, namely the chitonoidosides of group A (such chains are considered as linear). The attachment of glucose as the third sugar unit to C-4 Xyl1, followed by the addition of glycosylation with different monosaccharide residues (3-*O*-methylxylose or 3-*O*-methylglucose) and sulfation, leads to the formation of the chitonoidosides of groups C and F (Figure 2). The elongation of the bottom semi-chain in chitonoidoside F (by C-4 Qui2) results in chitonoidoside H formation. The further elongation of the sugar chains of the chitonoidosides belonging to the group A and additional sulfation lead to the formation of chitonoidosides of the group D, followed by the subsequent formation of chitonoidosides belonging to group G. When the elongation of the sugar chains of the chitonoidosides of group A occurs without sulfation, the chitonoidosides of the group B are biosynthesized.

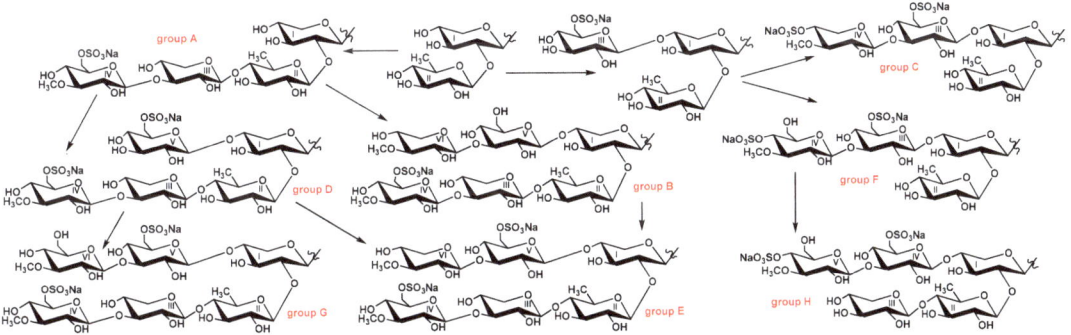

Figure 2. Biosynthetic network of carbohydrate chains of chitonoidosides of the groups A–H.

Noticeably, that the sulfation of terminal monosaccharide in the upper semi-chain of tetraosides—the chitonoidosides of groups C and F—precedes the subsequent elongation of the bottom semi-chain. Therefore, these glycosides cannot be the precursors of the chitonoidosides of group E containing non-sulfated terminal 3-*O*-methylxylose in the upper semi-chain. Similarly, hexaosides—chitonoidosides of group B—with the only sulfate group at C-6 MeGlc4 cannot be formed from pentaosides, the chitonoidosides of group D because, of the sulfation of Glc5 in the latter. Additionally, the carbohydrate chain of the chitonoidosides of group E can be formed through the sulfation of the chain of chitonoidosides of group B or through the glycosylation of the chain of chitonoidosides of group D. All these data demonstrate that glycosylation and sulfation are competitive and parallel/simultaneous processes in carbohydrate chain biosynthesis.

3. Materials and Methods

3.1. General Experimental Procedures

Specific rotation, PerkinElmer 343 Polarimeter (PerkinElmer, Waltham, MA, USA); NMR, Bruker AMX 500 (Bruker BioSpin GmbH, Rheinstetten, Germany) (500.12/125.67 MHz (^{1}H/^{13}C) spectrometer; ESI MS (positive and negative ion modes), Agilent 6510 Q-TOF apparatus (Agilent Technology, Santa Clara, CA, USA), sample concentration 0.01 mg/mL; HPLC, Agilent 1260 Infinity II with a differential refractometer (Agilent Technology, Santa Clara, CA, USA); columns Supelcosil LC-Si (4.6 × 150 mm, 5 µm) and Ascentis RP-Amide (10 × 250 mm, 5 µm) (Supelco, Bellefonte, PA, USA).

3.2. Animals and Cells

The specimens of the holothurian *Psolus chitonoides* (family Psolidae; order Dendrochirotida) were harvested in the Bering Sea during the 14th expedition cruise on board the r/v "Akademik Oparin" on August 24, 1991, north of Bering Island (Commander Islands). The harvesting was carried out by the Sigsbee trawl at depths of 100–150 m. The animals were taxonomically determined by Dr. Alexey V. Smirnov, Zoological Institute of the Russian Academy of Sciences. Voucher specimens are kept at the Zoological Institute of RAS, St. Petersburg, Russia.

The human erythrocytes were purchased from the Station of Blood Transfusion in Vladivostok. The human adenocarcinoma cell line HeLa cells were provided by the N.N. Blokhin National Medicinal Research Center of Oncology of the Ministry of Health Care of the Russian Federation, (Moscow, Russia). The human colorectal adenocarcinoma cell line DLD-1 CCL-221™ cells and the human monocytes THP-1 TIB-202TM, as well as the human promyeloblast cell line HL-60 CCL-240, were received from ATCC (Manassas, VA, USA). The HeLa cell line was cultured in the medium of DMEM (Gibco Dulbecco's Modified Eagle Medium), with a 1% penicillin/streptomycin sulfate (Biolot, St. Petersburg, Russia) and 10% fetal bovine serum (FBS) (Biolot, St. Petersburg, Russia). The cells from the DLD-1, HL-60, and THP-1 lines were cultured in an RPMI medium composed of 1% penicillin/streptomycin (Biolot, St. Petersburg, Russia) and 10% fetal bovine serum (FBS) (Biolot, St. Petersburg, Russia). All the cells were incubated at 37 °C in a humidified atmosphere at 5% (v/v) CO_2.

The study was conducted according to the guidelines of the Declaration of Helsinki, and approved by the Ethics Committee of the Pacific Institute of Bioorganic Chemistry (Protocol No. 0037.12.03.2021).

3.3. Extraction and Isolation

The sea cucumbers were minced and kept in EtOH at +10 °C. Next, they were extracted twice with refluxing 60% EtOH. The combined extracts were concentrated to dryness in a vacuum, dissolved in H2O, and chromatographed on a Polychrom-1 column (powdered Teflon, Biolar, Latvia). Eluting first the inorganic salts and impurities with H2O and then the glycosides with 50% EtOH produced 3200 mg of crude glycoside fraction, which was submitted to stepwise column chromatography on Si gel using $CHCl_3$/EtOH/H2O (100:75:10), (100:100:17) and (100:125:25) as mobile phases to produce fractions I–IV. The HPLC of fraction III on the silica-based column Supelcosil LC-Si (4.6 × 150 mm, 5 µm) with $CHCl_3$/MeOH/H2O (60/25/4) as the mobile phase resulted in the isolation of six subfractions (III.1–III.6). The subsequent HPLC of subfraction III.4 on Supelco Ascentis RP-Amide (10 × 250 mm) with CH_3CN/H_2O/NH_4OAc (1 M water solution) (40/59/1) as the mobile phase resulted in the isolation of seven fractions (III.4.1–III.4.7). Repeated chromatography of III.4.3 on the same column but with MeOH/H_2O/NH_4OAc (1 M water solution) (67/31/2) as the mobile phase produced 9.2 mg of chitonoidoside E_1 (**1**). Rechromatography of III.4.6 using mobile phase MeOH/H_2O/NH_4OAc (1 M water solution) (68/30/2) produced 4.3 mg of chitonoidoside F (**2**). Fraction IV obtained after Si gel column chromatography was submitted to HPLC on Supelcosil LC-Si (4.6 × 150 mm, 5 µm) with $CHCl_3$/MeOH/H_2O (63/27/4) as the mobile phase to produce a set of subfractions

(IV.1–IV.6). Chitonoidoside G (**3**) (3.7 mg) was isolated as a result of HPLC of subfraction IV.3 on Supelco Ascentis RP-Amide (10 × 250 mm) with MeOH/H_2O/NH_4OAc (1 M water solution) (72/26/2) as the mobile phase. Chitonoidoside H (**4**) (4.7 mg) was obtained after HPLC of subfraction IV.1 on Supelco Ascentis RP-Amide (10 × 250 mm) with MeOH/H_2O/NH_4OAc (1 M water solution) (70/28/2) as the mobile phase.

3.3.1. Chitonoidoside E_1 (1)

Colorless powder; $(\alpha)_D^{20} -35°$ (c 0.1, 50% MeOH). NMR: See Table S1 and Table 1, Figures S1–S7. (−)HR-ESI-MS m/z: 1543.5315 (calc. 1543.5339) $[M_{2Na}-Na]^-$, 760.2734 (calc. 760.2723) $[M_{2Na}-2Na]^{2-}$. (−)ESI-MS/MS m/z: 1423.6 $[M_{2Na}-Na-NaHSO_4]^-$, 1266.5 $[M_{2Na}-Na-C_7H_{12}O_8SNa\ (MeGlcOSO_3Na)+H]^-$, 1133.5 $[M_{2Na}-Na-C_7H_{12}O_8SNa\ (MeGlcOSO_3Na)-C_5H_8O_4\ (Xyl)+H]^-$, 987.4 $[M_{2Na}-Na-C_7H_{12}O_8SNa\ (MeGlcOSO_3Na)-C_5H_8O_4\ (Xyl)-C_6H_{10}O_4\ (Qui)+H]^-$, 841.4 $[M_{2Na}-Na-C_7H_{12}O_8SNa\ (MeGlcOSO_3Na)-C_5H_8O_4\ (Xyl)-C_6H_{10}O_4\ (Qui)-C_6H_{11}O_4\ (MeXyl)+2H]^-$, 665.1 $[M_{2Na}-Na-C_{30}H_{44}O_4\ (Agl)-C_6H_{11}O_4\ (MeXyl)-C_6H_9O_8SNa\ (GlcOSO_3Na)+H]^-$, 533.1 $[M_{2Na}-Na-C_{30}H_{44}O_4\ (Agl)-C_6H_{11}O_4\ (MeXyl)-C_6H_9O_8SNa\ (GlcOSO_3Na)-C_5H_8O_4\ (Xyl)+H]^-$, 387.0 $[M_{2Na}-Na-C_{30}H_{44}O_4\ (Agl)-C_6H_{11}O_4\ (MeXyl)-C_6H_9O_8SNa\ (GlcOSO_3Na)-C_5H_8O_4\ (Xyl)-C_6H_{10}O_4\ (Qui)+H]^-$, 255.0 $[M_{2Na}-Na-C_{30}H_{44}O_4\ (Agl)-C_6H_{11}O_4\ (MeXyl)-C_6H_9O_8SNa\ (GlcOSO_3Na)-C_5H_8O_4\ (Xyl)-C_6H_{10}O_4\ (Qui)-C_5H_8O_4\ (Xyl)+H]^-$ (Figure S8).

3.3.2. Chitonoidoside F (2)

Colorless powder; $(\alpha)_D^{20} -19°$ (c 0.1, 50% MeOH). NMR: See Table S2 and Table 2, Figures S9–S15. (−)HR-ESI-MS m/z: 1265.4337 (calc. 1265.4337) $[M_{2Na}-Na]^-$, 621.2244 (calc. 621.2269) $(M_{2Na}-2Na)^{2-}$; (−)ESI-MS/MS m/z: 1146.5 $[M_{2Na}-Na-NaSO_4]^-$, 987.4 $[M_{2Na}-Na-C_7H_{12}O_8SNa\ (MeGlcOSO_3Na)+H]^-$, 841.4, $[M_{2Na}-Na-C_7H_{12}O_8SNa\ (MeGlcOSO_3Na)-C_6H_{10}O_4\ (Qui)+H]^-$ (Figure S16).

3.3.3. Chitonoidoside G (3)

Colorless powder; $(\alpha)_D^{20} -48°$ (c 0.1, 50% MeOH). NMR: See Tables 3 and 4, Figures S17–S23. (−)HR-ESI-MS m/z: 1559.5646 (calc. 1559.5652) $[M_{2Na}-Na]^-$, 768.2895 (calc. 768.2880) $[M_{2Na}-2Na]^{2-}$; (−)ESI-MS/MS m/z: 1439.6 $[M_{2Na}-Na-NaHSO_4]^-$, 1383.6 $[M_{2Na}-Na-C_7H_{13}O_5\ (MeGlc)+H]^-$, 1281.6 $[M_{2Na}-Na-C_7H_{12}O_8SNa\ (MeGlcOSO_3Na)+H]^-$, 1149.5 $[M_{2Na}-Na-C_7H_{12}O_8SNa\ (MeGlcOSO_3Na)-C_5H_8O_4\ (Xyl)+H]^-$, 1003.5 $[M_{2Na}-Na-C_7H_{12}O_8SNa\ (MeGlcOSO_3Na)-C_5H_8O_4\ (Xyl)-C_6H_{10}O_4\ (Qui)+H]^-$, 533.1 $[M_{2Na}-Na-C_{30}H_{46}O_3\ (Agl)-C_7H_{13}O_5\ (MeGlc)-C_7H_{12}O_8SNa\ (MeGlcOSO_3Na)-C_5H_8O_4\ (Xyl)+H]^-$, 387.0 $[M_{2Na}-Na-C_{30}H_{46}O_3\ (Agl)-C_7H_{13}O_5\ (MeGlc)-C_7H_{12}O_8SNa\ (MeGlcOSO_3Na)-C_5H_8O_4\ (Xyl)-C_6H_{10}O_4\ (Qui)+H]^-$, 255.0 $[M_{2Na}-Na-C_{30}H_{46}O_3\ (Agl)-C_7H_{13}O_5\ (MeGlc)-C_7H_{12}O_8SNa\ (MeGlcOSO_3Na)-C_5H_8O_4\ (Xyl)-C_6H_{10}O_4\ (Qui)-C_5H_8O_4\ (Xyl)+H]^-$ (Figure S24).

3.3.4. Chitonoidoside H (4)

Colorless powder; $(\alpha)_D^{20} -28°$ (c 0.1, 50% MeOH). NMR: See Tables S3 and 5, Figures S25–S32. (−)HR-ESI-MS m/z: 1397.4749 (calc. 1397.4760) $[M_{2Na}-Na]^-$, 687.2442 (calc. 687.2434) $[M_{2Na}-2Na]^{2-}$; (−)ESI-MS/MS m/z: 1277.5 $[M_{2Na}-Na-NaHSO_4]^-$, 1119.5 $[M_{2Na}-Na-C_7H_{12}O_8SNa\ (MeGlcOSO_3Na)+H]^-$, 1119.5 $[M_{2Na}-Na-C_5H_8O_4\ (Xyl)-C_6H_{10}O_4\ (Qui)]^-$, 987.4 $[M_{2Na}-Na-C_7H_{12}O_8SNa\ (MeGlcOSO_3Na)-C_5H_8O_4\ (Xyl)+H]^-$, 841.4 $[M_{2Na}-Na-C_7H_{12}O_8SNa\ (MeGlcOSO_3Na)-C_5H_8O_4\ (Xyl)-C_6H_{10}O_4\ (Qui)+H]^-$, 519.0 $[M_{2Na}-Na-C_{30}H_{44}O_4\ (Agl)-C_7H_{12}O_8SNa\ (MeGlcOSO_3Na)-C_5H_8O_4\ (Xyl)+H]^-$, 399.0 $[M_{2Na}-Na-C_{30}H_{44}O_4\ (Agl)-C_7H_{12}O_8SNa\ (MeGlcOSO_3Na)-C_5H_8O_4\ (Xyl)-NaHSO_4]^-$, 373.0 $[M_{2Na}-Na-C_{30}H_{44}O_4\ (Agl)-C_5H_8O_4\ (Xyl)-C_6H_{10}O_4\ (Qui)-C_7H_{12}O_8SNa\ (MeGlcOSO_3Na)+H]^-$, 255.0 $[M_{2Na}-Na-C_{30}H_{46}O_3\ (Agl)-C_7H_{12}O_8SNa\ (MeGlcOSO_3Na)-C_6H_9O_8SNa\ (GlcOSO_3Na)-C_5H_8O_4\ (Xyl)+H]^-$ (Figure S33).

3.4. Cytotoxic Activity (MTT Assay Applied for HeLa Cells)

All the studied substances (including the chitonoidoside A and cisplatin, used as positive controls) were tested in concentrations from 0.1 µM to 100 µM using twofold dilution in d-H2O. The cell suspension (180 µL) and solutions (20 µL) of the tested compounds in different concentrations were injected in wells of 96 well plates (1 × 10^4 cells/well) and incubated at 37 °C for 24 h in 5% CO_2. After incubation, the tested substances with medium were replaced by 100 µL of fresh medium. Next, 10 µL of MTT (3-(4,5-dimethylthiazol-2-yl)-2,5-diphenyltetrazolium bromide) (Sigma-Aldrich, St. Louis, MO, USA) stock solution (5 mg/mL) was added to each well, followed by the incubation of the microplate for 4 h. Subsequently, 100 µL of SDS-HCl solution (1 g SDS/10 mL d-H2O/17 µL 6 N HCl) was added to each well and incubated for 18 h. The absorbance of the converted dye, formazan, was measured with a Multiskan FC microplate photometer (Thermo Fisher Scientific, Waltham, MA, USA) at 570 nm. The cytotoxic activity of the tested compounds was calculated as the concentration that caused 50% cell metabolic activity inhibition (IC50). The experiments were carried out in triplicate, $p < 0.05$.

3.5. Cytotoxic Activity (MTS Assay Applied for DLD-1, THP-1 and HL-60 Cells)

The cells of the HL-60 line (6 × 10^3/200 µL) were placed in 96 well plates at 37 °C for 24 h in a 5% CO_2 incubator. The cells were treated with tested substances and chitonoidoside A and cisplatin were used as positive controls at concentrations from 0 to 100 µM for an additional 24 h of incubation. Next, the cells were incubated with 10 µL MTS (3-(4,5-dimethylthiazol-2-yl)-5-(3-carboxymethoxyphenyl)-2-(4-sulfophenyl)-2H-tetrazolium) for 4 h, and the absorbance in each well was measured at 490/630 nm with plate reader PHERA star FS (BMG Labtech, Ortenberg, Germany). The experiments were carried out in triplicate and the mean absorbance values were calculated. The results were presented as the percentage of inhibition that produced a reduction in absorbance after the tested compound treatment compared to the non-treated cells (negative control), $p < 0.01$.

3.6. Hemolytic Activity

The erythrocytes were isolated from human blood through centrifugation with phosphate-buffered saline (PBS) (pH 7.4) at 4 °C for 5 min by 450× g on centrifuge LABOFUGE 400R (Heraeus, Hanau, Germany) three times. Next, the residue of the erythrocytes was resuspended in an ice-cold phosphate saline buffer (pH 7.4) to a final optical density of 1.5 at 700 nm, and kept on ice. For the hemolytic assay, 180 µL of erythrocyte suspension was mixed with 20 µL of test compound solution (including chitonoidoside A used as positive control) in V-bottom 96 well plates. After 1 h of incubation at 37 °C, the plates were exposed to centrifugation for 10 min at 900× g on laboratory centrifuge LMC-3000 (Biosan, Riga, Latvia). Next, 100 µL of supernatant was carefully selected and transferred into new flat-plates, respectively. The lysis of the erythrocytes was determined by measuring of the concentration of hemoglobin in the supernatant with microplate photometer Multiskan FC (Thermo Fisher Scientific, Waltham, MA, USA), λ = 570 nm. The effective dose causing 50% hemolysis of erythrocytes (ED50) was calculated using the computer program SigmaPlot 10.0. All the experiments were performed in triplicate, $p < 0.01$.

4. Conclusions

The continuation of the research into triterpene glycosides from the sea cucumber *Psolus chitonoides* resulted in the isolation of four previously unknown chitonoidosides E_1 (**1**), F (**2**), G (**3**) and H (**4**). The compounds characterized by two types of the aglycones (holotoxinogenin and its structural analog with 18(20)-epoxy-cycle instead of a lactone) were also found earlier in the series of chitonoidosides A–E. The compounds **1**–**4** differed in the number of monosaccharides in their sugar chains (from four to six), the architecture of these chains (for tetra- and pentaosides), their monosaccharide composition, and the positions of their sulfate groups. Terminal 3-O-methylglucose unit was sulfated by C-4 in chitonoidosides F (**2**) and H (**4**), which is a rare position for a sulfate group from sea cucumber glycosides. Notably, in the first series of the studied glycosides from *P. chitonoides* [15] 3-*O*-methylxylose residue sulfated by C-4 was found. This indicates the presence of specific sulfatase in this species of the sea cucumber, capable of attaching the sulfate group to C-4 of monosaccharides in pyranose form. The observed "structure-activity relationships" were as follows: tetraosides with a shortened bottom semi-chain displayed the weakest membranolytic effect; and the activity of the glycosides with the new-type aglycone with a 18(20)-ether bond instead of 18(20)-lactone was comparable with that of the substances with holostane-type aglycones. Hexaosides and tetraosides with linear carbohydrate chains (having bottom semi-chain) were the most active in the series of the glycosides from *P. chitonoides*. The pathways of the biosynthetic transformations were analyzed based on the structures of eight types of carbohydrate chains found in the glycosides of *P. chitonoides*. The analysis revealed and confirmed that glycosylation and sulfation are parallel and competitive processes. All the discussed data broaden knowledge about structural diversity of triterpene glycosides from the sea cucumbers and help us to the understand the complicated biosynthesis process of this class of metabolites, which is currently a large gap in knowledge for scientists.

Supplementary Materials: The following are available online at https://www.mdpi.com/article/10.3390/md19120696/s1. Figure S1. The ^{13}C NMR (125.67 MHz) spectrum of chitonoidoside E$_1$ (**1**) in C$_5$D$_5$N/D$_2$O (4/1); Figure S2. The ^{1}H NMR (500.12 MHz) spectrum of chitonoidoside E$_1$ (**1**) in C$_5$D$_5$N/D$_2$O (4/1); Figure S3. The COSY (500.12 MHz) spectrum of chitonoidoside E$_1$ (**1**) in C$_5$D$_5$N/D$_2$O (4/1); Figure S4. The HSQC (500.12 MHz) spectrum of chitonoidoside E$_1$ (**1**) in C$_5$D$_5$N/D$_2$O (4/1); Figure S5. The ROESY (500.12 MHz) spectrum of chitonoidoside E$_1$ (**1**) in C$_5$D$_5$N/D$_2$O (4/1); Figure S6. The HMBC (500.12 MHz) spectrum of chitonoidoside E$_1$ (**1**) in C$_5$D$_5$N/D$_2$O (4/1); Figure S7. 1 D TOCSY (500.12 MHz) spectra of Xyl1, Qui2, Xyl3, MeGlc4, Glc5 and MeXyl6 of chitonoidoside E$_1$ (**1**) in C$_5$D$_5$N/D$_2$O (4/1); Figure S8. HR-ESI-MS and ESI-MS/MS spectra of chitonoidoside E$_1$ (**1**); Table S1. ^{13}C and ^{1}H NMR chemical shifts, HMBC and ROESY correlations of aglycone moiety of chitonoidoside E$_1$ (**1**); Figure S9. The ^{13}C NMR (125.67 MHz) spectrum of chitonoidoside F (**2**) in C$_5$D$_5$N/D$_2$O (4/1); Figure S10. The ^{1}H NMR (500.12 MHz) spectrum of chitonoidoside F (**2**) in C$_5$D$_5$N/D$_2$O (4/1); Figure S11. The COSY (500.12 MHz) spectrum of chitonoidoside F (**2**) in C$_5$D$_5$N/D$_2$O (4/1); Figure S12. The HSQC (500.12 MHz) spectrum of chitonoidoside F (**2**) in C$_5$D$_5$N/D$_2$O (4/1); Figure S13. The HMBC (500.12 MHz) spectrum of chitonoidoside F (**2**) in C$_5$D$_5$N/D$_2$O (4/1); Figure S14. The ROESY (500.12 MHz) spectrum of chitonoidoside F (**2**) in C$_5$D$_5$N/D$_2$O (4/1); Figure S15. 1D TOCSY (500.12 MHz) spectra of Xyl1, Qui2, Glc3 and MeGlc4 of chitonoidoside F (**2**) in C$_5$D$_5$N/D$_2$O (4/1); Figure S16. HR-ESI-MS and ESI-MS/MS spectra of chitonoidoside F (**2**); Table S2. ^{13}C and ^{1}H NMR chemical shifts, HMBC and ROESY correlations of the aglycone part of chitonoidoside F (**2**); Figure S17. The ^{13}C NMR (125.67 MHz) spectrum of chitonoidoside G (**3**) in C$_5$D$_5$N/D$_2$O (4/1); Figure S18. The ^{1}H NMR (500.12 MHz) spectrum of chitonoidoside G (**3**) in C$_5$D$_5$N/D$_2$O (4/1); Figure S19. The COSY (500.12 MHz) spectrum of chitonoidoside G (**3**) in C$_5$D$_5$N/D$_2$O (4/1); Figure S20. The HSQC (500.12 MHz) spectrum of chitonoidoside G (**3**) in C$_5$D$_5$N/D$_2$O (4/1); Figure S21. The HMBC (500.12 MHz) spectrum of chitonoidoside G (**3**) in C$_5$D$_5$N/D$_2$O (4/1); Figure S22. The ROESY (500.12 MHz) spectrum of chitonoidoside G (**3**) in C$_5$D$_5$N/D$_2$O (4/1); Figure S23. 1 D TOCSY (500.12 MHz) spectra of Xyl1, Qui2, Xyl3, MeGlc4, Glc5 and MeGlc6 of chitonoidoside G (**3**) in C$_5$D$_5$N/D$_2$O (4/1); Figure S24. HR-ESI-MS and ESI-MS/MS spectra of chitonoidoside G (**3**); Figure S25. The ^{13}C NMR (125.67 MHz) spectrum of chitonoidoside H (**4**) in C$_5$D$_5$N/D$_2$O (4/1); Figure S26. The ^{1}H NMR (500.12 MHz) spectrum of chitonoidoside H (**4**) in C$_5$D$_5$N/D$_2$O (4/1); Figure S27. The COSY (500.12 MHz) spectrum of chitonoidoside H (**4**) in C$_5$D$_5$N/D$_2$O (4/1); Figure S28. The HSQC (500.12 MHz) spectrum of chitonoidoside H (**4**) in C$_5$D$_5$N/D$_2$O (4/1); Figure S29. The ROESY (500.12 MHz) spectrum of chitonoidoside H (**4**) in C$_5$D$_5$N/D$_2$O (4/1); Figure S30. The HMBC (500.12 MHz) spectrum of chitonoidoside H (**4**) in C$_5$D$_5$N/D$_2$O (4/1); Figure S31. 1D TOCSY (500.12 MHz) spectra of Xyl1, Qui2, Xyl3, Glc4 and MeGlc5 of chitonoidoside H (**4**) in C$_5$D$_5$N/D$_2$O (4/1); Figure S32. 2D TOCSY (500.12 MHz) spectrum of chitonoidoside H (**4**) in C$_5$D$_5$N/D$_2$O (4/1); Figure S33. HR-ESI-MS and ESI-MS/MS spectra of chitonoidoside H (**4**); Table S3. ^{13}C and ^{1}H NMR chemical shifts, HMBC and ROESY correlations of the aglycone part of chitonoidoside H (**4**).

Author Contributions: Conceptualization, A.S.S., V.I.K.; methodology, A.S.S., S.A.A., V.I.K.; investigation, A.S.S., V.I.K., A.I.K., S.A.A., R.S.P., P.S.D., E.A.C., P.V.A.; writing—original draft preparation, A.S.S., V.I.K. writing—review and editing, A.S.S., V.I.K. All authors have read and agreed to the published version of the manuscript.

Funding: The investigation was carried out with the financial support of a grant from the Ministry of Science and Higher Education, Russian Federation, Grant No. 13.1902.21.0012, Contract No. 075-15-2020-796.

Institutional Review Board Statement: The study was conducted according to the guidelines of the Declaration of Helsinki, and approved by the Ethics Committee of the Pacific Institute of Bioorganic Chemistry (Protocol No. 0037.12.03.2021).

Informed Consent Statement: Not applicable.

Acknowledgments: The study was carried out using the equipment of the Collective Facilities Center "The Far Eastern Center for Structural Molecular Research (NMR/MS) PIBOC FEB RAS". The authors are grateful to Valentin Stonik for reading the manuscript and providing useful comments.

Conflicts of Interest: The authors declare no conflict of interest.

References

1. Aminin, D.L.; Menchinskaya, E.S.; Pislyagin, E.A.; Silchenko, A.S.; Avilov, S.A.; Kalinin, V.I. Sea cucumber triterpene glycosides as anticancer agents. In *Studies in Natural Product Chemistry*; Rahman, A.U., Ed.; Elsevier B.V.: Amsterdam, The Netherlands, 2016; Volume 49, pp. 55–105.
2. Khotimchenko, Y. Pharmacological potential of sea cucumbers. *Int. J. Mol. Sci.* **2020**, *19*, 1342. [CrossRef] [PubMed]
3. Menchinskaya, E.S.; Gorpenchenko, T.Y.; Silchenko, A.S.; Avilov, S.A.; Aminin, D.L. Modulation of doxorubicin intracellular accumulation and anticancer activity by triterpene glycoside cucumarioside A2-2. *Mar. Drugs* **2019**, *17*, 597. [CrossRef] [PubMed]
4. Zhao, Y.-C.; Xue, C.-H.; Zhang, T.T.; Wang, Y.-M. Saponins from sea cucumber and their biological activities. *Agric. Food Chem.* **2018**, *66*, 7222–7237. [CrossRef] [PubMed]
5. Gomes, A.R.; Freitas, A.C.; Duarte, A.C.; Rocha-Santos, T.A.P. Echinoderms: A review of bioactive compounds with potential health effects. In *Studies in Natural Products Chemistry*; Rahman, A.U., Ed.; Elsevier B.V.: Amsterdam, The Netherlands, 2016; Volume 49, pp. 1–54.
6. Aminin, D.; Pisliagin, E.; Astashev, M.; Es'kov, A.; Kozhemyako, V.; Avilov, S.; Zelepuga, E.; Yurchenko, E.; Kaluzhskiy, L.; Kozlovskaya, E.; et al. Glycosides from edible sea cucumbers stimulate macrophages via purinergic receptors. *Sci. Rep.* **2016**, *6*, 39683. [CrossRef] [PubMed]
7. Dyshlovoy, S.A.; Madanchi, R.; Hauschild, J.; Otte, K.; Alsdorf, W.H.; Schumacher, U.; Kalinin, V.I.; Silchenko, A.S.; Avilov, S.A.; Honecker, F.; et al. The marine triterpene glycoside frondoside A induces p53-independent apoptosis and inhibits autophagy in urothelial carcinoma cells. *BMC Cancer* **2017**, *17*, 93. [CrossRef] [PubMed]
8. Yun, S.-H.; Sim, E.-H.; Han, S.-H.; Kim, T.-R.; Ju, M.-H.; Han, J.-Y.; Jeong, J.-S.; Kim, S.-H.; Silchenko, A.S.; Stonik, V.A.; et al. In vitro and in vivo anti-leukemic effects of cladoloside C2 are mediated by activation of Fas/ceramide syntase 6/P38 kinase/C-Jun NH2-terminal kinase/caspase-8. *Oncotarget* **2018**, *9*, 495–511. [CrossRef] [PubMed]
9. Omran, N.E.; Salem, H.K.; Eissa, S.H.; Kabbash, A.M.; Kandeil, M.A.; Salem, M.A. Chemotaxonomic study of the most abundant Egyptian sea-cucumbers using ultra-performance liquid chromatography (UPLC) coupled to high-resolution mass spectrometry (HRMS). *Chemoecology* **2020**, *30*, 35–48. [CrossRef]
10. Kalinin, V.I.; Silchenko, A.S.; Avilov, S.A. Taxonomic significance and ecological role of triterpene glycosides from holothurians. *Biol. Bull.* **2016**, *43*, 532–540. [CrossRef]
11. Kalinin, V.I.; Avilov, S.A.; Silchenko, A.S.; Stonik, V.A. Triterpene Glycosides of Sea Cucumbers (Holothuroidea, Echinodermata) as Taxonomic Markers. *Nat. Prod. Commun.* **2015**, *10*, 21–26. [CrossRef] [PubMed]
12. Silchenko, A.S.; Kalinovsky, A.I.; Avilov, S.A.; Andrijaschenko, P.V.; Popov, R.S.; Dmitrenok, P.S.; Chingizova, E.A.; Kalinin, V.I. Triterpene Glycosides from the Far Eastern Sea Cucumber *Thyonidium (=Duasmodactyla) kurilensis* (Levin): The Structures, Cytotoxicities, and Biogenesis of Kurilosides A3, D1, G, H, I, I1, J, K, and K1. *Mar. Drugs* **2021**, *19*, 187. [CrossRef] [PubMed]
13. Silchenko, A.S.; Kalinovsky, A.I.; Avilov, S.A.; Kalinin, V.I.; Andrijaschenko, P.V.; Dmitrenok, P.S.; Popov, R.S.; Chingizova, E.A.; Ermakova, S.P.; Malyarenko, O.S. Structures and bioactivities of six new triterpene glycosides, psolusosides E, F, G, H, H_1 and I and the corrected structure of psolusoside B from the sea cucumber *Psolus fabricii*. *Mar. Drugs* **2019**, *17*, 358. [CrossRef]
14. Zelepuga, E.A.; Silchenko, A.S.; Avilov, S.A.; Kalinin, V.I. Structure-activity relationships of holothuroid's triterpene glycosides and some in silico insights obtained by molecular dynamics study on the mechanisms of their membranolytic action. *Mar. Drugs* **2021**, *19*, 604. [CrossRef] [PubMed]
15. Silchenko, A.S.; Kalinovsky, A.I.; Avilov, S.A.; Andrijaschenko, P.V.; Popov, R.S.; Dmitrenok, P.S.; Chingizova, E.A.; Kalinin, V.I. Unusual Structures and Cytotoxicities of Chitonoidosides A, A_1, B, C, D, and E, Six Triterpene Glycosides from the Far Eastern Sea Cucumber *Psolus chitonoides*. *Mar. Drugs* **2021**, *19*, 449. [CrossRef] [PubMed]

16. Maltsev, I.I.; Stonik, V.A.; Kalinovsky, A.I.; Elyakov, G.B. Triterpene glycosides from sea cucumber *Stichopus japonicus* Selenka. *Comp. Biochem. Physiol.* **1984**, *78B*, 421–426. [CrossRef]
17. Silchenko, A.S.; Kalinovsky, A.I.; Avilov, S.A.; Andrijaschenko, P.V.; Popov, R.S.; Dmitrenok, P.S.; Chingizova, E.A.; Ermakova, S.P.; Malyarenko, O.S.; Dautov, S.S.; et al. Structures and bioactivities of quadrangularisosides A, A_1, B, B_1, B_2, C, C_1, D, D_1–D_4, and E from the sea cucumber *Colochirus quadrangularis*: The first discovery of the glycosides, sulfated by C-4 of the terminal 3-*O*-methylglucose residue. Synergetic effect on colony formation of tumor HT-29 cells of these glycosides with radioactive irradiation. *Mar. Drugs* **2020**, *18*, 394.
18. Silchenko, A.S.; Kalinovsky, A.I.; Avilov, S.A.; Andrijaschenko, P.V.; Popov, R.S.; Dmitrenok, P.S.; Chingizova, E.A.; Kalinin, V.I. Kurilosides A_1, A_2, C_1, D, E and F-triterpene glycosides from the Far Eastern sea cucumber *Thyonidium* (=*Duasmodactyla*) *kurilensis* (Levin): Structures with unusual non-holostane aglycones and cytotoxicities. *Mar. Drugs* **2020**, *18*, 551. [CrossRef] [PubMed]
19. Aminin, D.L.; Pislyagin, E.A.; Menchinskaya, E.S.; Silchenko, A.S.; Avilov, S.A.; Kalinin, V.I. Immunomodulatory and anticancer activity of sea cucumber triterpene glycosides. In *Studies in Natural Products Chemistry*; Rahman, A.U., Ed.; Elsevier Science, B.V.: Amsterdam, The Netherlands, 2014; Volume 41, pp. 75–94.
20. Kim, C.G.; Kwak, J.-Y. Anti-cancer effects of triterpene glycosides, frondoside A and cucumarioside A_2-2 isolated from sea cucumbers. In *Handbook of Anticancer Drugs from Marine Origin*; Kim, S.K., Ed.; Springer International Publishing: Cham, Switzerland, 2015; pp. 673–682.
21. Careaga, V.P.; Maier, M.S. Cytotoxic triterpene glycosides from sea cucumbers. In *Handbook of Anticancer Drugs from Marine Origin*; Kim, S.K., Ed.; Springer International Publishing: Cham, Switzerland, 2015; pp. 515–528.
22. Kalinin, V.I.; Silchenko, A.S.; Avilov, S.A.; Stonik, V.A. Non-holostane aglycones of sea cucumber triterpene glycosides. Structure, biosynthesis, evolution. *Steroids* **2019**, *147*, 42–51. [CrossRef] [PubMed]
23. Kalinin, V.I.; Silchenko, A.S.; Avilov, S.A.; Stonik, V.A. Progress in the studies of triterpene glycosides from sea cucumbers (Holothuroidea, Echinodermata) Between 2017 and 2021. *Nat. Prod. Commun.* **2021**, *16*. [CrossRef]

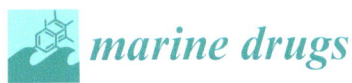

Article

Structure-Activity Relationships of Holothuroid's Triterpene Glycosides and Some In Silico Insights Obtained by Molecular Dynamics Study on the Mechanisms of Their Membranolytic Action

Elena A. Zelepuga, Alexandra S. Silchenko, Sergey A. Avilov and Vladimir I. Kalinin *

G.B. Elyakov Pacific Institute of Bioorganic Chemistry, Far Eastern Branch of the Russian Academy of Sciences, Pr. 100-letya Vladivostoka 159, Vladivostok 690022, Russia; zel@piboc.dvo.ru (E.A.Z.); silchenko_als@piboc.dvo.ru (A.S.S.); avilov_sa@piboc.dvo.ru (S.A.A.)
* Correspondence: kalininv@piboc.dvo.ru; Tel./Fax: +7-(423)2-31-40-50

Abstract: The article describes the structure-activity relationships (SAR) for a broad series of sea cucumber glycosides on different tumor cell lines and erythrocytes, and an in silico modulation of the interaction of selected glycosides from the sea cucumber *Eupentacta fraudatrix* with model erythrocyte membranes using full-atom molecular dynamics (MD) simulations. The in silico approach revealed that the glycosides bound to the membrane surface mainly through hydrophobic interactions and hydrogen bonds. The mode of such interactions depends on the aglycone structure, including the side chain structural peculiarities, and varies to a great extent. Two different mechanisms of glycoside/membrane interactions were discovered. The first one was realized through the pore formation (by cucumariosides A_1 (**40**) and A_8 (**44**)), preceded by bonding of the glycosides with membrane sphingomyelin, phospholipids, and cholesterol. Noncovalent intermolecular interactions inside multimolecular membrane complexes and their stoichiometry differed for **40** and **44**. The second mechanism was realized by cucumarioside A_2 (**59**) through the formation of phospholipid and cholesterol clusters in the outer and inner membrane leaflets, correspondingly. Noticeably, the glycoside/phospholipid interactions were more favorable compared to the glycoside/cholesterol interactions, but the glycoside possessed an agglomerating action towards the cholesterol molecules from the inner membrane leaflet. In silico simulations of the interactions of cucumarioside A_7 (**45**) with model membrane demonstrated only slight interactions with phospholipid polar heads and the absence of glycoside/cholesterol interactions. This fact correlated well with very low experimental hemolytic activity of this substance. The observed peculiarities of membranotropic action are in good agreement with the corresponding experimental data on hemolytic activity of the investigated compounds in vitro.

Keywords: triterpene glycosides; sea cucumber; membranolytic action; hemolytic; cytotoxic activity; molecular dynamic simulation

1. Introduction

The majority of triterpene glycosides from sea cucumbers possess strong hemolytic and cytotoxic actions against different cells, including cancer cells [1–4]. However, the mechanism of their membranolytic action is not yet fully understood at the molecular level, particularly in relation to the structural diversity of these compounds. Some trends of SAR of sea cucumber glycosides have been discussed [5,6], but the molecular interactions of different functional groups with the components of biomembranes which affect the membranotropic action of the glycosides remain unexplored.

The broad spectrum of bioactivity of sea cucumber triterpene glycosides derives from their ability to interact with the lipid constituents of the membrane bilayer, changing the functional properties of the plasmatic membrane. Sterols are very important structural

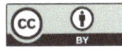

components influencing the properties and functions of eukaryotic cell membranes. The selective bonding to the sterols of the cell membranes underlines the molecular mechanisms of action of many natural toxins, including triterpene glycosides of the sea cucumbers. The formation of complexes with 5,6-unsaturated sterols of target cell membranes is the basis of their biological activity including ichthyotoxic action that may protect sea cucumbers against fish predation. In fact, some experimental data indicated the interaction of the aglycone part of the glycosides with cholesterol [7,8]. The saturation of ascites cell membranes with cholesterol increased the cytotoxicity of the sea cucumber glycosides [9]. This complexing reaction of both the animal and plant saponins leads to the formation of pores, the permeabilization of cells, and in the case of red blood cells for which the membranes are known to be enriched in cholesterol [10], the subsequent loss of hemoglobin in the extracellular medium [11]. Malyarenko et al. tested a series of triterpene glycosides isolated from the starfish *Solaster pacificus* that had exogenic origin from a sea cucumber eaten by this starfish [12]. The authors showed that the addition of cholesterol to corresponding tumor cell culture media significantly decreases the cytotoxicity of these glycosides. It clearly confirmed the cholesterol-dependent character of the membranolytic action of sea cucumber triterpene glycosides. It is of special interest that the activity of a glycoside with 18(16)-lactone instead of 18(20)-lactone, and a shortened side chain, was also decreased by the adding of cholesterol.

The sea cucumber glycosides may be active in subtoxic concentrations, and such a kind of activity is cholesterol-independent. Aminin et al. showed that the immunostimulatory action of cucumarioside A_2-2 from *Cucumaria japonica* resulted from the specific interaction of the glycoside with a P2X receptor and was cholesterol-independent [13]. The addition of cholesterol to the medium or to the mixture of substances may decrease the cytotoxic properties of the glycosides while preserving their other activities. This property of cholesterol has been applied to the development of ISCOMs (immune-stimulating complexes) and subunit protein antigen-carriers, composed of cholesterol, phospholipid, and glycosides [14,15]. Moreover, the immunomodulatory lead–"Cumaside" as a complex of monosulfated glycosides of the Far Eastern Sea cucumber *Cucumaria japonica* with cholesterol, has been created [16]. It possesses significantly less cytotoxic activity against sea urchin embryos and Ehrlich carcinoma cells than the corresponding glycosides, but has an antitumor activity against different forms of experimental mouse Ehrlich carcinoma in vivo [17].

Therefore, cholesterol seems to be the main molecular target for the majority of glycosides in the cell membranes. However, the experimental data for some plant saponins indicate that saponin-membrane binding can occur independently of the presence of cholesterol, cholesterol can even delay the cytotoxicity, such as for ginsenoside Rh2, and phospholipids or sphingomyelin play an important role in these interactions [7,18]. Thus, different mechanisms exist, cholesterol-dependent and -independent, that are involved in saponin-induced membrane permeabilization, depending on the structure of saponins [11]. However, recent in vitro experiments and the monolayer simulations of membrane binding of the sea cucumber glycoside frondoside A, confirmed previous findings that suggest the presence of cholesterol is essential to the strong membranolytic activity of saponins. However, the cholesterol-independent, weak binding of the glycoside to the membrane phospholipids, driven by the lipophilic character of the aglycone, was discovered. Then saponins assemble into complexes with membrane cholesterol followed by the accumulation of saponin-sterol complexes into clusters that finally induce curvature stress, resulting in membrane permeabilization and pore formation [7].

The aims of this study were: the analysis of SAR data for a broad series of sea cucumber glycosides, mainly obtained by our research team over recent years on different tumor cell lines and erythrocytes and additionally the explanation for these data by modelling the interactions of the glycosides from the sea cucumber *Eupentacta fraudatrix* with the constituents of model red blood cell membrane through the full-atom molecular dynamics (MD) simulation. Such an investigation appears even more relevant since different molecules and their complexes composing of cell membranes, for example, cholesterol-enriched lipid rafts, have continued to attract attention as the factors involved in tumorigenesis and a number of cellular pathways related to cell survival, proliferation, and apoptosis [19]. Therefore, it may be of great advantage to modulate the interactions of the membrane constituents by membrane-active compounds, such as triterpene glycosides. An in silico technique was applied to reinforce the numerous experimental observations (SAR) by modelling a multitude of inter-molecular interactions at a high spatial (atomic level) and temporal (nanosecond) resolution within a simulation framework that can reconstitute the natural behavior on the basis of physical interactions [20,21]. Such in silico MD simulations can be regarded as a "computational microscope" capable of visualizing molecular behavior with unprecedented precision [22].

2. Results and Discussion

2.1. Structure-Activity Relationships (SAR) Observed in the Glycosides from Sea Cucumbers

The triterpene glycosides of sea cucumbers are natural compounds that have been investigated for a long time. Several hundred structures of the glycosides are now known from the representatives of different orders of the class Holothuroidea. The finding of a significant number of new glycosides by our research team, especially over recent years, led to the broadening of the knowledge of their great structural diversity. This facilitated SAR highlighting through the comparative analysis of their structural features, including both carbohydrate chain composition and architecture, aglycone structures, and their bioactivity (cytotoxic and hemolytic action).

It became obvious that glycosides cytotoxic activity depends not only on their structures, but also on the type of processed cells differing by composition and functional peculiarities of their membranes [1]. Analyzing the majority of tested compounds, it has been revealed that the membranes of erythrocytes are more sensitive to the glycoside membranolytic action than the other tested cells such as mouse spleen lymphocytes, ascites of mouse Ehrlich carcinoma, and neuroblastoma Neuro 2a or normal epithelial JB-6 cells. This regularity was observed in the glycosides of the *Actinocucumis typica* [23], *Colochirus robustus* [24], *Massinium magnum* [25,26], *Eupentacta fraudatrix* [27–29], *Psolus fabricii* [30,31], and *Colochirus quadrangularis* [32] sea cucumbers. One of the explanations for this phenomenon may be the enrichment of red blood cell membranes with cholesterol [10].

The structures of holothuroids' triterpene glycosides vary in a number of structural features while retaining the general plan of molecular structure. The influence of structural signs such as the monosaccharide composition and architecture of carbohydrate chains, the quantity and positions of sulfate groups, the type of aglycone, and the structure of a side chain on the activity of the glycosides is significant.

2.1.1. The Dependence of the Glycosides Hemolytic Activity on Their Carbohydrate Chain Structure

It was earlier noticed that the presence of a linear tetrasaccharide chain is necessary for the membranolytic action of the glycosides, that glycosides with quinovose as the second sugar unit in the chain are more active than those with glucose or xylose, and that the sulfate group at C-4 Xyl1 increases the activity of tetraosides and pentaosides with sugar parts branched by C-2 Qui2, however the sulfate groups at C-6 Glc3 and C-6 MeGlc4 of such pentaosides significantly decrease the activity [4,33,34].

In fact, the comparison of the hemolytic activities (Table 1) of cucumariosides B_1 (**1**) and B_2 (**2**) from *E. fraudatrix* with a trisaccharide chain with the monosaccharide residues attached to each other by β-(1→2)-glycosidic bonds [35], and the activity of cucumariosides H_5 (**3**) and H (**4**) (Figure 1) with pentasaccharide monosulfated chains [36] revealed the significance of the linear tetrasaccharide fragment with terminal O-methylated sugar residue, as the compounds **1**, **2** were almost not active.

Table 1. The hemolytic activities (synoptic data from the corresponding publications) of the glycosides 1–59 against mouse erythrocytes.

Glycoside	ED$_{50}$, µM/mL	Glycoside	ED$_{50}$, µM/mL	Glycoside	ED$_{50}$, µM/mL
Cucumarioside B$_1$ (1)	>100	Psolusoside K (21)	>100	Cucumarioside A$_{10}$ (41)	20.00
Cucumarioside B$_2$ (2)	18.8	Typicoside B$_1$ (22)	0.33	Cucumarioside I$_1$ (42)	23.24
Cucumarioside H$_5$ (3)	3.2	Typicoside C$_2$ (23)	0.18	Cucumarioside I$_4$ (43)	75.00
Cucumarioside H (4)	3.8	Cladoloside I$_1$ (24)	1.10	Cucumarioside A$_8$ (44)	0.70
Magnumoside A$_2$ (5)	33.33	Cladoloside I$_2$ (25)	2.04	Cucumarioside A$_7$ (45)	>100
Magnumoside A$_3$ (6)	12.53	Cladoloside J$_1$ (26)	1.37	Cucumarioside A$_9$ (46)	>100
Magnumoside A$_4$ (7)	20.12	Cladoloside K$_1$ (27)	0.18	Cucumarioside A$_{11}$ (47)	>100
Magnumoside B$_1$ (8)	49.57	Cladoloside L$_1$ (28)	0.82	Cucumarioside A$_{14}$ (48)	>100
Magnumoside B$_2$ (9)	58.11	Psolusoside L (29)	2.42	Cucumarioside I$_3$ (49)	>100
Magnumoside B$_3$ (10)	8.49	Psolusoside M (30)	67.83	Colochiroside B$_1$ (50)	39.5
Magnumoside B$_4$ (11)	1.42	Psolusoside Q (31)	>100	Typicoside C$_1$ (51)	6.25
Magnumoside C$_1$ (12)	6.97	Psolusoside P (32)	10.92	Cladoloside D$_2$ (52)	10.40
Magnumoside C$_2$ (13)	16.20	Quadrangularisoside B$_2$ (33)	0.51	Cladoloside K$_2$ (53)	11.41
Magnumoside C$_3$ (14)	17.80	Quadrangularisoside D$_2$ (34)	3.31	Cladoloside D$_1$ (54)	0.67
Magnumoside C$_4$ (15)	6.52	Quadrangularisoside E (35)	2.04	Quadrangularisoside A (55)	1.57
Psolusoside A (16)	1.4	Colochiroside C (36)	2.5	Quadrangularisoside A$_1$ (56)	1.11
Psolusoside E (17)	0.23	Psolusoside F (37)	2.8	Psolusoside D$_3$ (57)	1.12
Psolusoside H (18)	2.5	Colochiroside B$_2$ (38)	37.02	Psolusoside D$_5$ (58)	12.37
Psolusoside H$_1$ (19)	2.7	Cucumarioside A$_3$-2 (39)	40.6	Cucumarioside A$_2$ (59)	4.70
Psolusoside J (20)	>100	Cucumarioside A$_1$ (40)	0.07		

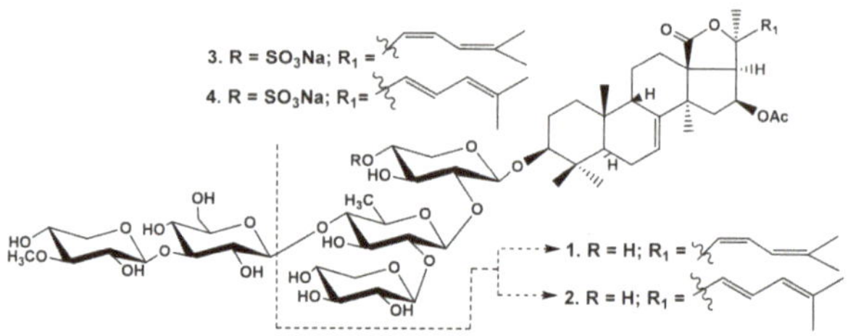

Figure 1. Structures of the glycosides 1–4 from *Eupentacta fraudatrix*.

The analysis of the data on the hemolytic activity of the glycosides from *M. magnum*, with identical aglycones and differing by the oligosaccharide chain structures, demonstrates that the influence of the carbohydrate chain structure indirectly depends on its combination with different aglycones. There were three groups of the glycosides in *M. magnum*: monosulfated biosides (magnumosides of the group A (5–7)), monosulfated tetraosides (magnumosides of the group B (8–11)) and disulfated tetraosides (magnumosides of the group C (12–15)) (Figure 2), all were attached to non-holostane aglycones with 18(16)-lactone differing by the side chain structures [25,26].

In the series of magnumosides B$_1$ (8) and C$_1$ (12) and magnumosides A$_2$ (5), B$_2$ (9), C$_2$ (13), with the hydroxyl group in the aglycone side chains, the disulfated tetraosides 12 and 13 were the most active compounds, while in the series of magnumosides A$_3$ (6), B$_3$ (10), C$_3$ (14) and magnumosides A$_4$ (7), B$_4$ (11), C$_4$ (15), which comprised the side chains with a double bond, the monosulfated tetraosides 10 and 11 showed the strongest effect (Table 1). Magnumosides of group A (5–7) demonstrated considerable hemolytic effects despite the absence of a tetrasaccharide linear fragment (Table 1). A compensation for the absence of two sugars by a sulfate at C-4 of the first xylose residue was earlier described for sea cucumber glycosides with 18(20)-lactone in aglycones. [5,33].

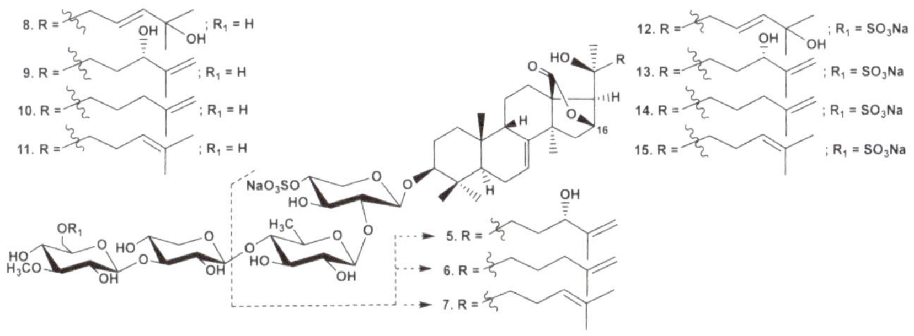

Figure 2. Structures of the glycosides **5–15** from *Massinum magnum*.

The interesting observations were made when the activity of the glycosides from the sea cucumber *Psolus fabricii* (Figure 3) was analyzed [30,31]. Psolusosides A (**16**) and E (**17**) having linear tetrasaccharide sugar moieties were the strongest cytotoxins in this series, but the activity of psolusosides H (**18**) and H$_1$ (**19**) (the glycosides with trisaccharide chains) was close to that of the linear tetraosides **16**, **17** (Table 1) despite the absence of tetrasaccharide linear moiety and the change in the second unit (quinovose) in the chain of **16**, **17** to glucose residue in **18**, **19**. However, psolusosides J (**20**) and K (**21**) with tetrasaccharide chains branched by C-4 Xyl1 and three sulfate groups were completely inactive despite the presence of holostane (i.e., with 18(20)-lactone) aglycones.

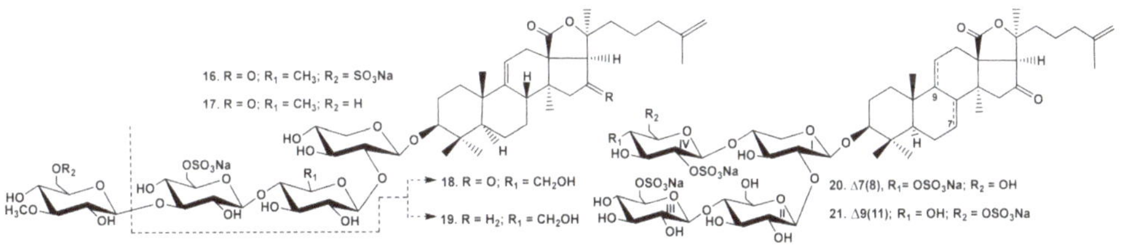

Figure 3. Structures of the glycosides **16–21** from *Psolus fabricii*.

The majority of the glycosides found in the sea cucumber, *Cladolabes schmeltzii*, and characterized by penta- or hexasaccharide moieties branched by C-4 Xyl1, demonstrated strong hemolytic action that was only slightly dependent on their monosaccharide composition. The general trend observed was that hexaosides are more active than pentaosides [37–41].

Therefore, the influence of carbohydrate chain structure on the activity of glycosides is mediated by its combination with the aglycone, however, the general trend is that more developed (tetra-, penta- and hexa-saccharide) sugar moieties provide higher membranolytic action.

2.1.2. The Dependence of Hemolytic Activity of the Gycosides on the Positions and Quantity of Sulfate Groups

The comparison of the hemolytic effects of typicosides B$_1$ (**22**) and C$_2$ (**23**) from *A. typica* [23] (Figure 4)–linear tetraosides differing by the quantity of sulfate groups showed that the disulfated compound **23** is more active than a monosulfated one (Table 1). High hemolytic activity was demonstrated by the sulfated glycosides from *C. shcmeltzii* [39]–cladolosides of groups I (**24**, **25**) and J$_1$ (**26**), with pentasaccharide chains branched by C-4 Xyl1 with the sulfate group at C-6 MeGlc in the bottom or upper semi-chains, correspondingly, as well as cladolosides K$_1$ (**27**) and L$_1$ (**28**)–with monosulfated hexasaccharide chains differing by the sulfate group position (Figure 4). This trend was also confirmed by SAR demonstrated by the glycosides from *P. fabricii* [31]. Psolusoside L (**29**) (Figure 5) was strongly hemolytic in spite of the presence of three sulfate groups at C-6 of two glucose and 3-O-methylglucose residues in the pentasaccharide chain branched by C-4 Xyl1. Thus, the presence of sulfate groups attached to C-6 of monosaccharide units did not decrease the activity of pentaosides branched by C-4 Xyl1 in comparison to that of pentaosides branched by C-2 Qui2 [4,33].

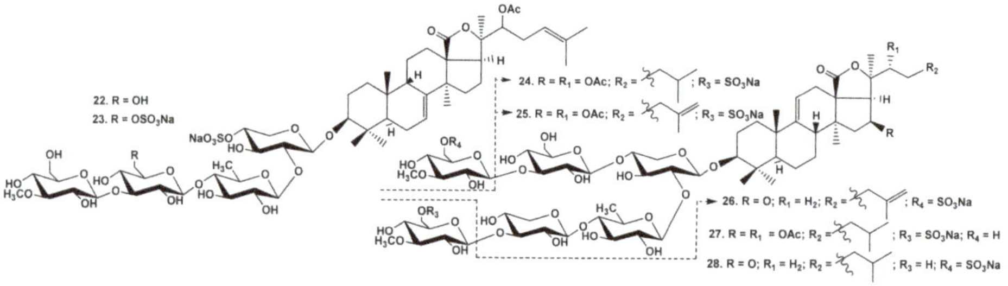

Figure 4. Structures of glycosides **22** and **23** from *Actinocucumis typica* and **24–28** from *Cladolabes shcmeltzii*.

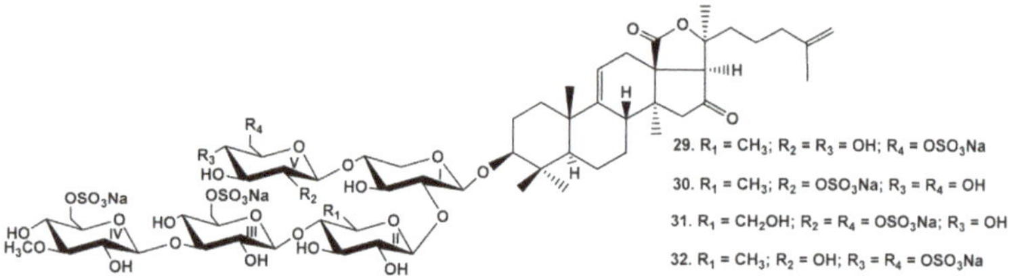

Figure 5. Structures of the glycosides **29–32** from *Psolus fabricii*.

The influence of sulfate position is clearly reflected through the comparison of the activity of psolusosides M (**30**) and Q (**31**). The latter glycoside was characterized by the sulfate position attached to C-2 Glc5 (the terminal residue), that caused an extreme decrease in its activity (Table 1). Even the tetrasulfated (by C-6 Glc3, C-6 MeGlc4, C-6 Glc5, and C-4 Glc5) psolusoside P (**32**) was much more active than trisulfated psolusoside M (**30**) containing the sulfate group at C-2 Glc5 (Figure 5).

The analysis of SAR in the raw of glycosides from the sea cucumbers *Colochirus quadrangularis* [32] (quadrangularisosides B_2 (**33**), D_2 (**34**), and E (**35**)), *C. robustus* [24] (colochiroside C (**36**)) (Figure 6) and *P. fabricii* [30] (psolusosides A (**16**), E (**17**) (Figure 3), and F (**37**)) (Figure 6) with the same holostane aglycone and linear tetrasaccharide chains and differing by the third monosaccharide residue and the number and positions of sulfate groups, showed that they all were strong hemolytics (Table 1). However, the presence of a sulfate group at C-4 or C-6 of terminal MeGlc residue resulted in approximately a tenfold decrease in activity, while the sulfation of C-3 Qui2 or C-6 Glc3 did not decrease the hemolytic action.

Hence, the influence of sulfate groups on the membranolytic action of triterpene glycosides depends on the architecture of their carbohydrate chains and the positions of attachment of these functional groups.

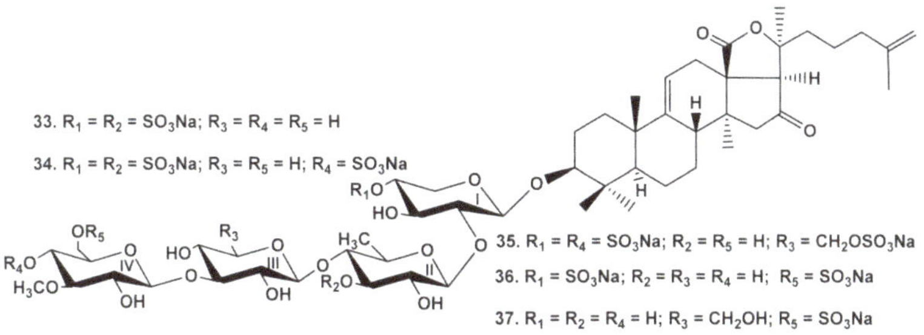

Figure 6. Structures of the glycosides **33**–**35** from *Colochirus quadrangularis*, **36** from *Colochirus robustus* and **37** from *Psolus fabricii*.

2.1.3. The Dependence of Hemolytic Activity of the Glycosides on Aglycone Structure

In the earlier studies of glycoside SAR, the necessity of the presence of a holostane-type aglycone (with 18(20)-lactone), was noticed for the compound to be active. The glycosides containing non-holostane aglycones (i.e., having 18(16)-lactone, without a lactone with a shortened or normal side chain), as a rule, demonstrate only weak membranolytic action [4,33]. However, different functional groups attached to polycyclic nucleus or the side chain of holostane aglycones can significantly influence the membranotropic activity of the glycosides.

All the glycosides isolated from *M. magnum* contain non-holostane aglycones with 18(16)-lactone, 7(8)-double bond and a normal (non-shortened) side chain. Despite this fact, the compounds demonstrated high or moderate hemolytic effects (Table 1) (except for the compounds containing OH-groups in the side chains) [25,26]. Nevertheless, the comparison of hemolytic activity of the pairs of compounds (Table 1) colochiroside B_2 (**38**) (Figure 7) and magnumoside B_1 (**8**), as well as colochiroside C (**36**) and magnumoside C_3 (**14**), and differing by the aglycones nuclei (holostane and non-holostane, correspondingly), showed that compounds **36** and **38**, which contained the holostane aglycones, were more active, and this is consistent with the earlier conclusions.

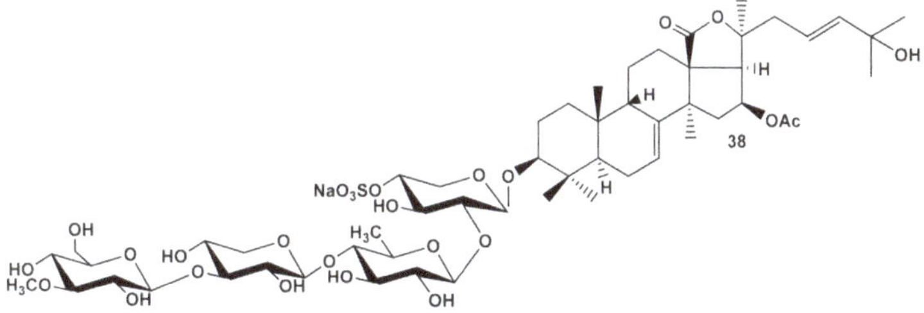

Figure 7. Structure of colochiroside B_2 (**38**) from *Colochirus robustus*.

Additionally, the glycosides of the sea cucumber, *Cucumaria fallax* [42], did not display any activity due to containing unusual hexa-*nor*-lanostane aglycones with an 8(9)-double bond and without a lactone. The only glycoside from this series, cucumarioside A_3-2 (**39**) (Figure 8), that was moderately hemolytic (Table 1) was characterized by hexa-*nor*-lanostane aglycone, but, as typical for the glycosides of sea cucumbers, having a 7(8)-double bond and 9β-H configuration, which demonstrates the significance of these structural elements for the membranotropic action of the glycosides.

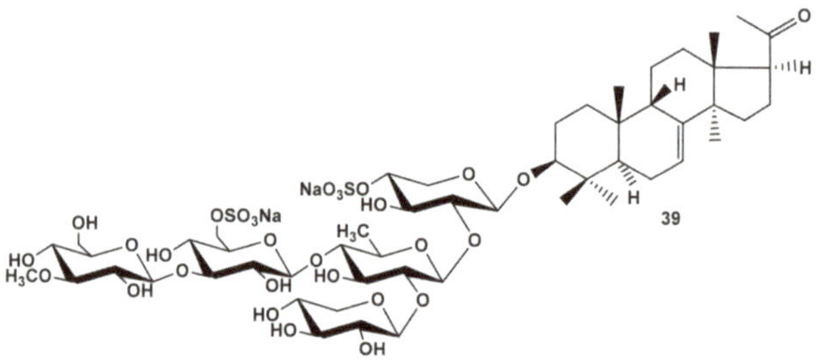

Figure 8. Structure of cucumarioside A$_3$-2 from *Cucumaria fallax*.

The influence of the side chain length and character of a lactone (18(20)- or 18(16)-) is nicely illustrated by the comparative analysis of the hemolytic activity of the series of glycosides from *E. fraudatrix* (cucumariosides A$_1$ (**40**) and A$_{10}$ (**41**) [28,29]; cucumariosides I$_1$ (**42**) and I$_4$ (**43**) [43]) (Figure 9), which indicates that the presence of a normal side chain is essential for the high membranolytic effect of the glycoside.

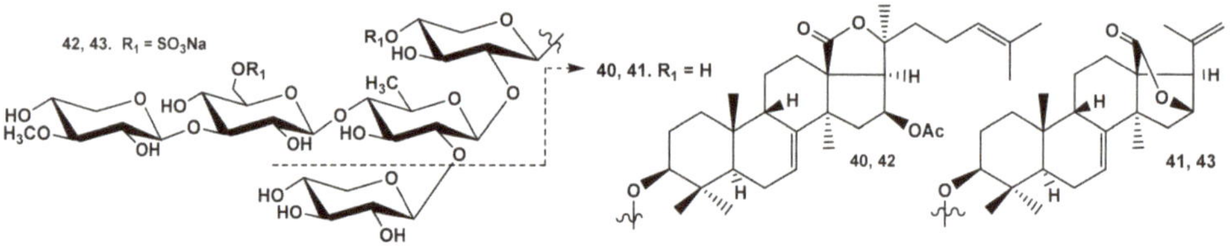

Figure 9. Structures of the glycosides **40–43** from *Eupentacta fraudatrix*.

Unexpectedly high hemolytic activity was displayed by cucumarioside A$_8$ (**44**) from *E. fraudatrix* [29] (Figure 10) with unique non-holostane aglycone and without lactone but with hydroxy-groups at C-18 and C-20, which can be considered as a biosynthetic precursor of the holostane aglycones. Its strong membranolytic action (Table 1) could be explained by the formation of an intramolecular hydrogen bond between the atoms of aglycone hydroxyls resulting in the spatial structure of the aglycone becoming similar to that of holostane-type aglycones. Noticeably, it is of special interest to check this issue by in silico calculations to clarify the molecular mechanism of membranotropic action of **44**.

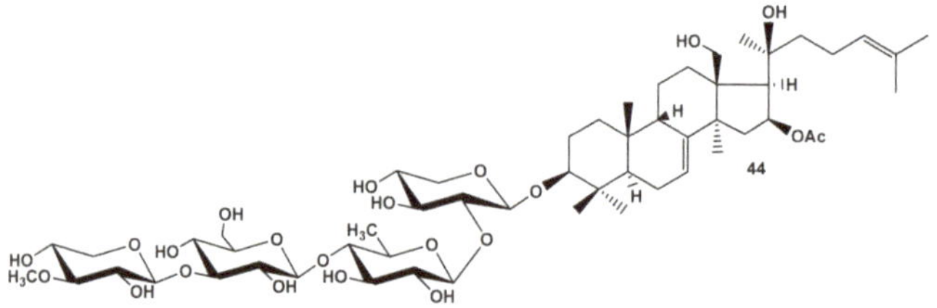

Figure 10. Structure of cucumarioside A$_8$ (**44**) from *Eupentacta fraudatrix*.

2.1.4. The Influence of Hydroxyl Groups in the Aglycones Side Chain to Hemolytic Activity of the Glycosides

A strong activity-decreasing effect of the hydroxyl groups in the aglycone side chains was revealed for the first time when the bioactivity of the glycosides from *E. fraudatrix* was studied [27–29,43]. In fact, cucumariosides A$_7$ (**45**), A$_9$ (**46**), A$_{11}$ (**47**), and A$_{14}$ (**48**), as well as I$_3$ (**49**), were not active against erythrocytes (Table 1) (Figure 11).

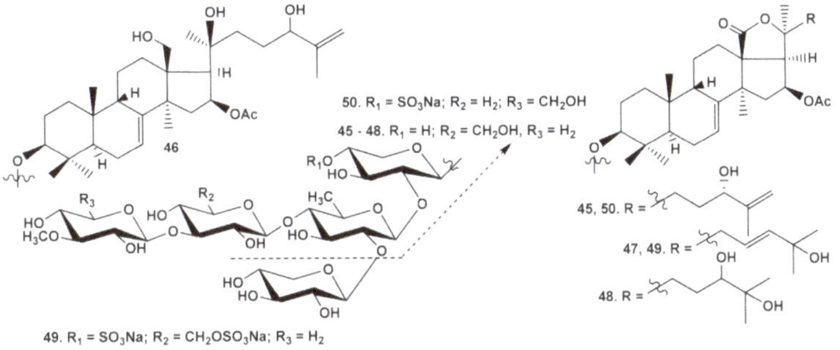

Figure 11. Structures of the glycosides **45–49** from *Eupentacta fraudatrix* and **50** from *Colochirus robustus*.

However, colochirosides B$_1$ (**50**) (Figure 11) and B$_2$ (**38**) from *C. robustus* [24], with the same aglycones as cucumariosides A$_7$ (**45**) and A$_{11}$ (**47**), correspondingly, but differing by the third (Xylose) and terminal monosaccharide residues (3-O-MeGlc) and the presence of sulfate group at C-4 Xyl1, demonstrated moderate hemolytic activity (Table 1). The activity of typicoside C$_1$ (**51**) from *A. typica* [23] as well as cladolosides D$_2$ (**52**) and K$_2$ (**53**) from *C. schmeltzii* [40,41], with a 22-OH group in the holostane aglycones, was significantly lower (Table 1) than that of typicoside C$_2$ (**23**) and cladolosides D$_1$ (**54**) (Figure 12) and K$_1$ (**27**), correspondingly, containing a 22-OAc group.

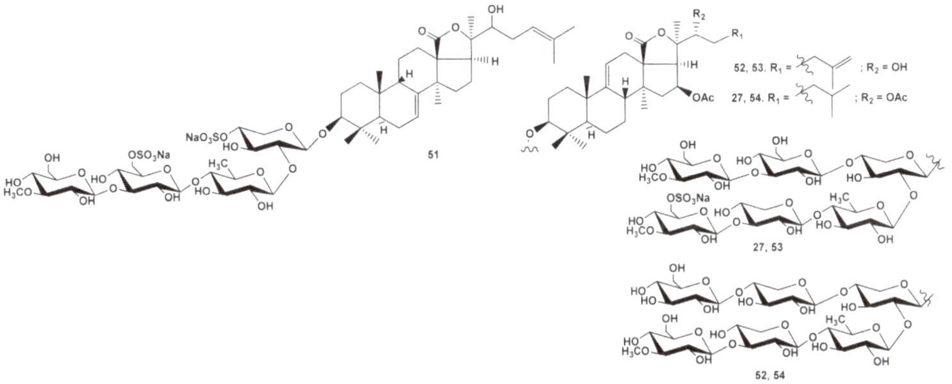

Figure 12. Structures of the glycosides **51–54** from *Cladolabes schmeltzii*.

The same activity-decreasing effect of the hydroxy-group in the side chain was observed for the glycosides of *M. magnum* with non-holostane aglycones (monosulfated glycosides (**5**, **8**, **9**)), however, the presence of additional sulfate groups in the carbohydrate chains of **12**, **13** compensated this influence to some extent (Table 1).

Recently, the glycosides containing hydroperoxyl groups in the aglycone side chains were found in sea cucumbers *C. quadrangularis* (quadrangularisosides A (**55**) and A$_1$ (**56**) [32]) and *P. fabricii* (psoluoside D$_3$ (**57**) [44]) (Figure 13). The comparative analysis of their hemolytic activity with that of their structural analogs that contained hydroxyl groups in the same positions (colochirosides B$_2$ (**38**), B$_1$ (**50**), and psoluoside D$_5$ (**58**), correspondingly) showed that the influence of OOH-functionalities was not so negative (Table 1).

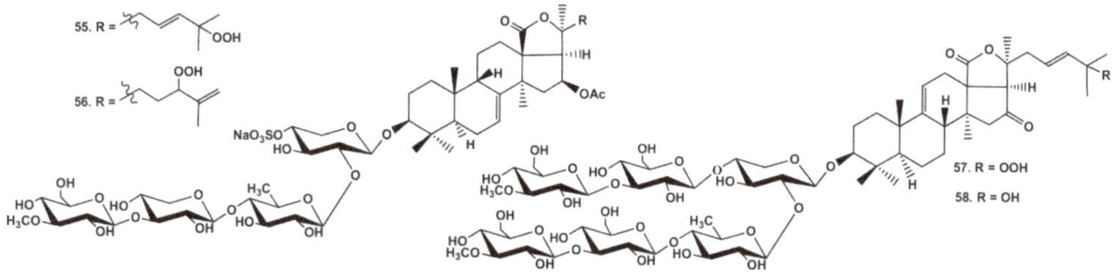

Figure 13. Structures of glycosides **55** and **56** from *Colochirus quadrangularis* and **57** and **58** from *Psolus fabricii*.

2.1.5. Correlation Analysis

To determine the structural elements of glycosides that might be responsible for membrane recognition, a set of physical properties of fifty-nine glycosides (represented in Table 1) were analyzed with MOE 2020.0901 CCG software [45]. Models of the spatial structure of the studied glycosides were built, protonated at pH 7.4, and subjected to energy minimization and a conformational search with MOE 2020.0901 CCG, and the dominant glycoside conformations were selected. The numerical descriptions or characterizations of the molecules that provide their physical properties such as the octanol/water partition coefficient, the polar surface area, the van der Waals (VDW) volume, the approximation to the sum of VDW surface areas of pure hydrogen bond acceptors/donors, the approximation to the sum of VDW surface areas of hydrophobic/polar atoms, etc. (296 in total), as well as their correlation matrix, were calculated with the QuaSAR-Descriptor tool of MOE 2020.0901 CCG software [45] (Figure S1). The correlation analysis did not reveal any strong direct correlation between the hemolytic activities of these compounds in vitro (Table 1) and certain calculated molecular 2D and 3D descriptors. Nevertheless, moderate positive correlations of their activity with the atomic contribution of the octanol/water partition coefficient [46], the total negative VDW surface area ($Å^2$), the number of oxygen atoms, the atomic valence connectivity index, the kappa shape indexes [47], which describe the different aspects of molecular shape, and the molecular VDW volume ($Å^3$) were disclosed. Therefore, an obvious joint effect of the molecular shape and volume (including the carbohydrate moiety shape and volume), the negative charge surface distribution, and the oxygen atom content on the membranotropic properties of the glycosides was observed. These results indicate the extremely complex nature of relationships between the structure of glycosides and their membranolytic action.

The analysis of SAR of the broad series of the glycosides from sea cucumbers also confirms the complicated and ambiguous character of these relationships because the impact in the membranotropic action of a certain structural element depends on the combination of such elements in the glycoside molecule. Nevertheless, there are some structural features causing the activity of the glycosides to be significant:

- The presence of a developed carbohydrate chain composed of four to six monosaccharide residues or a disaccharide chain with a sulfate group;
- The availability of 18(20)- or 18(16)-lactone and a normal (non-shortened) side chain;
- The presence of 9β-H, 7(8)-ene fragment, or 9(11)-double bond.

The influence of sulfate groups on the membranotropic action of the glycosides depends on the architecture of the sugar chain and the positions of sulfate groups. Hydroxyl groups attached to different positions of aglycone side chains extremely decrease the activity.

2.2. In Silico Analysis of the Interaction of the Glycosides from the Sea Cucumber Eupentacta fraudatrix with the Model Membrane

The molecular mechanisms of action of membranotropic compounds to the natural cell membranes are difficult to observe directly with any experimental techniques. Moreover, the lipid composition of membranes of diverse eukaryotic cell types varies to a great extent. The MD simulation providing information at the molecular level has become an increasingly popular "molecular-specific" technique for the study of issues related to bioactive molecule interactions with the membranes due to the rise of computing power, the development of methodologies, software, as well as the force field parameters. Nevertheless, artificial lipid bilayer membranes are suitable models for such investigations providing results consistent with the data obtained in the experiments with different cell lines. In this investigation the lipid composition of model membrane was chosen taking into account the balance between its complexity (resemblance to reality) and the feasibility of biophysical observations to interpret. The model of the symmetrical bilayer membrane containing two or three lipid types (phosphatidylcholine, sphingolipid, and sterol) is the most frequently used. Therefore, the artificial model of the erythrocyte-mimicking membrane constituting of phosphatidylcholine (POPC), cholesterol (CHOL), and palmitoyl-sphingomyelin (PSM) or 1-palmitoyl-2-oleoyl-sn-glycero-3-phosphoethanolamine (POPE) for the outer or inner leaflet, respectively, in a saline solution environment, was constructed based on the lipid composition of red blood cell membranes known to contain approximately 48% CHOL, 28% phosphatidylcholine and 24% sphingomyelin in the outer membrane leaflet, as well as phosphoethanolamine in the inner membrane leaflet [10,48].

To determine the membrane molecular targets of the binding glycosides, the simulations of full-atom molecular dynamic (MD) for the interactions of cucumariosides A_1 (**40**), A_2 (**59**), A_8 (**44**), and A_7 (**45**) from the sea cucumber *Eupentacta fraudatrix* (Figure 14) (hemolytic activities demonstrated by these compounds in vitro are presented in Table 1), differing from each other by the side chain or aglycone (for **44**) structures, with the model membrane for 600 ns time length (for each) were conducted (see Materials and Methods for details). The same MD simulations protocol was applied for the solvated bilayer system without the glycoside exposure, to be used as a control.

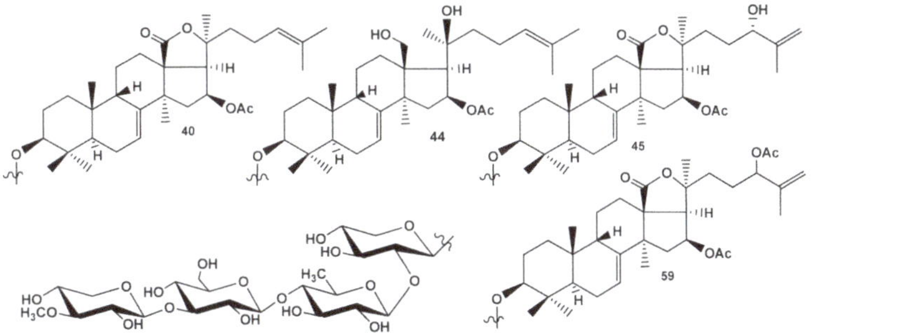

Figure 14. Structure of cucumariosides A_1 (**40**), A_8 (**44**), A_7 (**45**), and A_2 (**59**) used for in silico analysis of the interaction of the glycosides from the sea cucumber, *Eupentacta fraudatrix*, with the model membrane.

2.2.1. The Modelling of Cucumarioside A_1 (**40**) Membranotropic Action with MD Simulations

Our results derived from MD simulations of a model membrane system in the presence of cucumarioside A_1 (**40**) demonstrated that glycoside is able to interact specifically with the PSM of the outer membrane leaflet. The analysis of intermolecular interactions (Figure 15A) of cucumarioside A_1 (**40**), characterized by 24(25)-double bond, showed the attachment of its carbohydrate chain to membrane sphingomyelin (PSM) by hydrogen bonds (with the energy contribution of -11.94 kcal/M) (Table 2) enabling the anchoring of the glycoside at the interface of the membrane which is similar to dioscin behavior [49].

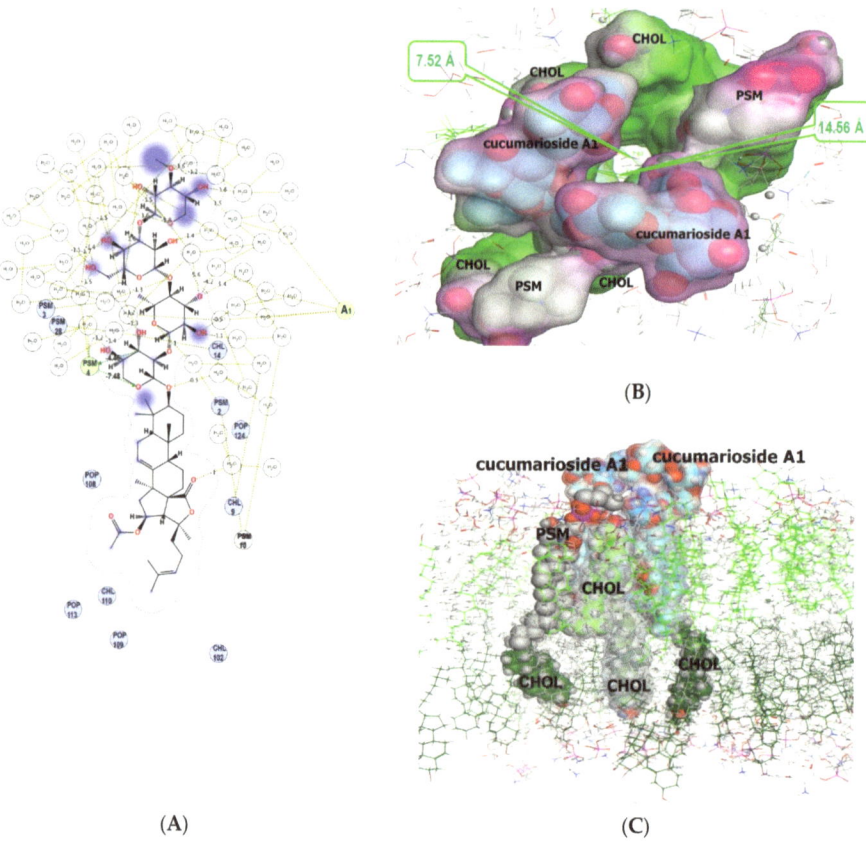

Figure 15. Spatial organization of multimolecular complex formed by two cucumarioside A_1 (**40**) molecules (I and II) and the model membrane components. (**A**) 2D diagram of noncovalent intermolecular interactions of the glycoside with water-lipid environment. (**B**) Multimolecular complex is presented as a semitransparent molecular surface, colored according to its lipophilicity: hydrophilic areas are pink, lipophilic areas are green, the view is perpendicular to membrane surface. The molecules of solvent and some membrane components are deleted for simplicity. (**C**) Multimolecular complex in membrane environment, the view parallel to membrane surface. The glycoside is presented as cyan "ball" model, POPC+PSM and CHOL molecules (6 Å surrounding glycoside-lipid complex) of outer membrane leaflet are grey and light-green "ball" models, respectively; POPC+PSM and CHOL of inner membrane leaflet, distant from molecular assembly, are presented as grey and dark-green "ball and stick" models, respectively.

Further MD simulations in the system CHOL/POPC/PSM/POPE which was exposed to cucumarioside A_1 (**40**) molecules demonstrated that glycoside integrates into the outer membrane leaflet leading to an asymmetrical pore formation with 7.52 Å diameter in the central part and 14.56 Å diameter in the entrance (Figure 15B,C). The stoichiometry of the pore forming components, glycoside/CHOL/POPC/PSM, is 2/4/5/6. Hence, cucumarioside A_1 (**40**) is capable of incorporating into the outer membrane leaflet predominantly through hydrophobic interactions of its aglycone with phospholipids, sphingomyelin, as well as cholesterol, that results in the membrane curvature, followed by its destabilization and permeability changing. It should be noted that during the formation of this multimolecular pore-like structure induced by cucumarioside A_1 (**40**), sphingomyelin molecules interact tightly with both glycosides and cholesterol through hydrogen-bonding as well as through hydrophobic interactions. Thus, sphingomyelin and cholesterol act as a functional pair to stabilize these complexes, similar to how they stabilize lipid rafts [22,50]. These data are in accordance with the high hemolytic effect of cucumarioside A_1 (**40**) (Table 1).

Table 2. Noncovalent intermolecular interactions inside the multimolecular complex formed by two molecules (I and II) of cucumarioside A_1 (**40**) and components of model lipid bilayer membrane.

Type of Bonding	Cucumarioside A_1 (40) Molecule	Membrane Component	Energy Contribution, kcal/mol	Distance, Å
Hydrogen bond	I	PSM4	−11.94	4.05
Hydrophobic	I	PSM4	−0.5	3.31
Hydrophobic	I	POPC108	−7.21	3.93
Hydrophobic	I	PSM2	−5.52	4.13
Hydrophobic	I	POP109	−4.69	3.92
Hydrophobic	I	PSM10	−3.71	4.19
Hydrophobic	I	CHOL9	−3.69	4.13
Hydrophobic	I	CHOL14	−2.18	4.01
Hydrophobic	I	POPC124	−1.59	4.02
Hydrophobic	I	POPC113	−0.55	4.13
Hydrophobic	II	CHOL38	−11.05	4.07
Hydrophobic	II	PSM31	−10.82	4.08
Hydrophobic	II	POPC124	−8.38	4.11
Hydrophobic	II	CHOL46	−4.77	4.06
Hydrophobic	II	CHOL14	−4.50	3.93
Hydrophobic	II	PSM28	−1.06	4.15
Hydrophobic	II	PSM74	0.05	3.95

The RMSD value of the heavy atoms of the model membrane phospholipids under cucumarioside A_1 (**40**) action was 2.89 Å, while for the lipid environment surrounding the glycoside at 10 Å (POPC, CHOL, PSM) it was 4.13 Å. Moreover, the deviation of CHOL heavy atoms in the outer leaflet did not exceed 1.89 Å, while in the inner leaflet the RMSD value was 4.97 Å and reached up to 6.99 Å for some of CHOL molecules (Figure 15C).

2.2.2. The Modelling of Cucumarioside A_8 (**44**) Membranotropic Action with MD Simulations

The in silico study of the action of cucumarioside A_8 (**44**) from *E. fraudatrix* [29] on a model erythrocyte membrane with MD simulations evidenced that the process apparently occurs in several stages: driven by electrostatic attracting, the glycoside reaches the membrane with its carbohydrate part and can anchor to phospholipid polar heads through hydrogen bonds (Figure 16C and Figure S2), after that its aglycone moiety completely immerses into the lipid layer, and the multimolecular assembly rearranges. Moreover, our computational results have disclosed the feasibility of the glycoside to induce the "pore-like" complex formation inside the membrane with stoichiometry of glycoside/CHOL/POPC/PSM (2/3/2/5) (Figure 16A,B, Table 3). Its assemblage is provided mainly through van der Waals bonds and hydrophobic interactions with PSM and contributes totally to complex formation up to −62.07 kcal/M. Simultaneously, the aglycone of one glycoside molecule (I) is anchored to a PSM head by a hydrogen bond (contributing −1 kcal/M), whereas the carbohydrate moiety of the other molecule (II) stabilizes this complex by another hydrogen bond generated with a POPC molecule (with a contribution of −3.10 kcal/M) (Table 3). This suggests that the mechanism of cucumarioside A_8 (**44**) hemolytic action is somewhat similar to that of cucumarioside A_1 (**40**).

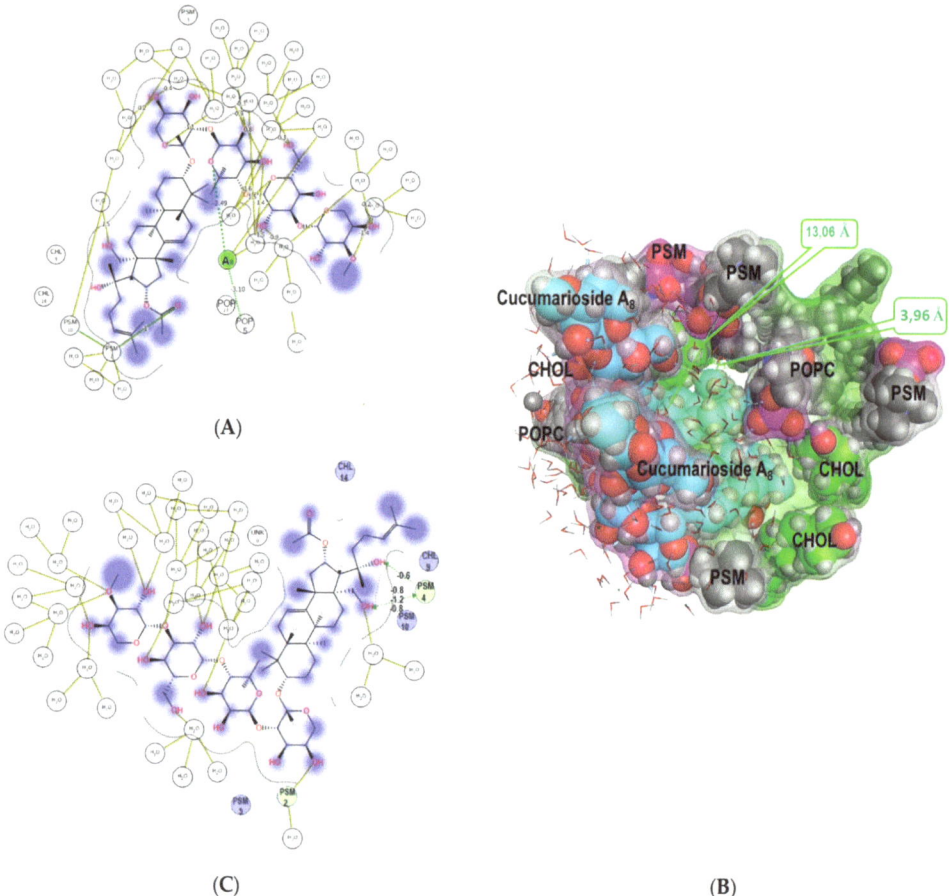

Figure 16. Spatial organization of multimolecular complex formed by two cucumarioside A_8 (**44**) molecules (I and II) and the model membrane components. (**A**) 2D diagram of noncovalent intermolecular interactions of the glycoside with water-lipid environment. (**B**) Multimolecular complex is presented as a semitransparent molecular surface, colored according to its lipophilicity: hydrophilic areas are pink, lipophilic areas are green, the view is perpendicular to membrane surface. The glycoside is presented as cyan "ball" model, POPC+PSM and CHOL molecules (6 Å surrounding glycoside-lipid complex) of the outer membrane leaflet are grey and light-green "ball" models. The molecules of solvent and some membrane components are deleted for simplicity. (**C**) 2D diagram of noncovalent intermolecular interactions of cucumarioside A_8 (**44**) with water-lipid environment at the initial stage of glycoside interaction with the model membrane.

The important functional role of hydroxy groups at C-18 and C-20 of cucumarioside A_8 (**44**) were found to promote an initial stage of glycoside integration into the lipid bilayer by the multiple hydrogen bond formations with sphingomyelin or phosphatidylcholine (Figure 16C). However, the extensive hydrophobic interactions became more energetically favorable at the subsequent stages of the glycoside engagement inside the outer membrane leaflet, allowing it to penetrate rather deeply into the bilayer (Figure S2B). Moreover, further MD simulations have revealed the inner membrane leaflet rearrangement under the influence of cucumarioside A_8 (**44**). Thus, the aglycone passed through the outer membrane leaflet and initiated the phosphatidylcholine molecule tails to move from the inner layer towards the "pore-like" assembly to generate hydrophobic interactions with the glycoside side chains (with a contribution of −3.72 kcal/M and −2.02 kcal/M) (Table 3, Figure S2D).

Table 3. Noncovalent intermolecular interactions inside multimolecular complex formed by two molecules (I, II) of cucumarioside A_8 (44) and the components of model lipid bilayer membrane.

Type of Bonding	Cucumarioside A_8 (44) Molecule	Membrane Component	Energy Contribution, kcal/mol	Distance, Å
Hydrogen bond	II	I	−3.49	3.36
Hydrophobic	II	I	−8.75	3.95
Hydrophobic	II	PSM20	−12.41	4.03
Hydrophobic	I	PSM2	−8.60	4.07
Hydrophobic	II	POPC13	−7.93	3.97
Hydrophobic	II	CHL7	−7.20	4.02
Hydrophobic	II	PSM2	−4.28	4.04
Hydrophobic	I	CHL9	−4.06	4.06
Hydrophobic	I	PSM10	−3.91	4.08
Hydrophobic	II	POPC108 *	−3.72	3.94
Hydrophobic	II	CHL14	−3.23	4.11
Hydrogen bond	II	POPC5	−3.10	2.60
Hydrophobic	I	PSM3	−2.31	3.96
Hydrophobic	II	POPC113 *	−2.02	4.21
Hydrophobic	I	POPC13	−1.39	3.59
Hydrophobic	II	PSM28	−1.01	4.26
Hydrogen bond	I	PSM2	−1.00	3.01

*—the inner membrane leaflet.

The analysis of noncovalent intermolecular interactions in this complex shows that, in contrast to the pore formed by cucumarioside A_1 (40), where the glycoside interacts predominantly with the lipid environment (CHOL/POPC/PSM) of the outer membrane layer (Table 2), the aglycone moieties of cucumarioside A_8 (44) molecules formed rather powerful hydrophobic contacts between each other (with a contribution of −8.75 kcal/M), as well as hydrogen bonds between their carbohydrate parts, contributing approximately −3.49 kcal/M to the complex formation. Apparently, these glycoside/glycoside interactions inside the pore led to a decrease in its diameter to 13.06 Å in the entrance and 3.96 Å in its narrowest part as compared to those for the cucumarioside A_1 (40)-induced pore (Figure 15). This finding suggests that the glycoside 44 is capable of forming pores in the erythrocyte membrane, similar to the glycoside 40, but their size and quantity would be more sensitive to the glycoside concentration. This result is in good agreement with the glycoside activities (Table 1), indicating an order of magnitude higher hemolytic activity of cucumarioside A_1 (40) compared to that of cucumarioside A_8 (44).

2.2.3. The Modelling of Cucumarioside A_2 (59) Membranotropic Action with MD Simulations

MD simulations of interactions of cucumarioside A_2 (59), with a 24-O-acetic group, demonstrated that glycoside bound to both the phospholipids and cholesterol of the outer membrane leaflet causing significant changes in the bilayer architecture and dynamics. The apolar aglycone part of the glycoside and the fatty acid residues of phospholipids interact with each other through hydrophobic bonds (with energy contribution from −1.23 kcal/M to −4.65 kcal/M) and hydrogen bonds (with energy contribution from −0.50 kcal/M to −8.20 kcal/M) (Table 4, Figure 17). The analysis of the energy contributions of different membrane components to the formation of multimolecular complexes including three molecules of cucumarioside A_2 (59) revealed that the glycoside/phospholipid interactions were more favorable compared to the glycoside/cholesterol interactions involving only the aglycone side chain area (Figure 17). One molecule of the glycoside interacted with 3–5 phospholipid molecules involving their polar heads being bound to the polycyclic nucleus and carbohydrate chains while fatty acid tales surrounded the aglycones side chain. Thus, a so-called "phospholipid cluster" is formed around the glycoside causing it to be partly embedded to the outer leaflet. A rather rigid "cholesterol cluster" is formed under the place of glycoside penetration to the outer membrane leaflet due to the lifting of cholesterol molecules from the inner leaflet attempting, to some extent to substitute the molecules of the outer leaflet which are bound with the glycoside (Figure 17).

Table 4. Noncovalent intermolecular interactions inside multimolecular complex formed by three molecules (I–III) of cucumarioside A_2 (**59**) and components of model lipid bilayer membrane.

Type of Bonding	Cucumarioside A_2 (59) Molecule	Membrane Component	Energy Contribution, kcal/mol	Distance, Å
Hydrophobic	I	PSM51	−4.63	4.21
Hydrophobic	I	POPC11	−3.34	3.99
Hydrophobic	I	CHOL92	−0.63	3.89
Hydrophobic	I	POPC49	−1.23	3.99
Hydrogen bond	II	PSM51	−0.49	3.18
Hydrophobic	II	PSM57	−6.19	4.14
Hydrophobic	II	CHOL104	−6.1	3.98
Hydrophobic	II	PSM55	−3.3	4.07
Hydrophobic	II	POPC11	−2.78	4.17
Hydrophobic	II	PSM51	−2.18	4.08
Hydrogen bond	III	POPC49	−8.2	2.49
Hydrophobic	III	POPC11	−3.08	4.20
Hydrophobic	III	POPC49	−1.43	3.91
Hydrophobic	III	CHOL99	−0.67	3.53

Therefore, the agglomerating action of cucumarioside A_2 (**59**) towards the cholesterol molecules not only in the immediate vicinity of the glycoside but involving the cholesterol molecules from the inner membrane leaflet became clear. However, since cholesterol, with its rather rigid structure, interacts mainly with the aglycone side chain, it continues to be embedded to the outer leaflet, while flexible phospholipid molecules, interacting with both the aglycone and carbohydrate chain, to some extent overlook the outer membrane leaflet. Hence, two so-called "lipid pools" are generated with one of them surrounding carbohydrate and polycyclic moieties of the glycoside and the second one located in the aglycone side chain area (Figure 17B).

Due to the asymmetric distribution of lipids between the membrane monolayers, their properties can differ significantly. POPC and PSM are characterized by saturated fatty acid tails, the asymmetry of leaflets is enhanced by different polar head properties of POPC, PSM, and POPE. Moreover, the presence of CHOL molecules in the bilayer, the content of which is close to 50% in the erythrocyte biomembrane, promotes the "elongation" and alignment of fatty tails of phospholipids parallel to the flat core of CHOL [51]. Our MD simulation results suggest that cucumarioside A_2 (**59**) apparently induced the disruption of tight CHOL/lipid and lipid/lipid interactions through an extensive hydrophobic area formation in the glycoside's immediate environment (Figure 17, Table 4). Additionally, the glycoside can provoke the process of CHOL release from the inner monolayer and its accumulation between monolayers or insertion to the outer one, because, unlike POPC, PSM and POPE, which have rather bulk polar heads, the small polar OH-group of CHOL is known to facilitate CHOL relocation between monolayers due to the low energy barrier of the "flip-flop" mechanism [51]. All these properties and forces led to the accumulation of CHOL molecules surround the glycoside, which resulted in an increase in layer viscosity. Simultaneously the CHOL outflow made the inner leaflet more fluid and unbalanced compared to the structured outer one that can cause the generation of non-bilayer disordered membrane architecture. These circumstances cause the inner membrane leaflet to be reorganized followed by the changing of the membrane barrier properties providing the hemolytic action of the glycoside.

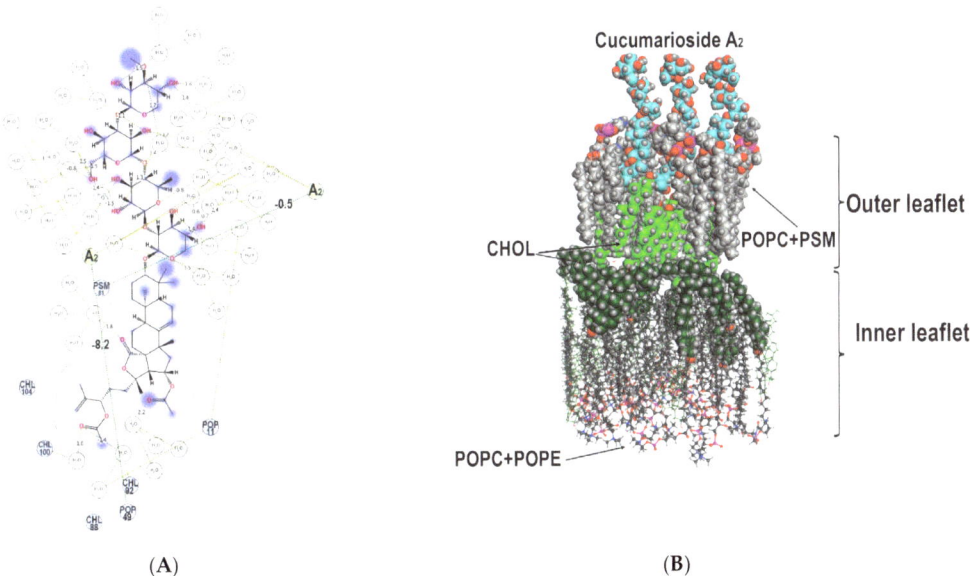

Figure 17. Spatial organization of multimolecular complex formed by three molecules (I–III) of cucumarioside A_2 (**59**) and the components of model membrane. (**A**) 2D diagram of intermolecular noncovalent interactions of three cucumarioside A_2 (**59**) molecules and the components of model water/lipid bilayer environment. Hydrogen bonds are green dotted lines. (**B**) Front view to the cucumarioside A_2 (**59**) multimolecular complex with a model membrane. The glycoside is presented as cyan "ball" model, POPC+PSM and CHOL (6 Å surrounding glycoside) of the outer membrane leaflet are presented as grey and light-green "ball" models, respectively; POPC+POPE and CHOL of inner membrane leaflet, distant from multimolecular assembly, are presented as grey and dark-green "ball and stick" models, respectively; CHOL molecules of the inner membrane leaflet at 5 Å distant from multimolecular complex are presented as a dark-green "ball" model. The molecules of solvent and some membrane components are deleted for simplicity.

Thus, according to our MD simulations, cucumarioside A_2 (**59**) exposure caused significant change in the architecture of the model membrane bilayer (Figure 17). It should be noted that although the dynamic behavior of the lipid environment of cucumarioside A_1 (**40**) and cucumarioside A_2 (**59**) was similar, there were a number of considerable differences. Despite the low RMSD value for all heavy atoms of membrane lipids (3.74 Å), which reflects the mobility of membrane components, the dynamic behavior of those located in the immediate environment of the glycoside molecules was changed to a great extent. So, their RMSD value (10 Å surrounding the glycoside) was 7.47 Å, and for some CHOL molecules, predominantly those forming the inner membrane leaflet, this value reached 17.68 Å.

2.2.4. The Modelling of Cucumarioside A_7 (**45**) Membranotropic Action with MD Simulations

Cucumarioside A_7 (**45**) differs from the compounds **40**, **44**, and **59** by the presence of an OH-group in the aglycone side chain that causes the extremal decreasing in its membranotropic activity (Table 1). In fact, in silico simulations of its interactions with model membrane demonstrated only slight interactions with phospholipid polar heads and the absence of glycoside/cholesterol interactions.

Moreover, MD simulations of cucumarioside A_7 (**45**) interactions showed RMSD values with neighboring lipids was comparable to those observed during MD simulations in the control membrane system and for both did not exceed 2.34 Å. This result indicated no significant changes in lipid packaging induced by cucumarioside A_7 (**45**); this is in good accordance with hemolytic activity, SAR data (Table 1), as well as other MD simulations which indicated the involvement of the aglycones side chain in the hydrophobic interactions with phospholipid fatty acid tails and cholesterol. It is obviously that hydroxyl groups in the side chain of **45** imped such interactions.

3. Materials and Methods

3.1. Model System for Artificial Plasma Membrane Mimicking the Erythrocyte Membrane

An asymmetric model bilayer comprising POPC (1-palmitoyl-2-oleoyl-sn-glycero-3-phosphocholine), CHOL (cholesterol), PSM (palmitoylshingomyeline for outer leaflet), or POPE (1-palmitoyl-2-oleoyl-sn-glycero-3-phosphoethanolamine) for the inner leaflet, respectively, in the ratio 1:2:1 was constructed by remote web resource CHARMM-GUIHMMM Builder [52,53], solvated, and equilibrated during 400 ns for optimal bilayer package.

3.2. Full Atom MD Simulations

Since we did not have any information on the possible orientation of glycosides during their interaction with the membrane, glycoside molecules were added to the previously equilibrated model membrane system and placed at a distance of 11 Å above the outer membrane leaflet. The orientation of the molecules was chosen arbitrarily provided that their long axis was located along the membrane surface (Figure S2A). The model membrane simulation system with the glycosides was resolvated with water (25 Å above and below the membrane) and neutralized with counterions for a simulating box of 200 × 200 × 90 Å, protonated at pH 7.4, and the total potential energy of the systems was minimized with the energy gradient of 0.01 kcal/mol/Å^{-1} to remove initial unfavorable contacts, then heated from 0 to 300 K for 100 ns and equilibrated at 300 K for another 200 ns.

The MD simulations of the free model membrane system or under the impact of glycosides in water environment were conducted with an Amber 14EHT force field. This was carried out with a checkpoint at 500 ps, a sample time of 10 ps, with Nosé-Poincaré–Andersen Hamiltonian equations of motion (NPA), and a time step of 0.001 ps, at a constant pressure (1 atm) and temperature (300 K) giving a total simulation time of 600 ns using MOE 2020.0901 CCG software [45]. Solvent molecules were treated as rigid. Computer simulations and theoretical studies were performed using cluster CCU "Far Eastern computing resource" FEB RAS (Vladivostok).

MD simulations of the control membrane system demonstrated RMSD value no higher than 2.34 Å.

The analysis of intramolecular interactions as well as the estimation of the interaction energy contribution was made with a ligand interaction suite from MOE 2020.0901 CCG software [45].

3.3. Triterpene Glycosides Chosen for MD Simulations

Cucumarioside A_1 (**40**): 3β-O-{3-O-methyl-β-D-xylopyranosyl-(1→3)-β-D-glucopyranosyl-(1→4)-β-D-quinovopyranosyl-(1→2)-β-D-xylopyranosyl}-16β-acetoxyholosta-7,24-diene; mp 190 °C; $[\alpha]_D^{20}$ −15° (c 0.1, C$_5$H$_5$N).

Cucumarioside A_2 (**59**): 3β-O-{3-O-methyl-β-D-xylopyranosyl-(1→3)-β-D-glucopyranosyl-(1→4)-β-D-quinovopyranosyl-(1→2)-β-D-xylopyranosyl}-16β,24ξ-diacetoxyholosta-7,25-diene; mp 167°C; $[\alpha]_D^{20}$ −17 (c 0.1, C$_5$H$_5$N). HR ESI MS (+) m/z: 1179.5555 (calc 1179.5558) [M + Na]$^+$.

Cucumarioside A_7 (**45**) is 3β-O-{3-O-methyl-β-D-xylopyranosyl-(1→3)-β-D-glucopyranosyl-(1→4)-β-D-quinovopyranosyl-(1→2)-β-D-xylopyranosyl}-16β-acetoxyholosta-24S-hydroxy-7,25-diene; mp 183–185 °C; $[\alpha]_D^{20}$ −5 (c 0.1, C$_5$H$_5$N). HR ESI MS (+) m/z: 1137.5460 (calc 1137.5452) [M + Na]$^+$.

Cucumarioside A_8 (**44**) 3β-O-[3-O-methyl-β-D-xylopyranosyl-(1→3)-β-D-glucopyranosyl-(1→4)-β-D-quinovopyranosyl-(1→ 2)-β-D-xylopyranosyl]-16β-acetoxy-9β-H-lanosta-7,24-diene-18,20β-diol. mp 238–240 °C; $[\alpha]_D^{20}$ −3 (c 0.1, C$_5$H$_5$N), HR MALDI TOF MS (+) m/z: 1125.5812 (calc 1125.5816) [M + Na]$^+$.

4. Conclusions

The SAR for the sea cucumber triterpene glycosides illustrated by their action on mouse erythrocytes, is very complicated. Nevertheless, in our study, several clear trends were found, providing significant membranolytic activity for the glycosides, namely: the presence of a developed carbohydrate chain composed of four to six monosaccharide residues (with linear tetrasaccharide fragment) or a disaccharide chain with a sulfate group; the availability of 18(20)- or 18(16)-lactone and a normal (non-shortened) side chain; the presence of 9β-H, 7(8)-ene fragment or 9(11)-double bond. It was also observed that the influence of sulfate groups on the membranotropic action of the glycosides depends on the architecture of the sugar chain and the positions of sulfate groups. Hydroxyl groups attached to different positions of aglycone side chains extremely decrease the activity.

Using an in silico approach of full-atom MD simulations for the investigation of interactions of sea cucumber triterpene glycosides with the molecules composing the model lipid bilayer membrane has resulted in the clarification of several characteristics of the molecular mechanisms of membranolytic action of these compounds. It was revealed that the studied glycosides bound to the membrane surface mainly by hydrophobic interactions and hydrogen bonds, but the mode of such interactions depended on the aglycone side chain structure and varied to a great extent. The formation of multimolecular lipid/glycoside complexes led to membrane curvature followed by the subsequent membranolytic effects of the glycosides. Different mechanisms of glycoside/membrane interactions were discovered for cucumariosides A_1 (**40**), A_8 (**44**), and A_2 (**59**). The first mechanism, inherent for **40** and **44**, was realized through the pore's formation differed by the shape, stoichiometry, and the impact of diverse noncovalent interactions into complex assembling, depending on the glycoside structural peculiarities. The second mode of membranotropic action was realized by **59** through the formation of phospholipid and cholesterol clusters in the outer and inner membrane leaflets, correspondingly.

The observed peculiarities of membranotropic action are in good agreement with the corresponding data of in vitro hemolytic activity of the investigated compounds [28,29]. In fact, the hemolytic activity of pore-forming cucumariosides A_1 (**40**) and A_8 (**44**) were 0.07 and 0.70 µM/mL, correspondingly. The value for cluster-forming cucumarioside A_2 (**59**) was 4.70 µM/mL, and cucumarioside A_7 (**45**) demonstrating the weakest capacity to embed the membrane, was not active to the maximal studied concentration of 100.0 µM/mL.

Further in silico studies of the relationships of the membrane lipid composition and structural peculiarities of the glycosides demonstrating membranolytic activity are necessary to ascertain the molecular targets of glycoside/membrane bonding and to deepen the understanding of these complex multistage mechanisms.

Supplementary Materials: The following are available online at https://www.mdpi.com/article/10.3390/md19110604/s1. Figure S1: The Correlation matrix of the hemolytic activities of glycosides in vitro (ED50, µM/mL, Table 1) and certain calculated molecular 2D and 3D descriptors conducted with the QuaSAR-Descriptor tool of MOE 2020.0901 CCG software [45]. Moderate positive correlation of their activity with the atomic contribution to Log of the octanol/water partition coefficient (h_logP) [46], the total negative VDW surface area (Å2), the number of oxygen atoms (a_no), the atomic valence connectivity index (chi0v), kappa shape indexes (Kier) [47], describing different aspects of molecular shape, the molecular VDW volume (Vol, vdw_vol, VSA_acc, (Å3)) were disclosed. Figure S2: (A) Initial conformation of cucumarioside A8 (**44**) for MD simulations, where the A8 (**44**) molecules are placed at a distance of 11 Å above the outer membrane leaflet with their long axis is directed along the membrane surface. (B) The snapshot of 85 ns MD simulations indicating the cucumarioside A8 carbohydrate parts come up to the phospholipid heads of the outer membrane leaflet. (C) The snapshot of 130 ns MD simulations indicating the cucumarioside A8 aglycone pass through the outer membrane leaflet. (D) The last snapshot of MD simulations indicating the aglycone moieties of two cucumarioside A8 molecules induce the "pore-like" complex formation inside the membrane. The glycoside is presented as cyan "ball" model, POPC+PSM +CHOL are presented as grey stick models. The solvent molecules and some membrane components are deleted for simplicity.

Author Contributions: Conceptualization, A.S.S., V.I.K., and S.A.A.; methodology, E.A.Z.; investigation, A.S.S., E.A.Z., and S.A.A.; writing—original draft preparation, A.S.S., E.A.Z.; writing—review and editing, A.S.S., V.I.K. All authors have read and agreed to the published version of the manuscript.

Funding: Grant from the Russian Foundation for Basic Research No. 19-04-000-14.

Institutional Review Board Statement: Not applicable.

Informed Consent Statement: Not applicable.

Data Availability Statement: Not applicable.

Acknowledgments: The study was carried out with the equipment of the Collective Facilities Center "The Far Eastern Center for Structural Molecular Research (NMR/MS) PIBOC FEB RAS".

Conflicts of Interest: The authors declare no conflict of interest.

References

1. Aminin, D.L.; Menchinskaya, E.S.; Pisliagin, E.A.; Silchenko, A.S.; Avilov, S.A.; Kalinin, V.I. Sea cucumber triterpene glycosides as anticancer agents. In *Studies in Natural Product Chemistry*; Atta-ur-Rahman, Ed.; Elsevier B.V.: Amsterdam, The Netherlands, 2016; Volume 49, pp. 55–105.
2. Kalinin, V.I.; Prokofieva, N.G.; Likhatskaya, G.N.; Schentsova, E.B.; Agafonova, I.G.; Avilov, S.A.; Drozdova, O.A. Hemolytic activities of triterpene glycosides from the holothurian order Dendrochirotida: Some trends in the evolution of this group of toxins. *Toxicon* **1996**, *34*, 475–483. [CrossRef]
3. Careaga, V.P.; Maier, M.S. Cytotoxic triterpene glycosides from sea cucumbers. In *Handbook of Anticancer Drugs from Marine Origin*; Kim, S.-K., Ed.; Springer International Publishing: Cham, Switzerland, 2015; pp. 515–528.
4. Kalinin, V.I.; Aminin, D.L.; Avilov, S.A.; Silchenko, A.S.; Stonik, V.A. Triterpene glycosides from sea cucumbers (Holothuroidea, Echinodermata), biological activities and functions. In *Studies in Natural Product Chemistry (Bioactive Natural Products)*; Atta-ur-Rahman, Ed.; Elsevier Science Publisher: Amsterdam, The Netherlands, 2008; Volume 35, pp. 135–196.
5. Kalinin, V.I. System-theoretical (holistic) approach to the modelling of structural-functional relationships of Biomolecules and their evolution: An example of triterpene glycosides from sea cucumbers (Echinodermata, Holothurioidea). *J. Theor. Biol.* **2000**, *206*, 151–168. [CrossRef]
6. Park, J.-I.; Bae, H.-R.; Kim, C.G.; Stonik, V.A.; Kwak, J.Y. Relationships between chemical structures and functions of triterpene glycosides isolated from sea cucumbers. *Front. Chem.* **2014**, *2*, 77. [CrossRef]
7. Claereboudt, E.J.S.; Eeckhaut, I.; Lins, L.; Deleu, M. How different sterols contribute to saponin tolerant plasma membranes in sea cucumbers. *Sci. Rep.* **2018**, *8*, 10845. [CrossRef] [PubMed]
8. Likhatskaya, G.N.; Yarovaya, T.P.; Rudnev, V.V.; Popov, A.M.; Anisimov, M.M.; Rovin, Y.G. Formation of complex of triterpene glycoside of holothurine A with cholesterol in liposomal membranes. *Biofizika* **1985**, *30*, 358–359.
9. Popov, A.M. A Comparative study of the hemolytic and cytotoxic activities of triterpenoids isolated from ginseng and sea cucumbers. *Biol. Bull.* **2002**, *29*, 120–128. [CrossRef]
10. Deleu, M.; Crowet, J.M.; Nasir, M.N.; Lins, L. Complementary biophysical tools to investigate lipid specificity in the interaction between bioactive molecules and the plasma membrane: A review. *Biochim. Biophys. Acta* **2014**, *1838*, 3171–3190. [CrossRef] [PubMed]
11. Lorent, J.H.; Quetin-Leclercq, J.; Mingeot-Leclercq, M.-P. The amphiphilic nature of saponins and their effects on artificial and biological membranes and potential consequences for red blood and cancer cells. *Org. Biomol. Chem.* **2014**, *12*, 8803–8822. [CrossRef] [PubMed]
12. Malyarenko, T.V.; Kicha, A.A.; Kalinovsky, A.I.; Dmitrenok, P.S.; Malyarenko, O.S.; Kuzmich, A.S.; Stonik, V.A.; Ivanchina, N.V. New triterpene glycosides from the Far Eastern starfish *Solaster pacificus* and their biological activity. *Biomolecules* **2021**, *11*, 427. [CrossRef]
13. Aminin, D.; Pisliagin, E.; Astashev, M.; Es'kov, A.; Kozhemyako, V.; Avilov, S.; Zelepuga, E.; Yurchenko, E.; Kaluzhskiy, L.; Kozlovskaya, E.; et al. Glycosides from edible sea cucumbers stimulate macrophages via purinergic receptors. *Sci. Rep.* **2016**, *6*, 39683. [CrossRef]
14. Kersten, G.F.; Crommelin, D.J. Liposomes and ISCOMS as vaccine formulations. *Biochim. Biophys. Acta* **1995**, *1241*, 117–138. [CrossRef]
15. Mazeyka, A.N.; Popov, A.M.; Kalinin, V.I.; Avilov, S.A.; Silchenko, A.S.; Kostetsky, E.Y. Complexation between triterpene glycosides of holothurians and cholesterol is the basis of lipid-saponin carriers of subunit protein antigens. *Biophysics* **2008**, *53*, 826–835.
16. Stonik, V.A.; Aminin, D.L.; Boguslavski, V.M.; Avilov, S.A.; Agafonova, I.G.; Silchenko, A.S.; Ponomarenko, L.P.; Prokofieva, N.G.; Chaikina, E.L. Immunostimulatory means Cumaside and pharmaceutical composition on its base. Patent of the Russian Federation No. 2271820, 20 March 2005. Appl. No. 2004120434/17, 2 July 2004.
17. Aminin, D.L.; Chaykina, E.L.; Agafonova, I.G.; Avilov, S.A.; Kalinin, V.I.; Stonik, V.A. Antitumor activity of the immunomodulatory lead Cumaside. *Intern. Immunopharm.* **2010**, *10*, 648–654. [CrossRef] [PubMed]

18. Verstraeten, S.L.; Deleu, M.; Janikowska-Sagan, M.; Claereboudt, E.J.S.; Lins, L.; Tyteca, D.; Mingeot-Leclercq1, M.P. The activity of the saponin ginsenoside Rh2 is enhanced by the interaction with membrane sphingomyelin but depressed by cholesterol. *Sci. Rep.* **2019**, *9*, 7285. [CrossRef] [PubMed]
19. Mollinedo, F.; Gajate, C. Lipid rafts as major platforms for signaling regulation in cancer. *Adv Biol Regul.* **2015**, *57*, 130–146. [CrossRef] [PubMed]
20. Guariento, S.; Bruno, O.; Fossa, P.; Cichero, E. New insights into PDE4B inhibitor selectivity: CoMFA analyses and molecular docking studies. *Mol. Divers.* **2016**, *20*, 77–92. [CrossRef]
21. Rusnati, M.; Sala, D.; Orro, A.; Bugatti, A.; Trombetti, G.; Cichero, E.; Urbinati, C.; Di Somma, M.; Millo, E.; Galietta, L.J.V.; et al. Speeding Up the Identification of Cystic Fibrosis Transmembrane Conductance Regulator-Targeted Drugs: An Approach Based on Bioinformatics Strategies and Surface Plasmon Resonance. *Molecules* **2018**, *23*, 120. [CrossRef]
22. Sezgin, E.; Levental, I.; Mayor, S.; Eggeling, C. The mystery of membrane organization: Composition, regulation and roles of lipid rafts. *Nat. Rev. Mol. Cell Biol.* **2017**, *18*, 361–374. [CrossRef]
23. Silchenko, A.S.; Kalinovsky, A.I.; Avilov, S.A.; Andryjaschenko, P.V.; Dmitrenok, P.S.; Martyyas, E.A.; Kalinin, V.I.; Jayasandhya, P.; Rajan, G.C.; Padmakumar, K.P. Structures and biological activities of typicosideds A_1, A_2, B_1, C_1 and C_2, triterpene glycosides from the sea cucumbers *Actinocucumis typica*. *Nat. Prod. Commun.* **2013**, *8*, 301–310.
24. Silchenko, A.S.; Kalinovsky, A.I.; Avilov, S.A.; Andryjaschenko, P.V.; Dmitrenok, P.S.; Kalinin, V.I.; Yurchenko, E.V.; Dolmatov, I.Y. Colochirosides B_1, B_2, B_3 and C, novel sulfated triterpene glycosides from the sea cucumber *Colochirus robustus* (Cucumariidae, Dendrochirotida). *Nat. Prod. Commun.* **2015**, *10*, 1687–1694. [CrossRef]
25. Silchenko, A.S.; Kalinovsky, A.I.; Avilov, S.A.; Andryjaschenko, P.V.; Dmitrenok, P.S.; Chingizova, E.A.; Ermakova, S.P.; Malyarenko, O.S.; Dautova, T.N. Nine new triterpene glycosides, magnumosides A_1–A_4, B_1, B_2, C_1, C_2 and C_4, from the Vietnamese sea cucumber *Neothyonidium* (=*Massinum*) *magnum*: Structures and activities against tumor cells independently and in synergy with radioactive irradiation. *Mar. Drugs* **2017**, *15*, 256. [CrossRef]
26. Silchenko, A.S.; Kalinovsky, A.I.; Avilov, S.A.; Kalinin, V.I.; Andrijaschenko, P.V.; Dmitrenok, P.S.; Chingizova, E.A.; Ermakova, S.P.; Malyarenko, O.S.; Dautova, T.N. Magnumosides B_3, B_4 and C_3, mono- and disulfated triterpene tetraosides from the Vietnamese sea cucumber *Neothyonidium* (=*Massinum*) *magnum*. *Nat. Prod. Commun.* **2017**, *12*, 1577–1582.
27. Silchenko, A.S.; Kalinovsky, A.I.; Avilov, S.A.; Andryjaschenko, P.V.; Dmitrenok, P.S.; Yurchenko, E.A.; Kalinin, V.I. Structures and cytotoxic properties of cucumariosides H_2, H_3 and H_4 from the sea cucumber *Eupentacta fraudatrix*. *Nat. Prod. Res.* **2012**, *26*, 1765–1774. [CrossRef]
28. Silchenko, A.S.; Kalinovsky, A.I.; Avilov, S.A.; Andryjashenko, P.V.; Dmitrenok, P.S.; Martyyas, E.A.; Kalinin, V.I. Triterpene glycosides from the sea cucumber *Eupentacta fraudatrix*. Structure and biological actions of cucumariosides A_1, A_3, A_4, A_5, A_6, A_{12} and A_{15}, seven new minor non-sulfated tetraosides and unprecedented 25-keto,25-norholostane aglycone. *Nat. Prod. Commun.* **2012**, *7*, 517–525. [CrossRef] [PubMed]
29. Silchenko, A.S.; Kalinovsky, A.I.; Avilov, S.A.; Andryjaschenko, P.V.; Dmitrenok, P.S.; Martyyas, E.A.; Kalinin, V.I. Triterpene glycosides from the sea cucumber *Eupentacta fraudatrix*. Structure and cytotoxic action of cucumariosides A_2, A_7, A_9, A_{10}, A_{11}, A_{13} and A_{14}, seven new minor non-sulated tetraosides and an aglycone with an uncommon 18-hydroxy group. *Nat. Prod. Commun.* **2012**, *7*, 845–852. [CrossRef]
30. Silchenko, A.S.; Kalinovsky, A.I.; Avilov, S.A.; Kalinin, V.I.; Andrijaschenko, P.V.; Dmitrenok, P.S.; Popov, R.S.; Chingizova, E.A.; Ermakova, S.P.; Malyarenko, O.S. Structures and bioactivities of six new triterpene glycosides, psolusosides E, F, G, H, H_1 and I and the corrected structure of psoluoside B from the sea cucumber *Psolus fabricii*. *Mar. Drugs* **2019**, *17*, 358. [CrossRef] [PubMed]
31. Silchenko, A.S.; Kalinovsky, A.I.; Avilov, S.A.; Kalinin, V.I.; Andrijaschenko, P.V.; Dmitrenok, P.S.; Popov, R.S.; Chingizova, E.A. Structures and bioactivities of psolusosides B_1, B_2, J, K, L, M, N, O, P, and Q from the sea cucumber *Psolus fabricii*. The first finding of tetrasulfated marine low molecular weight metabolites. *Mar. Drugs* **2019**, *17*, 631. [CrossRef] [PubMed]
32. Silchenko, A.S.; Kalinovsky, A.I.; Avilov, S.A.; Andrijaschenko, P.V.; Popov, R.S.; Dmitrenok, P.S.; Chingizova, E.A.; Ermakova, S.P.; Malyarenko, O.S.; Dautov, S.S.; et al. Structures and bioactivities of quadrangularisosides A, A_1, B, B_1, B_2, C, C_1, D, D_1–D_4, and E from the sea cucumber *Colochirus quadrangularis*: The first discovery of the glycosides, sulfated by C-4 of the terminal 3-O-methylglucose residue. Synergetic effect on colony formation of tumor HT-29 cells of these glycosides with radioactive irradiation. *Mar. Drugs* **2020**, *18*, 394. [CrossRef]
33. Kalinin, V.I.; Volkova, O.V.; Likhatskaya, G.N.; Prokofieva, N.G.; Agafonova, I.G.; Anisimov, M.M.; Kalinovsky, A.I.; Avilov, S.A.; Stonik, V.A. Hemolytic activity of triterpene glycosides from Cucumariidae family holothurians and evolution of this group of toxins. *J. Nat. Toxins* **1992**, *1*, 17–30.
34. Kim, S.-K.; Himaya, S.W.A. Triterpene glycosides from sea cucumbers and their biological activities. *Adv. Food Nutr. Res.* **2012**, *63*, 297–319.
35. Silchenko, A.S.; Kalinovsky, A.I.; Avilov, S.A.; Adnryjaschenko, P.V.; Dmitrenok, P.S.; Martyyas, E.A.; Kalinin, V.I. Triterpene glycosides from sea cucumber *Eupentacta fraudatrix*. Structure and biological activity of cucumariosides B_1 and B_2, two new minor non-sulfated unprecedented triosides. *Nat. Prod. Commun.* **2012**, *7*, 1157–1162. [CrossRef]
36. Silchenko, A.S.; Kalinovsky, A.I.; Avilov, S.A.; Andryjaschenko, P.V.; Dmitrenok, P.S.; Yurchenko, E.A.; Kalinin, V.I. Structure of cucumariosides H_5, H_6, H_7 and H_8. Glycosides from the sea cucumber *Eupentacta fraudatrix* and unprecedented aglycone with 16,22-epoxy-group. *Nat. Prod. Commun.* **2011**, *6*, 1075–1082. [CrossRef]

37. Silchenko, A.S.; Kalinovsky, A.I.; Avilov, S.A.; Andryjascchenko, P.V.; Dmitrenok, P.S.; Yurchenko, E.A.; Dolmatov, I.Y.; Kalinin, V.I.; Stonik, V.A. Structure and biological action of cladolosides B_1, B_2, C, C_1, C_2 and D, six new triterpene glycosides from the sea cucumber *Cladolabesschmeltzii*. *Nat. Prod. Commun.* **2013**, *8*, 1527–1534. [CrossRef]
38. Silchenko, A.S.; Kalinovsky, A.I.; Avilov, S.A.; Andryjaschenko, P.V.; Dmitrenok, P.S.; Yurchenko, E.A.; Dolmatov, I.Y.; Kalinin, V.I. Structures and biological activities of cladolosides C_3, E_1, E_2, F_1, F_2, G, H_1 and H_2, eight triterpene glycosides from the sea cucumber *Cladolabes schmeltzii* with one known and four new carbohydrate chains. *Carb. Res.* **2015**, *414*, 22–31. [CrossRef] [PubMed]
39. Silchenko, A.S.; Kalinovsky, A.I.; Avilov, S.A.; Andryjaschenko, P.V.; Dmitrenok, P.S.; Chingizova, E.A.; Dolmatov, I.Y.; Kalinin, V.I. Cladolosides I_1, I_2, J_1, K_1, K_2 and L_1, monosulfated triterpene glycosides with new carbohydrate chains from the sea cucumber *Cladolabes schmeltzii*. *Carb. Res.* **2017**, *445*, 80–87. [CrossRef] [PubMed]
40. Silchenko, A.S.; Kalinovsky, A.I.; Avilov, S.A.; Andryjaschenko, P.V.; Dmitrenok, P.S.; Yurchenko, E.A.; Ermakova, S.P.; Malyarenko, O.S.; Dolmatov, I.Y.; Kalinin, V.I. Cladolosides C_4, D_1, D_2, M, M_1, M_2, N and Q, new triterpene glycosides with diverse carbohydrate chains from sea cucumber *Cladolabes schmeltzii*. An uncommon 20,21,22,23,24,25,26,27-okta-*nor*-lanostane aglycone. The synergism of inhibitory action of non-toxic dose of the glycosides and radioactive irradiation on colony formation of HT-29 cancer cells. *Carb. Res.* **2018**, *468*, 36–44.
41. Silchenko, A.S.; Kalinovsky, A.I.; Avilov, S.A.; Andryjaschenko, P.V.; Dmitrenok, P.S.; Yurchenko, E.A.; Ermakova, S.P.; Malyarenko, O.S.; Dolmatov, I.Y.; Kalinin, V.I. Cladolosides O, P, P_1–P_3 and R, triterpene glycosides with two novel types of carbohydrate chains from the sea cucumber *Cladolabes schmeltzii*. Inhibition of cancer cells colony formation and its synergy with radioactive irradiation. *Carb. Res.* **2018**, *468*, 73–79. [CrossRef] [PubMed]
42. Silchenko, A.S.; Kalinovsky, A.I.; Avilov, S.A.; Adnryjaschenko, P.V.; Dmitrenok, P.S.; Kalinin, V.I.; Martyyas, E.A.; Minin, K.V. Fallaxosides C_1, C_2, D_1 and D_2, unusual oligosulfated triterpene glycosides from the sea cucumber *Cucumaria fallax* (Cucumariidae, Dendrochirotida, Holothuroidea) and a taxonomic status of this animal. *Nat. Prod. Commun.* **2016**, *11*, 939–945.
43. Silchenko, A.S.; Kalinovsky, A.I.; Avilov, S.A.; Andryjaschenko, P.V.; Dmitrenok, P.S.; Martyyas, E.A.; Kalinin, V.I. Triterpene glycosides from sea cucumber *Eupentacta fraudatrix*. Structure and biological action of cucumariosides I_1, I_3, I_4, three new minor didulfated pentaosides. *Nat. Prod. Commun.* **2013**, *8*, 1053–1058.
44. Silchenko, A.S.; Avilov, S.A.; Kalinovsky, A.I.; Kalinin, V.I.; Andrijaschenko, P.V.; Dmitrenok, P.S.; Popov, R.S.; Chingizova, E.A.; Kasakin, M.F. Psolusosides C_3 and D_2–D_5, five novel triterpene hexaosides from the sea cucumber *Psolus fabricii* (Psolidae, Dendrochirotida): Chemical structures and bioactivities. *Nat. Prod. Commun.* **2019**, *14*, 7. [CrossRef]
45. Molecular Operating Environment (MOE), 2019.01; Chemical Computing Group ULC, 1010 Sherbooke St. West, Suite #910, Montreal, QC, Canada, H3A 2R7, 2021.
46. Wildman, S.A.; Crippen, G.M. Prediction of Physiochemical Parameters by Atomic Contributions. *J. Chem. Inf. Comput. Sci.* **1999**, *39*, 868–873. [CrossRef]
47. Hall, L.H.; Kier, L.B. The Molecular Connectivity Chi Indices and Kappa Shape Indices in Structure-Property Modeling. *Rev. Comput. Chem.* **1991**, *2*, 367–422. [CrossRef]
48. Moroz, V.V.; Golubev, A.M.; Afanasyev, A.V.; Kuzovlev, A.N.; Sergunova, V.A.; Gudkova, O.E.; Chernysh, A.M. The structure and function of a red blood cell in health and critical conditions. *Gen. Reanimatol.* **2012**, *8*, 52–60. (In Russian) [CrossRef]
49. Lin, F.; Wang, R. Hemolytic mechanism of dioscin proposed by molecular dynamics simulations. *J. Mol. Model* **2010**, *16*, 107–118. [CrossRef] [PubMed]
50. Guan, X.L.; Souza, C.M.; Pichler, H.; Dewhurst, G.; Schaad, O.; Kajiwara, K.; Wakabayashi, H.; Ivanova, T.; Castillon, G.A.; Piccolis, M.; et al. Functional Interactions between Sphingolipids and Sterols in Biological Membranes Regulating Cell Physiology. *Mol. Biol. Cell.* **2009**, *20*, 2083–2095. [CrossRef]
51. Rabinovich, A.L.; Kornilov, V.V.; Balabaev, N.K.; Leermakers, F.A.M.; Filippov, A.V. Properties of unsaturated phospholipid bilayers: Effect of cholesterol. *Biol. Membr.* **2007**, *24*, 490–505. [CrossRef]
52. Lee, J.; Cheng, X.; Swails, J.M.; Yeom, M.S.; Eastman, P.K.; Lemkul, J.A.; Wei, S.; Buckner, J.; Jeong, J.C.; Qi, Y.; et al. CHARMM-GUI input generator for NAMD, GROMACS, AMBER, OpenMM, and CHARMM/OpenMM simulations using the CHARMM36 additive force field. *J. Chem. Theory Comput.* **2016**, *12*, 405–413. [CrossRef]
53. Lee, D.S.; Patel, J.; Ståhle, S.-J.; Park, N.R.; Kern, S.; Kim, J.; Lee, X.; Cheng, M.A.; Valvano, O.; Holst, Y.; et al. Im CHARMM-GUI Membrane Builder for Complex Biological Membrane Simulations with Glycolipids and Lipoglycans. *J. Chem. Theory Comput.* **2019**, *15*, 775–786. [CrossRef]

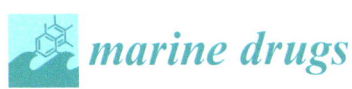

Article

Triterpene Glycosides from the Far Eastern Sea Cucumber *Thyonidium (=Duasmodactyla) kurilensis* (Levin): The Structures, Cytotoxicities, and Biogenesis of Kurilosides A_3, D_1, G, H, I, I_1, J, K, and K_1

Alexandra S. Silchenko, Anatoly I. Kalinovsky, Sergey A. Avilov, Pelageya V. Andrijaschenko, Roman S. Popov, Pavel S. Dmitrenok, Ekaterina A. Chingizova and Vladimir I. Kalinin *

G.B. Elyakov Pacific Institute of Bioorganic Chemistry, Far Eastern Branch of the Russian Academy of Sciences, Pr. 100-letya Vladivostoka 159, 690022 Vladivostok, Russia; silchenko_alexandra_s@piboc.dvo.ru (A.S.S.); kaaniv@piboc.dvo.ru (A.I.K.); avilov_sa@piboc.dvo.ru (S.A.A.); andrijashchenko_pv@piboc.dvo.ru (P.V.A.); popov_rs@piboc.dvo.ru (R.S.P.); paveldmt@piboc.dvo.ru (P.S.D.); chingizova_ea@piboc.dvo.ru (E.A.C.)
* Correspondence: kalininv@piboc.dvo.ru; Tel./Fax: +7-(423)2-31-40-50

Citation: Silchenko, A.S.; Kalinovsky, A.I.; Avilov, S.A.; Andrijaschenko, P.V.; Popov, R.S.; Dmitrenok, P.S.; Chingizova, E.A.; Kalinin, V.I. Triterpene Glycosides from the Far Eastern Sea Cucumber *Thyonidium (=Duasmodactyla) kurilensis* (Levin): The Structures, Cytotoxicities, and Biogenesis of Kurilosides A_3, D_1, G, H, I, I_1, J, K, and K_1. *Mar. Drugs* **2021**, *19*, 187. https://doi.org/10.3390/md19040187

Academic Editors: Vassilios Roussis and Hitoshi Sashiwa

Received: 25 February 2021
Accepted: 24 March 2021
Published: 27 March 2021

Publisher's Note: MDPI stays neutral with regard to jurisdictional claims in published maps and institutional affiliations.

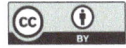

Copyright: © 2021 by the authors. Licensee MDPI, Basel, Switzerland. This article is an open access article distributed under the terms and conditions of the Creative Commons Attribution (CC BY) license (https://creativecommons.org/licenses/by/4.0/).

Abstract: Nine new mono-, di-, and trisulfated triterpene penta- and hexaosides, kurilosides A_3 (**1**), D_1 (**2**), G (**3**), H (**4**), I (**5**), I_1 (**6**), J (**7**), K (**8**), and K_1 (**9**) and two desulfated derivatives, DS-kuriloside L (**10**), having a trisaccharide branched chain, and DS-kuriloside M (**11**), having hexa-*nor*-lanostane aglycone with a 7(8)-double bond, have been isolated from the Far-Eastern deep-water sea cucumber *Thyonidium (=Duasmodactyla) kurilensis* (Levin) and their structures were elucidated based on 2D NMR spectroscopy and HR-ESI mass-spectrometry. Five earlier unknown carbohydrate chains and two aglycones (having a 16β,(20S)-dihydroxy-fragment and a 16β-acetoxy,(20S)-hydroxy fragment) were found in these glycosides. All the glycosides **1**–**9** have a sulfate group at C-6 Glc, attached to C-4 Xyl1, while the positions of the other sulfate groups vary in different groups of kurilosides. The analysis of the structural features of the aglycones and the carbohydrate chains of all the glycosides of *T. kurilensis* showed their biogenetic relationships. Cytotoxic activities of the compounds **1**–**9** against mouse neuroblastoma Neuro 2a, normal epithelial JB-6 cells, and erythrocytes were studied. The highest cytotoxicity in the series was demonstrated by trisulfated hexaoside kuriloside H (**4**), having acetoxy-groups at C(16) and C(20), the latter one obviously compensated the absence of a side chain, essential for the membranolytic action of the glycosides. Kuriloside I_1 (**6**), differing from **4** in the lacking of a terminal glucose residue in the bottom semi-chain, was slightly less active. The compounds **1**–**3**, **5**, and **8** did not demonstrate cytotoxic activity due to the presence of hydroxyl groups in their aglycones.

Keywords: *Thyonidium kurilensis*; triterpene glycosides; kurilosides; sea cucumber; cytotoxic activity

1. Introduction

The investigations of the triterpene glycosides from different species of sea cucumbers have a range of goals. Among them are the drug discoveries based on the promising candidates, demonstrating the target bioactivity [1–6], the solving of some taxonomic problems of the class Holothuroidea based on the specificity of the glycosides having characteristic structural peculiarities for the certain systematic groups [7–10], the ascertaining of biologic and ecologic functions of these metabolites [11–15], and the discovery of novel compounds, especially minor ones, that can be the "hot metabolites" clarifying the biosynthetic pathways of triterpene glycosides [16–18].

As a continuation of our investigation of glycoside composition of the sea cucumber *Thyonidium (=Duasmodactuyla) kurilensis* (Levin), we report herein the isolation and structure elucidation of nine glycosides, kurilosides A_3 (**1**), D_1 (**2**), G (**3**), H (**4**), I (**5**), I_1 (**6**), J (**7**), K (**8**), and K_1 (**9**) as well as two desulfated derivatives, DS-kuriloside L (**10**) and DS-kuriloside

M (**11**). The animals were collected near Onekotan Island in the Sea of Okhotsk. The structures of the compounds **1–11** were established by the analyses of the ^{1}H, ^{13}C NMR, 1D TOCSY, and 2D NMR (^{1}H,^{1}H-COSY, HMBC, HSQC, ROESY) spectra as well as HR-ESI mass spectra. All the original spectra are presented in Figures S1–S85 in the Supplementary Materials. The hemolytic activities against mouse erythrocytes, cytotoxic activities against mouse neuroblastoma Neuro 2a, and normal epithelial JB-6 cells have been reported.

2. Results and Discussion

2.1. Structural Elucidation of the Glycosides

The concentrated ethanolic extract of the sea cucumber *Thyonidium* (=*Duasmodactyla*) *kurilensis* was chromatographed on a Polychrom-1 column (powdered Teflon, Biolar, Latvia). The glycosides were eluted with 50% EtOH and separated by repeated chromatography on Si gel columns using CHCl$_3$/EtOH/H$_2$O (100:100:17) and (100:125:25) as mobile phases to give five fractions (I–V). The glycosides **1–9** (Figure 1) were isolated as a result of subsequent HPLC of the fractions II–V on a reversed-phase semipreparative column Phenomenex Synergi Fusion RP (10 × 250 mm).

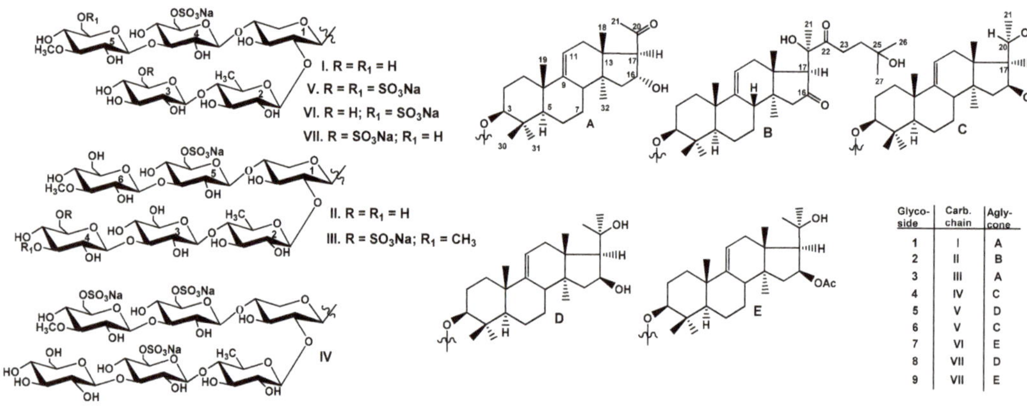

Figure 1. Chemical structures of glycosides isolated from *Thyonidium kurilensis*: **1**—kuriloside A$_3$; **2**—kuriloside D$_1$; **3**—kuriloside G; **4**—kuriloside H; **5**—kuriloside I; **6**—kuriloside I$_1$; **7**—kuriloside J, **8**—kuriloside K, **9**—kuriloside K$_1$.

The molecular formula of kuriloside A$_3$ (**1**) was determined to be C$_{54}$H$_{87}$O$_{29}$SNa from the [M$_{Na}$ − Na]$^-$ ion peak at *m/z* 1231.5063 (calc. 1231.5059) in the (−)HR-ESI-MS. Kuriloside A$_3$ (**1**) as well as the reported earlier kurilosides A, A$_1$, and A$_2$ [19] belong to the same group of glycosides, so these compounds have the identical monosulfated pentasaccharide chains that were confirmed by the coincidence of their ^{1}H and ^{13}C NMR spectra corresponding to the carbohydrate chains (Table S1). The presence of five characteristic doublets at δ_H = 4.64–5.18 (*J* = 7.1–7.6 Hz), and corresponding signals of anomeric carbons at δ_C = 102.3–104.7 in the ^{1}H and ^{13}C NMR spectra of the carbohydrate part of **1** indicate the presence of a pentasaccharide chain and β-configurations of the glycosidic bonds. Monosaccharide composition of **1**, established by the analysis of the ^{1}H,^{1}H-COSY, HSQC, and 1D TOCSY spectra, includes one xylose (Xyl1), one quinovose (Qui2), two glucoses (Glc3 and Glc4), and one 3-O-methylglucose (MeGlc5) residue. The signal of C-6 Glc4 was observed at δ_C = 67.1 due to α-shifting effect of a sulfate group at this position. The positions of interglycosidic linkages were established by the ROESY and HMBC spectra (Table S1). The analysis of NMR spectra of the aglycone part of **1** (Table S2) indicated the presence of 22,23,24,25,26,27-hexa-*nor*-lanostane aglycone with a 16α-hydroxy,20-oxo-fragment and 9(11)-double bond due to the characteristic signals: (δ_C 149.0 (C-9) and 114.2 (C-11), δ_C = 71.1 (C-16) and δ_H = 5.40 (brt, *J* = 7.5 Hz, H-16), δ_C = 208.8 (C-20)). The ROE correlations H-16/H-15β and H-16/H-18 indicated a 16α-OH orientation in the aglycone of kuriloside A$_3$ (**1**). 17αH-orientation, common for the sea cucumber glycosides, was deduced from the ROE-correlation H-17/H-32. The same aglycone was found earlier in kuriloside F [19].

The (−)ESI-MS/MS of **1** demonstrated the fragmentation of [M$_{Na}$ − Na]$^-$ ion at m/z 1231.5. The peaks of fragment ions were observed at m/z 1069.5 [M$_{Na}$ − Na − C$_6$H$_{10}$O$_5$ (Glc)]$^-$, 1055.4 [M$_{Na}$ − Na − C$_7$H$_{12}$O$_5$(MeGlc)]$^-$, 923.4 [M$_{Na}$ − Na − C$_6$H$_{10}$O$_5$(Glc) − C$_6$H$_{10}$O$_4$(Qui)]$^-$, 747.3 [M$_{Na}$ − Na − C$_6$H$_{10}$O$_5$(Glc) − C$_6$H$_{10}$O$_4$(Qui) − C$_7$H$_{12}$O$_5$(MeGlc)]$^-$, 695.1 [M$_{Na}$ −Na − C$_{24}$H$_{37}$O$_3$(Agl) − C$_6$H$_{10}$O$_5$ (Glc) − H]$^-$, 565.1 [M$_{Na}$ − Na − C$_{24}$H$_{37}$O$_2$ (Agl) − C$_6$H$_{10}$O$_5$(Glc) − C$_6$H$_{10}$O$_4$ (Qui) − H]$^-$, 549.1 [M$_{Na}$ − Na − C$_{24}$H$_{37}$O$_3$(Agl) − C$_6$H$_{10}$O$_5$(Glc) − C$_6$H$_{10}$O$_4$(Qui) − H]$^-$, 417.1 [M$_{Na}$ − Na − C$_{24}$H$_{37}$O$_3$(Agl) − C$_6$H$_{10}$O$_5$(Glc) − C$_6$H$_{10}$O$_4$(Qui) − C$_5$H$_8$O$_4$(Xyl) − H]$^-$, 241.0 [M$_{Na}$ − Na − C$_{24}$H$_{37}$O$_3$(Agl) − C$_6$H$_{10}$O$_5$(Glc) − C$_6$H$_{10}$O$_4$(Qui) − C$_5$H$_8$O$_4$(Xyl) − C$_7$H$_{12}$O$_5$(MeGlc) − H]$^-$, corroborating the structure of kuriloside A$_3$ (**1**).

All these data indicate that kuriloside A$_3$ (**1**) is 3β-O-{β-D-glucopyranosyl-(1→4)-β-D-quinovopyranosyl-(1→2)-[3-O-methyl-β-D-glucopyranosyl-(1→3)-6-O-sodium sulfate-β-D-glucopyranosyl-(1→4)]-β-D-xylopyranosyl}-22,23,24,25,26,27-hexa-nor-16α-hydroxy,20-oxo-lanost-9(11)-ene.

The molecular formula of kuriloside D$_1$ (**2**) was determined to be C$_{66}$H$_{107}$O$_{36}$SNa from the [M$_{Na}$ − Na]$^-$ ion peak at m/z 1507.6291 (calc. 1507.6268) in the (−)HR-ESI-MS. The hexasaccharide monosulfated carbohydrate chain of **2** was identical to that of previously reported kuriloside D [19] since their ^{1}H and ^{13}C NMR spectra corresponding to the carbohydrate moieties were coincident (Table S3). Actually, six signals of anomeric doublets at $δ_H$ = 4.70–5.28 (d, J = 7.5–8.2 Hz) and corresponding signals of anomeric carbons at $δ_C$ = 103.7–105.7 indicated the presence of a hexasaccharide chain in kuriloside D$_1$ (**2**). The presence of xylose (Xyl1), quinovose (Qui2), three glucose (Glc3, Glc4, Glc5), and 3-O-methylglucose (MeGlc6) residues were deduced from the analysis of the ^{1}H,^{1}H-COSY, HSQC, and 1D TOCSY spectra of **2**. The positions of the interglycosidic linkages were elucidated based on the ROESY and HMBC correlations (Table S3). The presence in the ^{13}C NMR spectrum of kuriloside D$_1$ (**2**) of the only signal of the O-methyl group at $δ_C$ 60.5 and the upfield shift of the signal of C-3 Glc4 to $δ_C$ 71.5 indicated the presence of a non-methylated terminal Glc4 residue. Analysis of the ^{1}H and ^{13}C NMR spectra of the aglycone part of **2** indicated the presence of a lanostane aglycone (the signals of lactone ring are absent and the signals of methyl group C-18 are observed at $δ_C$ 16.9 and $δ_H$ 1.30 (s, H-18) with normal side chain (30 carbons) and 9(11)-double bond (the signals at $δ_C$ 149.0 (C-9), 114.9 (C-11), and $δ_H$ 5.35 (brd, J = 6.2 Hz; H-11) (Table 1). The comparison of the ^{13}C NMR spectra of **2** and kuriloside D showed their great similarity, except for the signals of the side chain from C-23 to C-27. Two strongly deshielded signals at $δ_C$ 216.3 (C-16) and 217.6 (C-22) corresponded to carbonyl groups, whose positions were established on the base of the HMBC correlations H-15/C-16, H-21/C-22, H-23/C-22, and H-24/C-22. The signals of protons assigned to the methylene group adjacent to 22-oxo group were deshielded to $δ_H$ 3.67 (dd, J = 10.6; 18.2 Hz; H-23a) and 3.43 (dt, J = 7.8; 18.2 Hz; H-23b) and correlated in the ^{1}H,^{1}H-COSY spectrum of **2** with one signal only at $δ_H$ 2.27 (t, J = 7.8 Hz; H-24). These data, along with the deshielded signal of quaternary carbon at $δ_C$ 69.0 (C-25) and the almost coinciding signals of methyl groups C-26 and C-27 ($δ_C$ 30.0 and 29.5, $δ_H$ 1.42 and 1.41, correspondingly), indicated the attachment of the hydroxy-group to C-25. Therefore, the side chain of kuriloside D$_1$ (**2**) is characterized by the 22-oxo-25-hydroxy-fragment (Table 1).

The (−)ESI-MS/MS of **2** demonstrated the fragmentation of [M$_{Na}$ − Na]$^-$ ion at m/z 1507.6. The peaks of fragment ions were observed at m/z 1349.5 [M$_{Na}$ − Na − C$_8$H$_{15}$O$_3$ + H]$^-$, corresponding to the loss of the aglycone fragment from C(20) to C(27), 1187.5 [M$_{Na}$ − Na − C$_8$H$_{15}$O$_3$ − C$_6$H$_{10}$O$_5$(Glc) + H]$^-$, 1025.4 [M$_{Na}$ − Na − C$_8$H$_{15}$O$_3$ − C$_6$H$_{10}$O$_5$(Glc) − C$_6$H$_{10}$O$_5$ (Glc) + H]$^-$, 879.4 [M$_{Na}$ − Na − C$_8$H$_{15}$O$_3$ − C$_6$H$_{10}$O$_5$(Glc) − C$_6$H$_{10}$O$_5$ (Glc) − C$_6$H$_{10}$O$_4$(Qui) + H]$^-$, 565.1 [M$_{Na}$ − Na − C$_{30}$H$_{47}$O$_4$(Agl) − C$_6$H$_{10}$O$_5$(Glc) − C$_6$H$_{10}$O$_5$(Glc) − C$_6$H$_{10}$O$_4$(Qui) − H]$^-$, 417.1 [M$_{Na}$ − Na − C$_{30}$H$_{47}$O$_5$(Agl) − C$_6$H$_{10}$O$_5$(Glc)

− $C_6H_{10}O_5$(Glc) − $C_6H_{10}O_4$(Qui) − $C_5H_8O_4$(Xyl) − H]$^−$, 241.0 [M$_{Na}$ − Na − $C_{30}H_{47}O_5$ (Agl) − $C_6H_{10}O_5$(Glc) − $C_6H_{10}O_5$(Glc) − $C_6H_{10}O_4$(Qui) − $C_5H_8O_4$(Xyl) − $C_7H_{12}O_5$(MeGlc) − H]$^−$, corroborating the structure of kuriloside D$_1$ (2).

All these data indicate that kuriloside D$_1$ (2) is 3β-O-{β-D-glucopyranosyl-(1→3)-β-D-glucopyranosyl-(1→4)-β-D-quinovopyranosyl-(1→2)-[3-O-methyl-β-D-glucopyranosyl-(1→3)-6-O-sodium sulfate-β-D-glucopyranosyl-(1→4)]-β-D-xylopyranosyl}-16,22-dioxo-25-hydroxylanost-9(11)-ene.

Table 1. ^{13}C and ^{1}H NMR chemical shifts, HMBC, and ROESY correlations of the aglycone moiety of kuriloside D$_1$ (1).

Position	δ$_C$ mult. [a]	δ$_H$ mult. (J in Hz) [b]	HMBC	ROESY
1	36.0 CH$_2$	1.77 brd (12.8)		H-11, H-19
		1.39 m		H-3, H-5, H-11
2	26.9 CH$_2$	2.20 m		
		1.94 brdd (11.3; 12.8)		H-19
3	88.4 CH	3.20 dd (3.8; 11.3)	C: 4, 30, 31, C: 1 Xyl1	H-1, H-5, H-31, H-1 Xyl1
4	39.7 C			
5	52.7 CH	0.90 m	C: 6, 19, 30	H-1, H-3, H-7, H-31
6	21.0 CH$_2$	1.69 m		
		1.44 m		H-8, H-19
7	28.2 CH	1.49 m		
		1.28 m		H-5
8	40.2 CH	2.33 m		H-18, H-19
9	149.0 C			
10	39.4 C			
11	114.9 CH	5.36 brd (6.0)	C: 8, 10, 13	H-1
12	36.5 CH$_2$	2.43 brd (16.5)		H-17, H-32
		2.20 brdd (6.0; 16.5)	C: 9, 11, 14	H-18, H-21
13	43.7 C			
14	41.9 C			
15	48.1 CH$_2$	2.27 d (16.3)	C: 14, 16, 32	
		2.03 d (18.0)	C: 13, 16, 32	H-7, H-32
16	216.3 C			
17	63.8 CH	3.69 s	C: 22	H-12, H-21, H-32
18	16.9 CH$_3$	1.30 s	C: 17	H-8, H-12, H-15, H-19, H-21
19	22.2 CH$_3$	1.12 s	C: 1, 5, 9, 10	H-1, H-2, H-6, H-8
20	80.8 C			
21	24.7 CH$_3$	1.61 s	C: 17, 20, 22	H-12, H-17, H-18, H-23
22	217.6 C			
23	32.2 CH$_2$	3.67 dd (10.6; 18.2)	C: 22, 24	H-26, H-27
		3.43 dt (7.8; 18.2)	C: 22, 24	H-21, H-26, H-27
24	38.0 CH$_2$	2.27 t (7.8)	C: 22, 23, 25, 26, 27	
25	69.0 C			
26	30.0 CH$_3$	1.42 s	C: 24, 25, 27	H-23, H-24, H-27
27	29.5 CH$_3$	1.41 s	C: 24, 25, 26	H-23, H-24, H-26
30	16.5 CH$_3$	1.06 s	C: 3, 4, 5, 31	H-2, H-6, H-31
31	27.9 CH$_3$	1.26 s	C: 3, 4, 5, 30	H-3, H-5, H-6, H-30, H-1 Xyl1
32	18.6 CH$_3$	0.89 s	C: 8, 13, 14, 15	H-7, H-12, H-15, H-17

[a] Recorded at 176.03 MHz in C_5D_5N/D_2O (4/1). [b] Recorded at 700.00 MHz in C_5D_5N/D_2O (4/1).

The molecular formula of kuriloside G (3) was determined to be $C_{61}H_{98}O_{37}S_2Na_2$ from the [M$_{2Na}$ − Na]$^−$ ion peak at m/z 1509.5102 (calc. 1509.5132) and the [M$_{2Na}$ − 2Na]$^{2−}$ ion-peak at m/z 743.2624 (calc. 743.2626) in the (−)HR-ESI-MS. In the ^{1}H and ^{13}C NMR spectra of the carbohydrate part of kuriloside G (3), six characteristic doublets at δ$_H$ 4.65–5.19 (J = 7.0–8.1 Hz) and signals of anomeric carbons at δ$_C$ 102.1–104.8, correlated with each anomeric proton by the HSQC spectrum, were indicative of a hexasaccharide chain and β-configurations of glycosidic bonds (Table 2). The signals of each monosaccharide unit were found as an isolated spin system based on the ^{1}H,^{1}H-COSY, and 1D TOCSY spectra of 3. Further analysis of the HSQC and ROESY spectra resulted in the assigning of the monosaccharide residues as one xylose (Xyl1), one quinovose (Qui2), two glucoses (Glc3 and Glc5), and two 3-*O*-methylglucose (MeGlc4 and MeGlc6) residues.

Table 2. ^{13}C and ^{1}H NMR chemical shifts, HMBC, and ROESY correlations of carbohydrate moiety of kuriloside G (**3**).

Atom	δ_C mult.[a,b,c]	δ_H mult. (*J* in Hz)[d]	HMBC	ROESY
Xyl1 (1→C-3)				
1	104.7 CH	4.65 d (7.8)	C: 3	H-3; H-3, 5 Xyl1
2	**82.2** CH	3.95 t (8.8)	C: 1 Qui2	H-1 Qui2; H-4 Xyl1
3	75.1 CH	4.15 t (8.8)	C: 4 Xyl1	H-5 Xyl1
4	**77.6** CH	4.15 m		H-1 Glc5
5	63.5 CH$_2$	4.36 dd (5.4; 10.8)		
		3.61 m		H-1 Xyl1
Qui2 (1→2Xyl1)				
1	104.4 CH	5.03 d (7.8)	C: 2 Xyl1	H-2 Xyl1; H-3, 5 Qui2
2	75.2 CH	3.89 t (7.8)	C: 3 Qui2	
3	75.2 CH	3.99 t (9.3)	C: 4 Qui2	
4	**86.4** CH	3.56 t (9.3)	C: 1 Glc3	H-1 Glc3; H-2 Qui2
5	71.4 CH	3.69 dd (6.2; 9.3)		H-1 Qui2
6	17.9 CH$_3$	1.64 d (6.2)	C: 4, 5 Qui2	
Glc3 (1→4Qui2)				
1	104.0 CH	4.85 d (8.1)	C: 4 Qui2	H-4 Qui2; H-3, 5 Glc3
2	73.5 CH	3.90 t (8.1)		
3	**87.5** CH	4.12 t (8.1)	C: 4 Glc3	H-1 MeGlc4; H-1, 5 Glc3
4	69.3 CH	3.84 t (8.1)	C: 5 Glc3	
5	77.5 CH	3.90 t (8.1)		
6	61.6 CH$_2$	4.34 d (11.6)		
		4.03 dd (7.0; 11.6)		
MeGlc4 (1→3Glc3)				
1	104.8 CH	5.12 d (8.1)	C: 3 Glc3	H-3 Glc3; H-3, 5 MeGlc4
2	74.5 CH	3.79 t (8.1)		
3	86.3 CH	3.65 t (8.1)	C: 4 MeGlc4; OMe	H-1 MeGlc4
4	69.9 CH	3.98 t (8.1)	C: 3, 5 MeGlc4	
5	75.5 CH	4.04 t (8.1)		H-1 MeGlc4
6	*67.0* CH$_2$	4.97 d (11.6)		
		4.73 dd (4.7; 11.6)		
OMe	60.5 CH$_3$	3.76 s	C: 3 MeGlc4	
Glc5 (1→4Xyl1)				
1	102.1 CH	4.87 d (7.0)	C: 4 Xyl1	H-4 Xyl1; H-3, 5 Glc5
2	73.2 CH	3.84 t (8.1)	C: 1, 3 Glc5	
3	**85.9** CH	4.16 t (8.1)	C: 1 MeGlc6; C: 2, 4 Glc5	H-1 MeGlc6; H-1 Glc5
4	69.2 CH	3.91 t (9.3)	C: 5 Glc5	H-6 Glc5
5	75.5 CH	4.02 m		H-1 Glc5
6	*67.1* CH$_2$	4.93 d (11.6)		
		4.69 dd (5.8; 11.6)	C: 5 Glc5	
MeGlc6 (1→3Glc5)				
1	104.4 CH	5.19 d (8.1)	C: 3 Glc5	H-3 Glc5; H-3, 5 MeGlc6
2	74.3 CH	3.84 t (8.1)		
3	86.9 CH	3.66 t (8.1)	OMe	H-1 MeGlc6
4	70.2 CH	3.89 t (8.1)	C: 5 MeGlc6	
5	77.5 CH	3.90 t (8.1)		H-1 MeGlc6
6	61.7 CH$_2$	4.34 d (11.6)		
		4.06 dd (5.8; 11.6)		
OMe	60.5 CH$_3$	3.80 s	C: 3 MeGlc6	

[a] Recorded at 176.03 MHz in C$_5$D$_5$N/D$_2$O (4/1). [b] Bold = interglycosidic positions. [c] Italic = sulfate position. [d] Recorded at 700.00 MHz in C$_5$D$_5$N/D$_2$O (4/1). Multiplicity by 1D TOCSY.

The positions of interglycosidic linkages were established by the ROESY and HMBC spectra of **3** (Table 2) where the cross-peaks between H-1 Xyl1 and H-3 (C-3) of an aglycone,

H-1 Qui2 and H-2 (C-2) Xyl1; H-1 Glc3 and H-4 (C-4) Qui2; H-1 MeGlc4 and H-3 Glc3; H-1 Glc5 and H-4 Xyl1; H-1 MeGlc6 and H-3 (C-3) Glc5 were observed.

The signals of C-6 MeGlc4 and C-6 Glc5 in the ^{13}C NMR spectrum of **3** were observed at δ_C 67.0 and δ_C 67.1, correspondingly, due to α-shifting effects of the sulfate groups at these positions. Thus, the hexasaccharide disulfated chain of kuriloside G (**3**) was first found in the sea cucumber glycosides. The NMR spectra of the aglycone part of **3** coincided with that of kuriloside A$_3$ (**1**), indicating the identity of these aglycones (Table S2).

The (−)ESI-MS/MS of **3** demonstrated the fragmentation of [M$_{2Na}$ − Na]$^-$ ion at *m/z* 1509.5. The peaks of fragment ions were observed at *m/z* 1389.6 [M$_{2Na}$ − Na − NaHSO$_4$]$^-$, 1333.5 [M$_{2Na}$ − Na − C$_7$H$_{12}$O$_5$(MeGlc)]$^-$, 1231.5 [M$_{2Na}$ − Na − C$_7$H$_{11}$O$_8$SNa(MeGlcSO$_3$Na)]$^-$, 1069.4 [M$_{2Na}$ − Na − C$_7$H$_{11}$O$_8$SNa(MeGlcSO$_3$Na) − C$_6$H$_{10}$O$_5$(Glc)]$^-$, 923.4 [M$_{2Na}$ − Na − C$_7$H$_{11}$O$_8$SNa(MeGlcSO$_3$Na) − C$_6$H$_{10}$O$_5$(Glc)] − C$_6$H$_{10}$O$_4$(Qui)]$^-$.

All these data indicate that kuriloside G (**3**) is 3β-*O*-{6-*O*-sodium sulfate-3-*O*-methyl-β-D-glucopyranosyl-(1→3)-β-D-glucopyranosyl-(1→4)-β-D-quinovopyranosyl-(1→2)-[3-*O*-methyl-β-D-glucopyranosyl-(1→3)-6-*O*-sodium sulfate-β-D-glucopyranosyl-(1→4)]-β-D-xylopyranosyl}-22,23,24,25,26,27-hexa-*nor*-16α-hydroxy,20-oxo-lanost-9(11)-ene.

The molecular formula of kuriloside H (**4**) was determined to be C$_{64}$H$_{101}$O$_{42}$S$_3$Na$_3$ from the [M$_{3Na}$ − Na]$^-$ ion peak at *m/z* 1683.4701 (calc. 1683.4730), [M$_{3Na}$ − 2Na]$^{2-}$ ion peak at *m/z* 830.2425 (calc. 830.2419), and [M$_{3Na}$ − 3Na]$^{3-}$ ion peak at *m/z* 545.8332 (calc. 545.8315) in the (−)HR-ESI-MS. The presence of three-charged ions in the (−)HR-ESI-MS of kuriloside H (**4**) was indicative for the trisulfated glycoside.

The ^{1}H and ^{13}C NMR spectra corresponding to the carbohydrate chain of kuriloside H (**4**) (Table 3) demonstrated six signals of anomeric protons at δ_H 4.63–5.21 (d, *J* = 7.1–8.6 Hz) and the signals of anomeric carbons at δ_C 102.8–104.7 deduced by the HSQC spectrum, indicative of hexasaccharide moiety with β-glycosidic bonds. The signals of each sugar residue were assigned by the analysis of the ^{1}H,^{1}H-COSY, 1D TOCSY, ROESY, and HSQC spectra, enabling the identification of monosaccharide units in the chain of **4** as one xylose (Xyl1), one quinovose (Qui2), three glucoses (Glc3, Glc4 and Glc5), and one 3-*O*-methylglucose (MeGlc6). Therefore, the monosaccharide composition of **4** was the same as in kuriloside D$_1$ (**2**).

However, in the ^{13}C NMR spectrum of **4** three signals at δ_C 67.6 (C-6 Glc3), 67.4 (C-6 Glc5), and 67.0 (C-6 MeGlc6), characteristic for sulfated by C-6 hexose units, were observed instead of one signal at δ_C 67.0 (C-6 Glc5) in the spectrum of **2**. The signal of the OMe-group observed at δ_C 60.4 indicated one terminal monosaccharide residue was methylated. Actually, the protons of the OMe-group (δ_H 3.75, s) correlated in the HMBC spectrum with C-3 MeGlc6 (δ_C 86.1), which was, in turn, attached to C-3 Glc5 (ROE-correlation H-1 MeGlc6 (δ_H 5.13 (d, *J* = 7.4 Hz)/H-3 Glc5 (δ_H 4.13 (t, *J* = 8.6 Hz)). At the same time, the fourth (another terminal) monosaccharide unit was glucose (the signal of C-3 Glc4 was shielded to δ_C 77.7 due to the absence of *O*-methylation). The positions of all interglycosidic linkages were elucidated based on the ROESY and HMBC correlations (Table 3).

Hence, kuriloside H (**4**) has a hexasaccharide chain with a non-methylated terminal Glc4 residue and three sulfate groups. This carbohydrate chain is first found in the glycosides of the sea cucumbers and kuriloside H (**4**) is the most polar glycoside discovered so far as well as two tetrasulfated pentaosides isolated from *Psolus fabricii* [20].

The analysis of the ^{13}C NMR spectrum of the aglycone part of **4** demonstrated its identity to the aglycone of kurilosides A$_1$ and C$_1$, isolated earlier [19]. Therefore, kuriloside H (**4**) contains a 22,23,24,25,26,27-hexa-*nor*-lanostane aglycone with 9(11)-double bond and acetoxy-groups at C-16 and C-20. β-orientation of the acetoxy group at C-16 and (20*S*)-configuration were established on the base of coincidence of the coupling constants ($J_{16/17}$ = 7.7 Hz and $J_{17/20}$ = 10.6 Hz), observed in the ^{1}H NMR spectra of **4** and kuriloside A$_1$, and confirmed by the ROE-correlation H-16/H-32 in the spectrum of **4** (Table S4).

Table 3. ^{13}C and ^{1}H NMR chemical shifts, HMBC, and ROESY correlations of carbohydrate moiety of kuriloside H (**4**).

Atom	δ_C mult. [a,b,c]	δ_H mult. (J in Hz) [d]	HMBC	ROESY
Xyl1 (1→C-3)				
1	104.7 CH	4.63 d (8.3)	C: 3	H-3; H-3, 5 Xyl1
2	**82.6** CH	3.83 t (7.1)	C: 1 Qui2	H-1 Qui2; H-4 Xyl1
3	75.1 CH	4.05 m	C: 4 Xyl1	H-1, 5 Xyl1
4	**79.4** CH	4.04 m		H-1 Glc5
5	63.5 CH$_2$	4.34 brd (10.1)	C: 3 Xyl1	
		3.59 m		H-1 Xyl1
Qui2 (1→2Xyl1)				
1	104.5 CH	4.88 d (7.1)	C: 2 Xyl1	H-2 Xyl1; H-3, 5 Qui2
2	75.4 CH	3.88 t (8.9)	C: 1, 3 Qui2	H-4 Qui2
3	74.9 CH	3.98 t (8.9)		H-1, 5 Qui2
4	**86.5** CH	3.35 t (8.9)	C: 1 Glc3	H-1 Glc3; H-2 Qui2
5	71.4 CH	3.63 dd (5.9; 8.9)		H-1, 3 Qui2
6	17.6 CH$_3$	1.58 d (5.8)	C: 4, 5 Qui2	
Glc3 (1→4Qui2)				
1	104.1 CH	4.72 d (8.5)	C: 4 Qui2	H-4 Qui2; H-3, 5 Glc3
2	73.4 CH	3.83 t (8.5)		
3	**86.3** CH	4.18 t (8.5)	C: 1 Glc4; C: 2, 4 Glc3	H-1 Glc4; H-1, 5 Glc3
4	69.3 CH	3.76 t (8.5)	C: 5, 6 Glc3	
5	74.7 CH	4.10 m	C: 4 Glc3	H-1 Glc3
6	67.6 CH$_2$	4.96 d (11.0)		
		4.57 d (11.0)		
Glc4 (1→3Glc3)				
1	104.5 CH	5.21 d (8.5)	C: 3 Glc3	H-3 Glc3; H-3, 5 Glc4
2	74.7 CH	3.93 t (8.5)	C: 1, 3 Glc4	
3	77.7 CH	4.11 t (8.5)	C: 4 MeGlc4	H-1, 5 Glc4
4	71.0 CH	3.94 t (8.5)		
5	77.7 CH	3.89 m		H-1 Glc4
6	61.9 CH$_2$	4.37 d (12.3)		
		4.06 dd (6.2; 12.3)		
Glc5 (1→4Xyl1)				
1	102.8 CH	4.85 d (8.6)	C: 4 Xyl1	H-4 Xyl1; H-3, 5 Glc5
2	73.2 CH	3.83 t (8.6)	C: 1, 3 Glc5	
3	**86.3** CH	4.13 t (8.6)	C: 1 MeGlc6; C: 2 Glc5	H-1 MeGlc6; H-1 Glc5
4	69.2 CH	3.76 t (8.6)		H-6 Glc5
5	77.2 CH	4.09 t (8.6)		H-1 Glc5
6	67.4 CH$_2$	4.96 d (11.1)		
		4.56 d (11.1)		H-4 Glc5
MeGlc6 (1→3Glc5)				
1	104.4 CH	5.13 d (7.4)	C: 3 Glc5	H-3 Glc5; H-3, 5 MeGlc6
2	74.3 CH	3.78 t (7.4)	C: 1 MeGlc6	H-4 MeGlc6
3	86.1 CH	3.63 t (8.6)	C: 4 MeGlc6; OMe	H-1, 5 MeGlc6; OMe
4	69.8 CH	4.00 t (8.6)	C: 3, 5 MeGlc6	
5	75.6 CH	4.00 m		H-1, 3 MeGlc6
6	67.0 CH$_2$	4.93 d (9.9)		
		4.75 dd (3.7; 11.1)		H-4 MeGlc6
OMe	60.4 CH$_3$	3.75 s	C: 3 MeGlc6	

[a] Recorded at 176.04 MHz in C$_5$D$_5$N/D$_2$O (4/1). [b] Bold = interglycosidic positions. [c] Italic = sulfate position. [d] Recorded at 700.13 MHz in C$_5$D$_5$N/D$_2$O (4/1). Multiplicity by 1D TOCSY.

The (−)ESI-MS/MS of kuriloside H (**4**) demonstrated the fragmentation of the [M$_{3Na}$ − Na]$^−$ ion at *m/z* 1683.5. The peaks of fragment ions were observed at *m/z* 1503.5 [M$_{3Na}$ − Na − CH$_3$COOH − NaHSO$_4$]$^−$, 1443.5 [M$_{3Na}$ − Na − 2CH$_3$COOH − NaHSO$_4$]$^−$, 1281.4 [M$_{3Na}$ − Na − 2CH$_3$COOH − NaHSO$_4$ − C$_6$H$_{10}$O$_5$(Glc)]$^−$, 1165.4 [M$_{3Na}$ − Na − 2CH$_3$COOH − NaHSO$_4$ − C$_7$H$_{11}$O$_8$SNa(MeGlcOSO$_3$)]$^−$, and 1003.4 [M$_{3Na}$ − Na − 2CH$_3$COOH − NaHSO$_4$ − C$_7$H$_{11}$O$_8$SNa(MeGlcOSO$_3$) − C$_6$H$_{10}$O$_5$(Glc)]$^−$, corroborating its carbohydrate chain structure.

All these data indicate that kuriloside H (**4**) is 3β-*O*-{β-D-glucopyranosyl-(1→3)-6-*O*-sodium sulfate-β-D-glucopyranosyl-(1→4)-β-D-quinovopyranosyl-(1→2)-[6-*O*-sodium sulfate-3-*O*-methyl-β-D-glucopyranosyl-(1→3)-6-*O*-sodium sulfate-β-D-glucopyranosyl-(1→4)]-β-D-xylopyranosyl}-22,23,24,25,26,27-hexa-*nor*-16β,(20*S*)-diacetoxy-lanost-9(11)-ene.

The molecular formula of kuriloside I (**5**) was determined to be $C_{54}H_{87}O_{35}S_3Na_3$ from the $[M_{3Na} - Na]^-$ ion peak at *m/z* 1437.3952 (calc. 1437.3991), $[M_{3Na} - 2Na]^{2-}$ ion peak at *m/z* 707.2049 (calc. 707.2049), and $[M_{3Na} - 3Na]^{3-}$ ion peak at *m/z* 463.8076 (calc. 463.8069) in the (−)HR-ESI-MS, indicating the presence of three sulfate groups. The ^{1}H and ^{13}C NMR spectra corresponding to the carbohydrate part of kuriloside I (**5**) (Table 4) demonstrated five characteristic doublets at δ_H 4.63–5.13 (d, *J* = 6.6–7.8 Hz) and corresponding signals of anomeric carbons at δ_C 102.4–104.7 deduced by the HSQC spectrum, which indicated the presence of five monosaccharide residues in the carbohydrate chain of **5**. The signals at δ_C 67.0, 67.6, and 67.7 indicated the presence of three sulfate groups as in the carbohydrate chain of kuriloside H (**4**). Indeed, the comparison of the ^{13}C NMR spectra of kurilosides I (**5**) and H (**4**) showed that they differed by the absence in the spectrum of **5** of the signals corresponding to non-sulfated terminal glucose residue attached to C-3 Glc3 in the carbohydrate chain of **4**. The signal of C-3 Glc3 in the ^{13}C NMR spectrum of **5** was observed at δ_C 76.9 (instead of δ_C 86.3 in the spectrum of **4**), demonstrating the absence of a glycosylation effect. The presence of xylose (Xyl1), quinovose (Qui2), two glucose (Glc3, Glc4), and one 3-*O*-methylglucose (MeGlc5) residue was deduced from the analysis of the ^{1}H,^{1}H-COSY, HSQC and 1D TOCSY spectra of **5**. The positions of interglycosidic linkages were elucidated based on the ROESY and HMBC correlations (Table 4) and indicated the presence of the branched at the C-4 Xyl1 pentasaccharide chain in **5**, with the same architecture as in the other pentaosides of *T. kurilensis*. Thus, kuriloside I (**5**) contains a new pentasaccharide branched trisulfated chain.

The analysis of the ^{13}C and ^{1}H NMR spectra of the aglycone part of **5** indicated the presence of 22,23,24,25,26,27-hexa-*nor*-lanostane aglycone having a 9(11)-double bond (Table 5). The signals of methine group CH-16 were observed at c δ_C 72.8 (C-16) and at δ_H 4.82 (dd, *J* = 7.1; 14.9 Hz, H-16) due to the attachment of the hydroxyl group to this position. The HMBC correlations H-15/C-16 and H-20/C-16 confirmed this. The signals of C-20 and H-20 were shielded to δ_C 66.5 and δ_H 4.38 (dd, *J* = 6.0; 9.5 Hz), correspondingly, when compared with the same signals in the spectra of kuriloside H (**4**) (δ_{C-20} 69.4, δ_{H-20} 5.46 (dd, *J* = 6.1; 10.6 Hz)), containing (20*S*)-acetoxy-group. Hence, it was supposed that the attachment of the hydroxyl group to C-20 was in the aglycone of kuriloside I (**5**) instead of the acetoxy group in the aglycone of kuriloside H (**4**).

The ROE-correlations H-16/H-17 and H-16/H-32 indicated a 16β-OH orientation in the aglycone of kuriloside I (**5**). (20*S*)-configuration in **5** was determined on the base of the closeness of the coupling constant $J_{20/17}$ = 9.5 Hz to those in the spectra of kurilosides A_1, C_1 [19], and H (**4**) and corroborated by the observed ROE-correlations H-17/H-21, H-20/H-18 and biogenetic background. Hence, kuriloside I (**5**) has an aglycone with a 16β,(20*S*)-dihydroxy-fragment that is unique in marine glycosides.

The (−)ESI-MS/MS of kuriloside I (**5**) demonstrated the fragmentation of the $[M_{3Na} - Na]^-$ ion at *m/z* 1437.5. The peaks of fragment ions were observed at *m/z* 1317.4 $[M_{3Na} - Na - NaHSO_4]^-$, 1197.4 $[M_{3Na} - Na - 2NaHSO_4]^-$, 1173.4 $[M_{3Na} - Na - C_6H_9O_8SNa(GlcOSO_3)]^-$, 1039.4 $[M_{3Na} - Na - NaHSO_4 - C_7H_{11}O_8SNa(MeGlcOSO_3)]^-$, 1027.3 $[M_{3Na} - Na - C_6H_9O_8SNa(GlcOSO_3) - C_6H_{10}O_4(Qui)]^-$, 907.3 $[M_{3Na} - Na - NaHSO_4 - C_6H_9O_8SNa(GlcOSO_3) - C_6H_{10}O_4(Qui)]^-$, 895.4 $[M_{3Na} - Na - C_6H_9O_8SNa(GlcOSO_3) - C_7H_{11}O_8SNa(MeGlcOSO_3)]^-$, 667.4 $[M_{3Na} - Na - C_{24}H_{39}O_2(Agl) - C_6H_9O_8SNa(GlcOSO_3) - C_6H_{10}O_4(Qui) - H]^-$, 519.0 $[M_{3Na} - Na - C_{24}H_{39}O_3(Agl) - C_6H_9O_8SNa(GlcOSO_3) - C_6H_{10}O_4(Qui) - C_5H_8O_4(Xyl) - H]^-$, and 417.1 $[M_{3Na} - Na - C_{24}H_{39}O_3(Agl) - C_6H_9O_8SNa(GlcOSO_3) - C_6H_{10}O_4(Qui) - C_5H_8O_4(Xyl) - NaHSO_3]^-$, corroborating the structure of the glycoside.

Table 4. ^{13}C and ^{1}H NMR chemical shifts, HMBC, and ROESY correlations of carbohydrate moiety of kurilosides I (**5**) and I$_1$ (**6**).

Atom	δ_C mult. [a,b,c]	δ_H mult. (J in Hz) [d]	HMBC	ROESY
Xyl1 (1→C-3)				
1	104.7 CH	4.63 d (6.6)	C: 3	H-3; H-3, 5 Xyl1
2	**82.1** CH	3.90 t (6.6)	C: 1 Qui2	H-1 Qui2
3	75.1 CH	4.10 t (6.6)	C: 4 Xyl1	
4	**78.5** CH	4.10 t (6.6)		H-1 Glc4
5	63.4 CH$_2$	4.34 dd (9.6; 11.7)	C: 3 Xyl1	
		3.59 t (11.2)		H-1 Xyl1
Qui2 (1→2Xyl1)				
1	104.4 CH	4.96 d (7.1)	C: 2 Xyl1	H-2 Xyl1; H-5 Qui2
2	75.4 CH	3.84 t (8.3)	C: 1, 3 Qui2	H-4 Qui2
3	74.9 CH	3.93 t (8.3)	C: 2, 4 Qui2	H-1, 5 Qui2
4	**87.0** CH	3.36 t (8.3)	C: 1 Glc3; C: 5, 6 Qui2	H-1 Glc3
5	71.3 CH	3.65 dd (5.9; 9.5)	C: 6 Qui2	H-1, 3 Qui2
6	17.7 CH$_3$	1.59 d (5.9)	C: 4, 5 Qui2	
Glc3 (1→4Qui2)				
1	104.7 CH	4.69 d (7.8)	C: 4 Qui2	H-4 Qui2; H-5 Glc3
2	74.1 CH	3.80 t (8.6)	C: 1, 3 Glc3	
3	76.9 CH	4.11 t (8.6)	C: 2, 4 Glc3	
4	70.8 CH	3.89 t (8.6)	C: 3, 5, 6 Glc3	H-2, 6 Glc3
5	75.5 CH	4.09 t (8.6)		
6	*67.6* CH$_2$	5.05 brd (9.5)		
		4.64 dd (7.8; 12.1)	C: 5 Glc3	
Glc4 (1→4Xyl1)				
1	102.4 CH	4.85 d (7.8)	C: 4 Xyl1	H-4 Xyl1; H-5 Glc4
2	73.1 CH	3.82 t (8.6)	C: 1 Glc4	
3	**86.3** CH	4.12 t (8.6)	C: 1 MeGlc5; C: 4 Glc4	H-1 MeGlc5
4	69.2 CH	3.81 t (8.6)	C: 3, 5, 6 Glc4	
5	74.9 CH	4.06 t (8.6)		H-1 Glc4
6	*67.4* CH$_2$	4.95 d (10.3)		
		4.61 dd (5.2; 10.3)		
MeGlc5 (1→3Glc4)				
1	104.5 CH	5.13 d (7.8)	C: 3 Glc4	H-3 Glc4; H-3, 5 MeGlc5
2	74.2 CH	3.77 t (8.6)	C: 1, 3 MeGlc5	H-4 MeGlc5
3	86.3 CH	3.62 t (8.6)	C: 2, 4 MeGlc5; OMe	H-1, 5 MeGlc5; OMe
4	69.8 CH	4.00 t (8.6)	C: 3, 5 MeGlc5	H-2, 6 MeGlc5
5	75.4 CH	4.01 t (8.6)		H-1 MeGlc5
6	*67.0* CH$_2$	4.92 d (10.3)	C: 4, 5 MeGlc5	
		4.74 dd (3.5; 10.3)	C: 5 MeGlc5	
OMe	60.4 CH$_3$	3.75 s	C: 3 MeGlc5	

[a] Recorded at 176.04 MHz in C$_5$D$_5$N/D$_2$O (4/1). [b] Bold = interglycosidic positions. [c] Italic = sulfate position. [d] Recorded at 700.13 MHz in C$_5$D$_5$N/D$_2$O (4/1). Multiplicity by 1D TOCSY.

All these data indicate that kuriloside I (**5**) is 3β-O-{6-O-sodium sulfate-β-D-glucopyranosyl-(1→4)-β-D-quinovopyranosyl-(1→2)-[6-O-sodium sulfate-3-O-methyl-β-D-glucopyranosyl-(1→3)-6-O-sodium sulfate-β-D-glucopyranosyl-(1→4)]-β-D-xylopyranosyl}-22,23,24,25,26,27-hexa-nor-16β,(20S)-dihydroxy-lanost-9(11)-ene.

The molecular formula of kuriloside I$_1$ (**6**) was determined to be C$_{58}$H$_{91}$O$_{37}$S$_3$Na$_3$ from the [M$_{3Na}$ − 2Na]$^{2-}$ ion peak at *m/z* 749.2148 (calc. 747.2155) and [M$_{3Na}$ − 3Na]$^{3-}$ ion peak at *m/z* 491.8146 (calc. 491.8139) in the (−)HR-ESI-MS. Kuriloside I$_1$ (**6**) as well as kuriloside I (**5**) belong to one group because they have identical trisulfated pentasaccharide chains and, therefore, parts of the ^{1}H and ^{13}C NMR spectra corresponding to the carbohydrate chains are coincident (Table 4). 22,23,24,25,26,27-hexa-*nor*-lanostane aglycone of kuriloside I$_1$ (**6**) is identical to that of kurilosides H (**4**), A$_1$ and C$_1$ [19] (Table S4) and characterized by the presence of 16β,(20S)-diacetoxy-fragment.

Table 5. ^{13}C and ^{1}H NMR chemical shifts, HMBC, and ROESY correlations of the aglycone moiety of kurilosides I (5) and K (8).

Position	δ_C mult. ^{a}	δ_H mult. (J in Hz) ^{b}	HMBC	ROESY
1	36.2 CH$_2$	1.67 m		H-11, H-30
		1.28 m		H-3, H-11
2	26.8 CH$_2$	2.07 m		
		1.83 brd (11.3)		H-19, H-30
3	88.7 CH	3.09 dd (4.2; 11.3)	C: 31, C: 1 Xyl1	H-5, H-31, H1-Xyl1
4	39.6 C			
5	52.8 CH	0.75 brd (12.5)	C: 6, 7, 30	H-3, H-7, H-31
6	21.1 CH$_2$	1.56 m		H-31
		1.28 dt (2.4; 12.5)		H-8, H-30
7	28.0 CH$_2$	1.52 m		
		1.17 m		H-5, H-32
8	41.2 CH	2.14 m		H-18, H-19
9	148.6 C			
10	39.1 C			
11	114.3 CH	5.15 brd (6.0)	C: 10, 12, 14	H-1
12	36.4 CH$_2$	1.98 brdd (3.0; 16.7)		H-32
		1.68 brd (16.7)	C: 9, 11	H-8, H-18, H-21
13	45.1 C			
14	43.2 C			
15	45.0 CH$_2$	2.07 dd (7.8; 12.5)	C: 14, 17, 32	H-32
		1.70 d (6.0; 12.5)	C: 13, 14, 16, 32	
16	72.8 CH	4.82 dd (7.1; 14.9)	C: 14	H-17, H-32
17	57.2 CH	2.11 m	C: 14, 18, 20, 21	H-21, H-32
18	16.0 CH$_3$	0.86 s	C: 12, 14, 15, 17	H-8, H-12, H-20, H-21
19	22.2 CH$_3$	0.97 s	C: 1, 5, 9, 10	H-1, H-2, H-8, H-18
20	66.5 CH	4.38 dd (6.0; 9.5)	C: 16, 17	H-18, H-21
21	22.7 CH$_3$	1.40 d (6.0)	C: 17, 20	H-12, H-17, H-18, H-20
30	16.5 CH$_3$	0.96 s	C: 3, 4, 5, 31	H-2, H-6, H-31, H-6 Qui2
31	27.9 CH$_3$	1.12 s	C: 3, 4, 5, 30	H-3, H-5, H-6, H-30, H-1 Xyl1
32	18.8 CH$_3$	0.67 s	C: 8, 13, 14, 15	H-7, H-15, H-17

^{a} Recorded at 176.03 MHz in C$_5$D$_5$N/D$_2$O (4/1). ^{b} Recorded at 700.00 MHz in C$_5$D$_5$N/D$_2$O (4/1).

The (−)ESI-MS/MS of **6** demonstrated the fragmentation of the [M$_{3Na}$ − Na]$^-$ ion at m/z 1521.4 and [M$_{3Na}$ − 2Na]$^{2-}$ ion at m/z 749.2. The peaks of fragment ions were observed at m/z: 1281.4 [M$_{3Na}$ − Na − 2CH$_3$COOH − NaHSO$_4$]$^-$, 1197.4 [M$_{3Na}$ − Na − CH$_3$COOH − C$_6$H$_9$O$_8$SNa(GlcOSO$_3$)]$^-$, 1137.4 [M$_{3Na}$ − Na − 2CH$_3$COOH − C$_6$H$_9$O$_8$SNa(GlcOSO$_3$)]$^-$, 859.4 [M$_{3Na}$ − Na − 2CH$_3$COOH − C$_6$H$_9$O$_8$SNa(GlcOSO$_3$) − C$_7$H$_{11}$O$_8$SNa(MeGlcOSO$_3$)]$^-$, 719.2 [M$_{3Na}$ − 2Na − CH$_3$COOH]$^{2-}$, 629.2 [M$_{3Na}$ − 2Na − NaHSO$_4$]$^{2-}$, and 557.2 [M$_{3Na}$ − 2Na − 2CH$_3$COOH − C$_6$H$_9$O$_8$SNa(GlcOSO$_3$)]$^{2-}$, which confirmed its structure, established by the NMR data.

All these data indicate that kuriloside I$_1$ (**6**) is 3β-O-{6-O-sodium sulfate-β-D-glucopyranosyl-(1→4)-β-D-quinovopyranosyl-(1→2)-[6-O-sodium sulfate-3-O-methyl-β-D-glucopyranosyl-(1→3)-6-O-sodium sulfate-β-D-glucopyranosyl-(1→4)]-β-D-xylopyranosyl}-22,23,24,25,26,27-hexa-*nor*-16β,(20*S*)-diacetoxy-lanost-9(11)-ene.

The molecular formula of kuriloside J (**7**) was determined to be C$_{56}$H$_{90}$O$_{33}$S$_2$Na$_2$ from the [M$_{2Na}$−Na]$^-$ ion peak at m/z 1377.4687 (calc. 1377.4709) and [M$_{2Na}$ − 2Na]$^{2-}$ ion peak at m/z 677.2413 (calc. 677.2408) in the (−)HR-ESI-MS. In the ^{1}H and ^{13}C NMR spectra of the carbohydrate part of kuriloside J (**7**) (Table 6), five signals of anomeric protons at δ_H 4.65–5.12 (d, *J* = 7.2–7.9 Hz) and corresponding five signals of anomeric carbons at δ_C 102.0–104.7, deduced by the HSQC spectrum, were observed, which indicated the presence of a pentasaccharide chain similar to compounds **5** and **6**. Actually, the comparison of the ^{13}C NMR spectra of sugar parts of kurilosides I (**5**) and J (**7**) revealed the closeness of the signals of four monosaccharide residues, except the signals of the third unit, attached to C-4 Qui2. The analysis of the signals of this residue in the ^{1}H,^{1}H-COSY, HSQC, 1D TOCSY, and ROESY spectra of kuriloside J (7) showed that it is a glucose without a sulfate group ($\delta_{C-6\,Glc3}$ 61.8, $\delta_{C-5\,Glc3}$ 77.7), while in the carbohydrate chain of 5, this residue is sulfated. The other sulfate groups occupy the same positions at C-6 Glc4 ($\delta_{C-6\,Glc4}$ 67.1, $\delta_{C-5\,Glc4}$ 75.1) and at C-6 MeGlc5 ($\delta_{C-6\,MeGlc5}$ 66.7, $\delta_{C-5\,MeGlc5}$ 75.5) as in the sugar chains of kurilosides I (5) and I$_1$ (6). The positions of interglycosidic linkages in the carbohydrate chain of 7, elucidated by the ROESY and HMBC correlations (Table 6), were the same as in kurilosides of groups A [19] and I. Thus, kuriloside J (7) is a branched disulfated pentaoside with the sulfate groups bonding to C-6 Glc4 and C-6 MeGlc5 in the upper semi-chain.

Table 6. ^{13}C and ^{1}H NMR chemical shifts, HMBC, and ROESY correlations of carbohydrate moiety of kuriloside J (7).

Atom	δ_C mult. [a,b,c]	δ_H mult. (J in Hz) [d]	HMBC	ROESY
Xyl1 (1→C-3)				
1	104.4 CH	4.65 d (7.6)	C: 3	H-3; H-3, 5 Xyl1
2	**82.1** CH	3.97 t (7.6)	C: 1 Qui2	H-1 Qui2
3	75.1 CH	4.15 t (7.3)	C: 4 Xyl1	
4	**77.5** CH	4.15 t (7.3)	C: 3 Xyl1	H-1 Glc4
5	63.4 CH$_2$	4.36 brd (9.3)		
		3.60 m		H-1, 3 Xyl1
Qui2 (1→2Xyl1)				
1	104.5 CH	5.07 d (7.9)	C: 2 Xyl1	H-2 Xyl1; H-5 Qui2
2	75.5 CH	3.91 t (7.9)	C: 1 Qui2	H-4 Qui2
3	75.1 CH	4.04 t (8.8)	C: 2, 4 Qui2	H-1 Qui2
4	**86.3** CH	3.56 t (8.8)	C: 1 Glc3; C: 5, 6 Qui2	H-1 Glc3; H-2 Qui2
5	71.3 CH	3.71 m		H-1, 3 Qui2
6	17.8 CH$_3$	1.65 d (6.2)	C: 4, 5 Qui2	
Glc3 (1→4Qui2)				
1	104.6 CH	4.84 d (7.2)	C: 4 Qui2	H-4 Qui2; H-3, 5 Glc3
2	74.2 CH	3.91 t (7.9)	C: 1 Glc3	
3	77.3 CH	4.16 t (7.9)	C: 4 Glc3	H-1 Glc3
4	70.9 CH	3.98 t (7.9)		
5	77.7 CH	3.95 m		H-1, 3 Glc3
6	61.8 CH$_2$	4.44 dd (2.0; 11.9)		
		4.11 dd (5.8; 11.2)		
Glc4 (1→4Xyl1)				
1	102.0 CH	4.87 d (7.9)	C: 4 Xyl1	H-4 Xyl1; H-5 Glc4
2	72.9 CH	3.82 t (8.4)	C: 1 Glc4	
3	**86.3** CH	4.10 t (8.4)	C: 1 MeGlc5; C: 4 Glc4	H-1 MeGlc5; H-1 Glc4
4	69.0 CH	3.86 m		
5	75.1 CH	4.05 m		H-1 Glc4
6	67.1 CH$_2$	4.98 m		
		4.69 m		
MeGlc5 (1→3Glc4)				
1	104.7 CH	5.12 d (7.8)	C: 3 Glc4	H-3 Glc4; H-3, 5 MeGlc5
2	74.3 CH	3.78 t (7.8)		H-4 MeGlc5
3	86.3 CH	3.62 t (7.8)	C: 2, 4 MeGlc5; OMe	H-1, 5 MeGlc5; OMe
4	69.7 CH	4.04 m	C: 3, 5 MeGlc5	
5	75.5 CH	3.99 m		H-1, 3 MeGlc5
6	66.7 CH$_2$	4.96 d (10.5)		
		4.79 dd (4.2; 10.5)		
OMe	60.2 CH$_3$	3.75 s	C: 3 MeGlc5	

[a] Recorded at 176.04 MHz in C$_5$D$_5$N/D$_2$O (4/1). [b] Bold = interglycosidic positions. [c] Italic = sulfate position. [d] Recorded at 700.13 MHz in C$_5$D$_5$N/D$_2$O (4/1). Multiplicity by 1D TOCSY.

The analysis of the ^{1}H and ^{13}C NMR spectra of the aglycone part of kuriloside J (7) (Table 7) revealed the presence of the hexa-*nor*-lanostane aglycone having a 9(11)-double bond, similar to the majority of the other glycosides of *T. kurilensis* [19]. The signals at δ_C 171.2 and 21.1 were characteristic for the acetoxy group, bonded to C-16, that was deduced from the characteristic δ_C 75.1 value of C-16 and the ROE-correlation between the signal of *O*-acetyl methyl group (δ_H 2.17 (s)) and H-16 (δ_H 5.76 (m)). Actually, in the spectrum of **7**, the signal of C-16 was deshielded by 2.3 ppm due to the presence of the acetoxy-group when compared with the corresponding signal in the spectrum of kuriloside I (**5**), having a 16-hydroxy-group. The presence of hydroxyl group at C-20 was deduced from the characteristic signals at δ_C 64.8 (C-20) and δ_H 4.28 (dd, *J* = 6.4; 10.0 Hz, H-20). Hence, the hydroxyl group is attached to C-20 in the aglycones of kuriloside I (**5**) and J (**7**). The ROE-correlation H-16/H-32 indicated 16β-O-Ac orientation in the aglycone of kuriloside J (**7**), which was confirmed by the coupling constant $J_{16/17}$ = 7.9 Hz, indicating both protons, H-16 and H-17, to be α [21]. (20*S*)-configuration in **7** was corroborated by the coupling constant $J_{17/20}$ = 10.0 Hz and the ROE-correlations H-17/H-21, H-20/H-18. Hence, kuriloside J (**7**) is characterized by the new hexa-*nor*-lanostane aglycone with a 16β-acetoxy,(20*S*)-hydroxy-fragment.

Table 7. ^{13}C and ^{1}H NMR chemical shifts, HMBC, and ROESY correlations of the aglycone moiety of kuriloside J (**7**) and K$_1$ (**9**).

Position	δ_C mult. ^{a}	δ_H mult. (*J* in Hz) ^{b}	HMBC	ROESY
1	36.0 CH$_2$	1.71 m		H-11, H-19
		1.33 m		H-3, H-5, H-11
2	26.6 CH$_2$	2.10 m		
		1.86 m		H-30
3	88.5 CH	3.12 dd (4.2; 11.6)		H1-Xyl1
4	39.5 C			
5	52.6 CH	0.79 brd (11.8)		H-1, H-3, H-31
6	20.9 CH$_2$	1.61 m		
		1.40 m		
7	27.8 CH$_2$	1.51 m		
		1.18 m		H-5, H-32
8	41.1 CH	2.13 m		H-15, H-18, H-19
9	148.6 C			
10	39.0 C			
11	114.2 CH	5.19 m		H-1
12	35.8 CH$_2$	2.01 m		H-17, H-32
		1.77 brdd (5.3; 16.2)		
13	45.2 C			
14	43.3 C			
15	43.9 CH$_2$	2.15 m	C: 14	H-32
		1.36 m	C: 13	H-18
16	75.1 CH	5.76 m		H-32
17	56.2 CH	2.29 brt (7.9; 10.0)	C: 20	H-12, H-21, H-32
18	15.1 CH$_3$	0.77 s	C: 12, 13, 14, 17	H-8, H-12, H-15, H-20
19	22.0 CH$_3$	1.05 s	C: 1, 5, 9, 10	H-1, H-2, H-8, H-18
20	64.8 CH	4.28 dd (6.4; 10.0)		H-18, H-21
21	23.1 CH$_3$	1.42 d (6.4)	C: 17, 20	H-12, H-17, H-18, H-20
30	16.4 CH$_3$	1.01 s	C: 3, 4, 5, 31	H-2, H-6, H-31
31	27.8 CH$_3$	1.16 s	C: 3, 4, 5, 30	H-3, H-5, H-6, H-30
32	18.8 CH$_3$	0.67 s	C: 8, 13, 14, 15	H-7, H-17
OAc	21.1 CH$_3$	2.17 s	OAc	
	171.2 C			

^{a} Recorded at 176.03 MHz in C$_5$D$_5$N/D$_2$O (4/1). ^{b} Recorded at 700.00 MHz in C$_5$D$_5$N/D$_2$O (4/1).

The (−)ESI-MS/MS of kuriloside J (**7**) demonstrated the fragmentation of [M$_{2Na}$ − Na]$^-$ ion at *m/z* 1377.5. The peaks of fragment ions were observed at *m/z* 1317.4 [M$_{2Na}$ − Na − CH$_3$COOH]$^-$, 1257.4 [M$_{2Na}$ − Na − NaHSO$_4$]$^-$, 1197.5 [M$_{2Na}$ − Na − CH$_3$COOH − NaHSO$_4$]$^-$, 1155.4 [M$_{2Na}$ − Na − CH$_3$COOH − C$_6$H$_{10}$O$_5$ (Glc)]$^-$, 1039.4 [M$_{2Na}$ − Na − CH$_3$COOH − C$_7$H$_{11}$O$_8$SNa(MeGlcOSO$_3$)]$^-$, 1009.4 [M$_{2Na}$ − Na − CH$_3$COOH − C$_6$H$_{10}$O$_5$(Glc) − C$_6$H$_{10}$O$_4$(Qui)]$^-$, 889.4 [M$_{2Na}$ − Na − NaHSO$_4$ − CH$_3$COOH − C$_6$H$_{10}$O$_5$(Glc) − C$_6$H$_{10}$O$_4$(Qui)]$^-$, 667.4 [M$_{2Na}$ − Na − C$_{26}$H$_{41}$O$_3$(Agl) − C$_6$H$_{10}$O$_5$(Glc) −

$C_6H_{10}O_4(Qui) - H]^-$, 519.0 $[M_{2Na} - Na - C_{26}H_{41}O_3(Agl) - C_6H_{10}O_5(Glc) - C_6H_{10}O_4$ (Qui) $- C_5H_8O_4(Xyl) - H]^-$, 417.1 $[M_{2Na} - Na - C_{26}H_{41}O_3(Agl) - C_6H_{10}O_5(Glc) - C_6H_{10}O_4$ (Qui) $- C_5H_8O_4(Xyl) - NaHSO_3]^-$, corroborating the structure of its aglycone and the carbohydrate chain.

All these data indicate that kuriloside J (**7**) is 3β-O-{β-D-glucopyranosyl-(1→4)-β-D-quinovopyranosyl-(1→2)-[6-O-sodium sulfate-3-O-methyl-β-D-glucopyranosyl-(1→3)-6-O-sodium sulfate-β-D-glucopyranosyl-(1→4)]-β-D-xylopyranosyl}-22,23,24,25,26,27-hexa-*nor*-16β-acetoxy,(20S)-hydroxy-lanost-9(11)-ene.

The molecular formula of kuriloside K (**8**) was determined to be $C_{54}H_{88}O_{32}S_2Na_2$ from the $[M_{2Na} - Na]^-$ ion peak at *m/z* 1335.4573 (calc. 1335.4603) and the $[M_{2Na} - 2Na]^{2-}$ ion peak at *m/z* 656.2357 (calc. 656.2356) in the (−)HR-ESI-MS. In the ^{1}H and ^{13}C NMR spectra of the carbohydrate part of kuriloside K (**8**) (Table 8), five signals of anomeric protons at δ$_H$ 4.62–5.19 (d, *J* = 6.5–8.5 Hz) and five signals of anomeric carbons at δ$_C$ 102.7–104.8, deduced by the HSQC spectrum, were indicative for the pentasaccharide chain with the β-configuration of glycosidic bonds. The comparison of the ^{13}C NMR spectra of oligosaccharide parts of trisulfated kuriloside I (**5**) and kuriloside K (**8**) revealed the coincidence of the monosaccharide residues, except for the signals of a terminal, 3-O-methylglucose (MeGlc5) unit. The analysis of the signals of this residue in the ^{1}H,^{1}H-COSY, HSQC, 1D TOCSY, and ROESY spectra of kuriloside K (**8**) showed the absence of a sulfate group (δ$_{C-6\ MeGlc5}$ 61.6, δ$_{C-5\ MeGlc5}$ 77.5), in contrast with the carbohydrate chain of **5** (δ$_{C-6\ MeGlc5}$ 67.0, δ$_{C-5\ MeGlc5}$ 75.4). The positions of interglycosidic linkages in the carbohydrate chain of **8**, deduced by the ROESY and HMBC correlations (Table 8), showed that kuriloside K (**8**) has branching at C-4 Xyl1 in the disulfated pentasaccharide chain with the sulfate groups at C-6 Glc3 and C-6 Glc4.

The NMR spectra as well as the ROE-correlations of the aglycone part of kuriloside K (**8**) were coincident to that of kuriloside I (**5**), indicating the presence of a 22,23,24,25,26,27-hexa-*nor*-lanostane aglycone with 16β,(20S)-dihydroxy-fragment (Table 5).

The (−)ESI-MS/MS of **8** demonstrated the fragmentation of the $[M_{2Na} - Na]^-$ ion at *m/z* 1335.4 resulted in the fragment ions observed at *m/z*: 1215.4 $[M_{2Na} - Na - NaHSO_4]^-$, 1159.4 $[M_{2Na} - Na - C_7H_{12}O_5(MeGlc)]^-$, 1071.4 $[M_{2Na} - Na - C_6H_9O_8SNa(GlcOSO_3)]^-$, 925.4 $[M_{2Na} - Na - C_6H_9O_8SNa(GlcOSO_3) - C_6H_{10}O_4(Qui)]^-$, 895.4 $[M_{2Na} - Na - C_6H_9O_8SNa(GlcOSO_3) - C_7H_{12}O_5(MeGlc)]^-$, 713.3 $[M_{2Na} - Na - C_{24}H_{39}O_2(Agl) - C_6H_9O_8SNa(GlcOSO_3) - H]^-$, 417.1 $[M_{2Na} - Na - C_{24}H_{39}O_3(Agl) - C_6H_9O_8SNa(GlcOSO_3) - C_6H_{10}O_4(Qui) - C_5H_8O_4(Xyl) - H]^-$, 241.0 $[M_{2Na} - Na - C_{24}H_{39}O_3(Agl) - C_6H_9O_8SNa(GlcOSO_3) - C_6H_{10}O_4(Qui) - C_5H_8O_4(Xyl) - C_7H_{12}O_5(MeGlc) - H]^-$, which confirmed the chemical structure established by the NMR data.

All these data indicate that kuriloside K (**8**) is 3β-O-{6-O-sodium sulfate-β-D-glucopyranosyl-(1→4)-β-D-quinovopyranosyl-(1→2)-[3-O-methyl-β-D-glucopyranosyl-(1→3)-6-O-sodium sulfate-β-D-glucopyranosyl-(1→4)]-β-D-xylopyranosyl}-22,23,24,25,26,27-hexa-*nor*-16β,(20S)-dihydroxy-lanost-9(11)-ene.

The molecular formula of kuriloside K_1 (**9**) was determined to be $C_{56}H_{90}O_{33}S_2Na_2$ from the $[M_{2Na} - Na]^-$ ion peak at *m/z* 1377.4723 (calc. 1377.4709) and the $[M_{2Na} - 2Na]^{2-}$ ion peak at *m/z* 677.2426 (calc. 677.2408) in the (−)HR-ESI-MS. The comparison of the ^{1}H and ^{13}C NMR spectra of the carbohydrate chains of kuriloside K_1 (**9**) and kuriloside K (**8**) demonstrated their coincidence (Table 8) due to the presence of the same pentasaccharide, branched by C-4 Xyl1, sugar parts with the sulfate groups at C-6 Glc3 and C-6 Glc4. The analysis of the NMR spectra of the aglycone part of **9** indicated the presence of 22,23,24,25,26,27-hexa-*nor*-lanostane aglycone with 16β-acetoxy,(20S)-hydroxy-fragment (Table 7), identical to that of kuriloside J (**7**). Hence, kuriloside K_1 (**9**) is an isomer of kuriloside J (**7**) by the position of one of the sulfate groups, that was confirmed by the presence of the ion-peaks having coincident *m/z* values in their (−)ESI-MS/MS spectra.

Table 8. ^{13}C and ^{1}H NMR chemical shifts, HMBC, and ROESY correlations of the carbohydrate moiety of kurilosides K (8) and K$_1$ (9).

Atom	δ_C mult. ^{a,b,c}	δ_H mult. (J in Hz) ^{d}	HMBC	ROESY
Xyl1 (1→C-3)				
1	104.7 CH	4.62 d (6.8)	C: 3	H-3; H-3, 5 Xyl1
2	**82.2** CH	3.88 t (7.6)	C: 1 Qui2; C: 1 Xyl1	H-1 Qui2
3	75.0 CH	4.07 t (7.6)	C: 2, 4 Xyl1	H-1 Xyl1
4	**78.9** CH	4.06 m		H-1 Glc4
5	63.4 CH$_2$	4.32 dd (7.6; 11.4)		
		3.60 m		H-1 Xyl1
Qui2 (1→2Xyl1)				
1	104.5 CH	4.93 d (8.5)	C: 2 Xyl1	H-2 Xyl1; H-3, 5 Qui2
2	75.4 CH	3.84 t (8.5)	C: 1, 3 Qui2	H-4 Qui2
3	74.5 CH	3.93 t (8.5)	C: 2, 4 Qui2	H-5 Qui2
4	**86.9** CH	3.35 t (8.5)	C: 1 Glc3; C: 3, 5 Qui2	H-1 Glc3; H-2 Qui2
5	71.3 CH	3.65 m		H-1, 3 Qui2
6	17.7 CH$_3$	1.60 d (5.3)	C: 4, 5 Qui2	
Glc3 (1→4Qui2)				
1	104.8 CH	4.69 d (6.5)	C: 4 Qui2	H-4 Qui2; H-3, 5 Glc3
2	74.1 CH	3.81 t (8.4)	C: 1, 3 Glc3	
3	76.9 CH	4.11 t (8.4)	C: 2, 4 Glc3	
4	70.8 CH	3.88 t (8.4)	C: 3, 5, 6 Glc3	
5	75.4 CH	4.10 m		H-1 Glc3
6	*67.6* CH$_2$	5.08 brd (11.2)		
		4.64 dd (8.4; 11.2)	C: 5 Glc3	
Glc4 (1→4Xyl1)				
1	102.7 CH	4.84 d (7.5)	C: 4 Xyl1	H-4 Xyl1; H-3, 5 Glc4
2	73.2 CH	3.83 m	C: 1, 3 Glc4	
3	**86.0** CH	4.16 t (8.4)9	C: 1 MeGlc5; C: 2, 4 Glc4	H-1 MeGlc5
4	69.1 CH	3.83 m	C: 5, 6 Glc4	
5	74.8 CH	4.05 m		H-1 Glc4
6	*67.3* CH$_2$	4.96 d (10.9)		
		4.61 m		
MeGlc5 (1→3Glc4)				
1	104.4 CH	5.19 d (7.2)	C: 3 Glc4	H-3 Glc4; H-3, 5 MeGlc5
2	75.1 CH	3.85 t (8.9)	C: 1, 3 MeGlc5	
3	86.9 CH	3.66 t (8.9)	C: 2, 4 MeGlc5; OMe	H-1 MeGlc5; OMe
4	70.2 CH	3.90 t (8.9)	C: 5 MeGlc5	
5	77.5 CH	3.89 m	C: 6 MeGlc5	H-1 MeGlc5
6	61.6 CH$_2$	4.36 brd (12.5)		
		4.07 dd (5.4; 12.5)	C: 5 MeGlc5	
OMe	60.5 CH$_3$	3.79 s	C: 3 MeGlc5	

^{a} Recorded at 176.04 MHz in C$_5$D$_5$N/D$_2$O (4/1). ^{b} Bold = interglycosidic positions. ^{c} Italic = sulfate position. ^{d} Recorded at 700.13 MHz in C$_5$D$_5$N/D$_2$O (4/1). Multiplicity by 1D TOCSY.

The (−)ESI-MS/MS of **9** demonstrated the fragmentation of [M$_{2Na}$ − Na]$^-$ ion at m/z 1377.5. The peaks of fragment ions were observed at m/z 1317.4 [M$_{2Na}$ − Na − CH$_3$COOH]$^-$, 1197.5 [M$_{2Na}$ − Na − CH$_3$COOH − NaHSO$_4$]$^-$, 1069.5 [M$_{2Na}$ − Na − C$_6$H$_{10}$O$_5$(Glc)]$^-$, 1053.4 [M$_{2Na}$ − Na − CH$_3$COOH − C$_6$H$_9$O$_8$SNa(GlcOSO$_3$)]$^-$, 877.4 [M$_{2Na}$ − Na − CH$_3$COOH − C$_6$H$_9$O$_8$SNa(GlcOSO$_3$) − C$_7$H$_{12}$O$_5$(MeGlc)]$^-$, 731.3 [M$_{2Na}$ − Na − CH$_3$COOH − C$_6$H$_9$O$_8$SNa(GlcOSO$_3$) − C$_7$H$_{12}$O$_5$(MeGlc) − C$_6$H$_{10}$O$_4$(Qui)]$^-$, 565.1 [M$_{2Na}$ − Na − C$_{26}$H$_{41}$O$_3$(Agl) − C$_6$H$_9$O$_8$SNa(GlcOSO$_3$) − C$_6$H$_{10}$O$_4$(Qui) − H]$^-$, 417.1 [M$_{2Na}$ − Na − C$_{26}$H$_{41}$O$_4$(Agl) − C$_6$H$_9$O$_8$SNa(GlcOSO$_3$) − C$_6$H$_{10}$O$_4$(Qui) − C$_5$H$_8$O$_4$(Xyl)]$^-$.

All these data indicate that kuriloside K$_1$ (**9**) is 3β-O-{6-O-sodium sulfate-β-D-glucopyranosyl-(1→4)-β-D-quinovopyranosyl-(1→2)-[3-O-methyl-β-D-glucopyranosyl-(1→3)-6-O-sodium sulfate-β-D-glucopyranosyl-(1→4)]-β-D-xylopyranosyl}-22,23,24,25,26,27-hexa-*nor*-16β-acetoxy,(20S)-hydroxy-lanost-9(11)-ene.

When the studies on the glycosides of *T. kurilensis* were started [22], the complexity of glycosidic mixture became obvious. Therefore, the part of the glycosidic sum was subjected to solvolytic desulfation to facilitate the chromatographic separation and isolation of the glycosides. However, the obtained fraction of desulfated glycosides was separated only recently as part of the effort to discover some minor glycosides possessing interesting structural peculiarities. As a result, the compounds **10** and **11** were isolated (Figure 2). Their structures were elucidated by thorough analysis of 1D and 2D NMR spectra, similar to the natural compounds **1–9** and confirmed by the HR-ESI-MS.

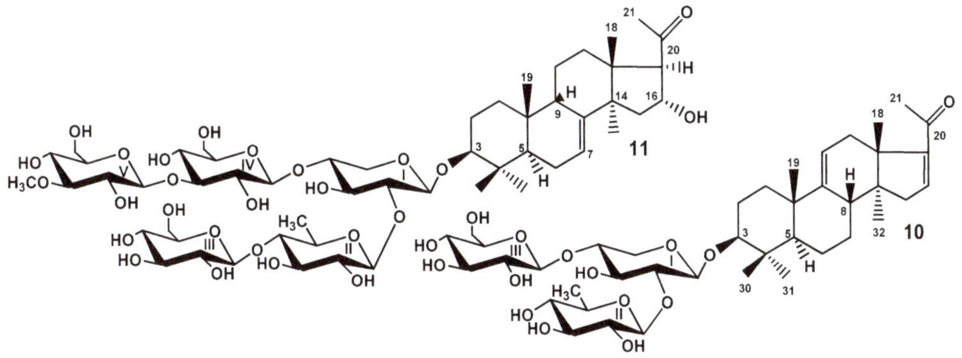

Figure 2. Chemical structures of desulfated glycosides isolated from *Thyonidium kurilensis*: **10**—DS-kuriloside L; **11**—DS-kuriloside M.

The molecular formula of DS-kuriloside L (**10**) was determined to be $C_{41}H_{64}O_{15}$ from the $[M − H]^−$ ion peak at *m/z* 795.4169 (calc. 795.4172) in the (−)HR-ESI-MS. Compound **10** has a trisaccharide sugar chain (for NMR data see Tables S5 and S6, for original spectra see Figures S69–S76) and a hexa-*nor*-lanostane-type aglycone identical to that of kuriloside A$_2$ [19].

The molecular formula of DS-kuriloside M (**11**) was determined to be $C_{54}H_{88}O_{26}$ from the $[M − H]^−$ ion peak at *m/z* 1151.5469 (calc. 1151.5491) in the (−)HR-ESI-MS. DS-kuriloside M (**11**), characterized by the 7(8)-double bond in the hexa-*nor*-lanostane nucleus and pentasaccharide chain, differed from the chains of kurilosides of the groups A, I, J, and K by the absence of sulfate groups (see Tables S7 and S8 for the NMR data, Figures S77–S85 for the original spectra). Noticeably, all of the isolated kurilosides, with the exception of **11**, contained a 9(11)-double bond in the polycyclic systems.

2.2. Bioactivity of the Glycosides

Cytotoxic activities of compounds **1–9** against mouse neuroblastoma Neuro 2a, normal epithelial JB-6 cells, and erythrocytes were studied (Table 9). Known earlier cladoloside C was used as a positive control because it demonstrated a strong hemolytic effect [23]. Erythrocytes are an appropriate model for the studying of structure–activity relationships of the glycosides, since, despite many of them demonstrate hemolytic activity, the effect strongly depends on the structure of the compound. Normal epithelial JB-6 cells were used to search the compounds, not cytotoxic against this cell line, but having selective activity against other cells. Triterpene glycosides of sea cucumbers are known modulators of P2X receptors of immunocompetent cells when acting in nanomolar concentrations [24]. Neuroblastoma Neuro 2a cells are convenient model for the study of agonists/antagonists of P2X receptors—the targets in the treatment of selected nervous system diseases. Therefore, the activators, modulators, and blockers of purinergic receptors are of great interest [4] and the compounds demonstrating high cytotoxicity against Neuro 2a cells could be more deeply studied with the models of neurodegenerative diseases.

Table 9. The cytotoxic activities of glycosides 1–9 and cladoloside C (positive control) against mouse erythrocytes, neuroblastoma Neuro 2a cells, and normal epithelial JB-6 cells.

Glycoside	ED$_{50}$, µM	Cytotoxicity EC$_{50}$, µM	
	Erythrocytes	JB-6	Neuro-2a
Kuriloside A$_3$ (1)	>100.00	>100.00	>100.00
Kuriloside D$_1$ (2)	>100.00	>100.00	>100.00
Kuriloside G (3)	76.26 ± 0.98	>100.00	>100.00
Kuriloside H (4)	6.85 ± 0.67	4.63 ± 0.08	38.28 ± 1.15
Kuriloside I (5)	>100.00	>100.00	>100.00
Kuriloside I$_1$ (6)	10.34 ± 0.28	11.48 ± 1.02	56.63 ± 0.98
Kuriloside J (7)	47.61 ± 1.73	77.75 ± 0.27	>100.00
Kuriloside K (8)	>100.00	>100.00	>100.00
Kuriloside K$_1$ (9)	20.97 ± 0.39	37.44 ± 0.13	>100.00
Cladoloside C (positive control)	0.54 ± 0.01	6.38 ± 0.08	9.54 ± 0.82

Kuriloside H (4), having a hexasaccharide trisulfated chain and the aglycone with acetoxy-groups at C(16) and C(20), was the most active compound in the series, demonstrating strong cytotoxicity against erythrocytes and JB-6 cells and a moderate effect against Neuro 2a cells. Kuriloside I$_1$ (6), differing from 4 by the lack of a terminal glucose residue in the bottom semi-chain, was slightly less active. The effect of this glycoside is obviously explained by the presence of the acetoxy-group at C(20) in their aglycones, which compensates for the absence of a side chain, essential for the demonstration of the membranolytic action of the glycosides. Kurilosides J (7) and K$_1$ (9), differing by the position of the second sulfate group attached to C(6) of different terminal monosaccharide residues, but having the same aglycones with 16β-acetoxy-group, were moderately cytotoxic against erythrocytes and JB-6 cells and had no any effect against Neuro 2a cells. However, the presence of the hydroxyl group in this position causes the loss of activity, so, the rest of compounds 1−3, 5, and 8 were not cytotoxic.

2.3. Biosynthetic Pathways of the Glycosides

The analysis of the structural peculiarities of the aglycones and carbohydrate chains of all the glycosides (kurilosides) found in the sea cucumber *T. kurilensis* allowed us to construct the metabolic network based on their biogenetic relationships. As a result, some biosynthetic pathways are taking shape (Figure 3).

Since the triterpene glycosides of sea cucumbers are the products of a mosaic type of biosynthesis [17], the carbohydrate chains and the aglycones are biosynthesized independently of each other. The main biosynthetic transformations of sugar parts of kurilosides are glycosylation and several rounds of sulfation that can be shifted in time relatively to each other (Figure 3). This has led to the formation of the set of compounds having 11 different oligosaccharide fragments. Meanwhile, there are some missing links (biosynthetic intermediates) in these biogenetic rows: biosides consisted of the glucose bonded to the xylose by β-(1→4)-glycosidic linkage, then triosides and tetraosides having glucose bonded to C(2) Xyl1—the precursors on kuriloside E, two types of disulfated hexaosides with a non-methylated terminal Glc4 unit that should biosynthetically appear between the carbohydrate chains of kurilosides of groups D and H; J and H; K and H, which have not so far been isolated. DS-kuriloside L (10) with a trisaccharide sugar chain is perfectly fit into the network as one of the initial stages of biosynthesis, illustrating the stepwise glycosylation of the synthesized chain. The structure of its sugar chain as well as the chain of kuriloside C$_1$ [19] suggests the glycosylation of C(4) Xyl1 and initialization of the growth of the upper semi-chain precedes the glycosylation of C(2) Xyl1. There are some branchpoints of the biosynthetic pathways where the processes of sulfation and glycosylation or sulfation and methylation are alternative/concurrent. The final product of such transformations is the trisulfated hexaoside kuriloside H (4), the most biologically active compound in the series

(Table 9), which can be formed by different pathways, and is a characteristic feature of a mosaic type of biosynthesis. However, this glycoside is minor (0.9 mg) in the glycosidic sum of *T. kurilensis*, while the main compounds are kurilosides of group A (~150 mg), and these carbohydrate chains can be considered as the most actively metabolized and resulted in the formation of at least three different types of sugar chains (kurilosides of the groups D, J, and K). Thus, their formation is a mainstream of the biosynthesis of carbohydrate chains of the glycosides of *T. kurilensis*.

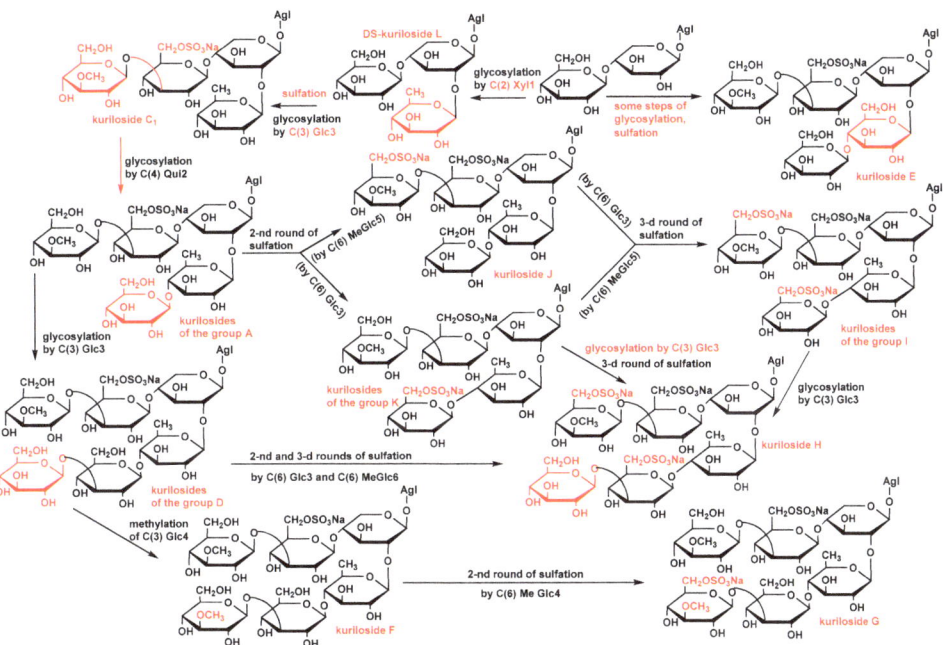

Figure 3. The metabolic network of the carbohydrate chains of the glycosides from *T. kurilensis*.

As for the directions of biosynthesis of the aglycone parts of kurilosides (Figure 4), the scheme presented earlier [19] was complemented by some structures found recently, representing intermediate biosynthetic stages. DS-kuriloside M (**11**) is the only glycoside from *T. kurilensis* characterized by the 7(8)-double bond in the lanostane nucleus, when all the other kurilosides contain a 9(11)-double bond in the polycyclic systems. This finding indicates the existence of two oxidosqualene cyclases (OSCs)—enzymes converted 2,3-oxidosqualene into different triterpene alcohols giving rise various skeletons of the aglycones—in this species of sea cucumbers. These data are in good agreement with the results of the investigations of the genes coding OSCs in the other species of the sea cucumbers—*Eupentacta fraudatrix* [25], *Stichopus horrens* [26], and *Apostichopus japonicus* [27], demonstrating that even when the glycosides preferably contain the aglycones with one certain position of intra-nucleus double bond (Δ7(8)-aglycones in *E. fraudatrix* [13,18] and *S. horrens* [28,29], and Δ9(11)-aglycones in *A. japonicus* [30,31]), the genes of at least two OSCs, producing aglycone precursors with different double bond positions, are expressed, albeit with different efficiency.

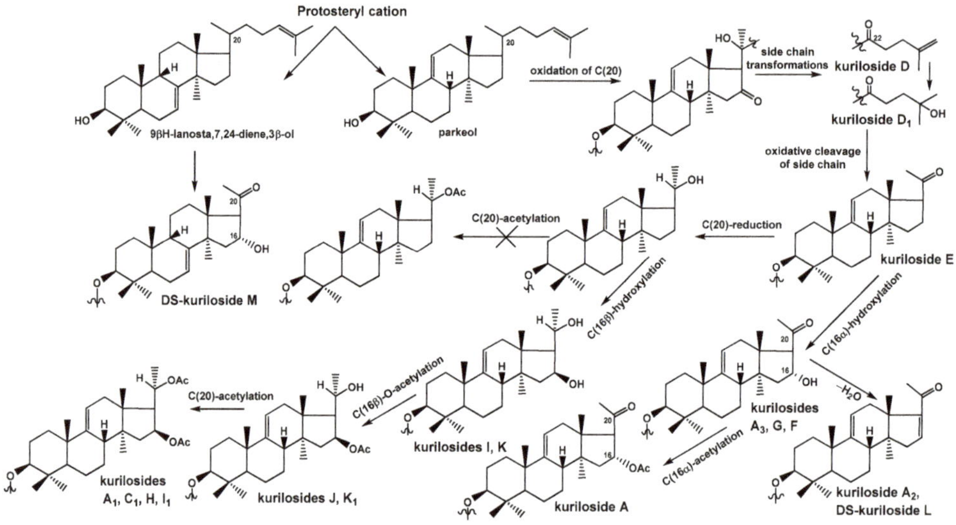

Figure 4. The biosynthetic pathways to aglycones of glycosides from *T. kurilensis*.

The constituent hexa-*nor*-lanostane aglycones of kurilosides are biosynthesized via the oxidative cleavage of the side chain from the precursors having normal side chains (for example, kurilosides D [19] and D_1 (**2**)) and oxygen-containing substituents at C-20 and C-22 (Figure 4). As result, the aglycone of kuriloside E [19] was formed. The subsequent biosynthetic transformations of the aglycones can occur in two directions. The first one started from the reduction of the C-20-oxo-group to the hydroxy-group, followed by the oxidation of C-16 to the hydroxy-group with the formation of the aglycones of kurilosides I (**5**) and K (**8**). It is important that the latter reaction is carried out by the cytochrome P450 monooxygenase selectively bonding to the β-hydroxy-group to C-16 in the derivatives containing the hydroxy-group at C-20. The next steps lead to the acetylation of hydroxyl group at C-16 (as in the aglycones of kurilosides J (**7**) and K_1 (**9**)) followed by the acetylation of the hydroxyl group at C-20 (the aglycones of kurilosides A_1, C_1, H (**4**), and I_1 (**6**) correspond to this conversion). Obviously, the oxidation of C-16 precedes the acetylation of C-20 since no aglycones with a 16-hydroxy,20-acetoxy-fragment have been found.

The second direction of the aglycone biosynthesis occurs through the introduction of the α-hydroxyl group to C-16, resulting in the formation of aglycone of kurilosides A_3 (**1**), G (**3**), and F [19]. Moreover, the transformation leading to hexa-*nor*-lanostane aglycones having a 16α-hydroxy,20-oxo-fragment is the same in the biosynthetic precursors with 7(8)- and 9(11)-double bonds, which is confirmed by the aglycone structure of **11**. Subsequent acetylation of the 16α-OH-group leads to the aglycone of kuriloside A, while intramolecular dehydration to the aglycone of kuriloside A_2 and DS-kuriloside L (**10**). Therefore, an α-hydroxy-group was selectively introduced to C-16 of the 20-oxo-lanostane precursors.

3. Materials and Methods

3.1. General Experimental Procedures

Specific rotation, Perkin-Elmer 343 Polarimeter (Perkin-Elmer, Waltham, MA, USA); NMR, Bruker Avance III 700 Bruker FT-NMR (Bruker BioSpin GmbH, Rheinstetten, Germany) (700.00/176.03 MHz) (^{1}H/^{13}C) spectrometer; ESI MS (positive and negative ion modes), Agilent 6510 Q-TOF apparatus (Agilent Technology, Santa Clara, CA, USA), sample concentration 0.01 mg/mL; HPLC, Agilent 1260 Infinity II with a differential refractometer

(Agilent Technology, Santa Clara, CA, USA); column Phenomenex Synergi Fusion RP (10 × 250 mm, 5 μm) (Phenomenex, Torrance, CA, USA).

3.2. Animals and Cells

Specimens of the sea cucumber *Thyonidium* (=*Duasmodactyla*) *kurilensis* (Levin) (family Cucumariidae; order Dendrochirotida) were collected in August 1990 using an industrial rake-type dredge in the waters of Onekotan Island (Kurile Islands, the Sea of Okhotsk) at a depth of 100 m by the medium fishing refrigerator trawler "Breeze" with a rear scheme of trawling during scallop harvesting. The sea cucumbers were identified by Prof. V.S. Levin; voucher specimens are preserved at the A.V. Zhirmunsky National Scientific Center of Marine Biology, Vladivostok, Russia.

CD-1 mice, weighing 18–20 g, were purchased from RAMS 'Stolbovaya' nursery (Stolbovaya, Moscow District, Russia) and kept at the animal facility in standard conditions. All experiments were performed following the protocol for animal study approved by the Ethics Committee of the Pacific Institute of Bioorganic Chemistry No. 0085.19.10.2020. All experiments were conducted in compliance with all of the rules and international recommendations of the European Convention for the Protection of Vertebrate Animals Used for Experimental Studies.

Mouse epithelial JB-6 cells Cl 41-5a and mouse neuroblastoma cell line Neuro 2a (ATCC® CCL-131) were purchased from ATCC (Manassas, VA, USA).

3.3. Extraction and Isolation

The extract of the glycosides, obtained by the standard procedure, and the initial stages of their separation were discussed in a previous paper [19]. As result of the chromatography on Si gel columns using $CHCl_3/EtOH/H_2O$ (100:125:25) as the mobile phase, the fractions II–V were obtained, which were subjected to HPLC on a Phenomenex Synergi Fusion RP (10 × 250 mm) column. The separation of fraction II with $MeOH/H_2O/NH_4OAc$ (1 M water solution) (63/35/2) as the mobile phase resulted in the isolation of individual kuriloside A_3 (**1**) (79.2 mg). HPLC of fraction III with $MeOH/H_2O/NH_4OAc$ (1 M water solution) (60/38/2) as the mobile phase gave 3.1 mg of kuriloside K_1 (**9**) and 0.9 mg of kuriloside K (**8**). Fraction IV was the result of the HPLC using $MeOH/H_2O/NH_4OAc$ (1 M water solution) (68/31/1) as the mobile phase was separated to the subfractions 1–7. Further rechromatography of subfraction 7 with $MeOH/H_2O/NH_4OAc$ (1 M water solution) (63/34/3) followed by (60/37/3) as the mobile phases gave 3.1 mg of kuriloside I_1 (**6**). The use of the ratio of $MeOH/H_2O/NH_4OAc$ (1 M water solution) (62/35/3) for subfraction 4 gave 2.3 mg of kuriloside J (**7**) and the ratio (58/39/3) for subfraction 3 gave 7 mg of kuriloside D_1 (**2**). For the HPLC of the most polar fraction V, obtained after Si gel chromatography, the ratio of the same solvents (60/39/1) was applied, which led to the isolation of 10 subfractions. Some of them were minor, thus only the main ones were submitted for further separation. For subfraction 10, the ratio (64/34/2) was applied to give 0.9 mg of kuriloside H (**4**). The ratio (54/43/3) used for HPLC of subfraction 4 gave 1.9 mg of kuriloside G (**3**) and 2.3 mg of kuriloside I (**5**).

The fraction of desulfated derivatives obtained earlier by the standard methodology (~350 mg) was submitted to column chromatography on Si gel using $CHCl_3/EtOH/H_2O$ (100:50:4) and $CHCl_3/MeOH/H_2O$ (250:75:3) as mobile phases to give subfractions DS-1–DS-8, which were subsequently subjected to HPLC on the same column as compounds **1–9**. Individual DS-kuriloside M (**11**) (3.8 mg) was isolated as a result of separating the subfraction DS-6 with 66% MeOH as the mobile phase which gave several fractions, followed by the HPLC of one of them with 32% CH_3CN as the mobile phase. HPLC of subfraction DS-2 with 50% CH_3CN as the mobile phase, followed by 46% CH_3CN as the mobile phase, gave 4.0 mg of DS-kuriloside L (**10**).

3.3.1. Kuriloside A$_3$ (1)

Colorless powder; $[\alpha]_D^{20}$ −1° (c 0.1, 50% MeOH). NMR: See Tables S1 and S2, Figures S1–S6. (−)HR-ESI-MS m/z: 1231.5063 (calc. 1231.5059) [M$_{Na}$ − Na]$^-$; (−)ESI-MS/MS m/z: 1069.5 [M$_{Na}$ − Na − C$_6$H$_{10}$O$_5$(Glc)]$^-$, 1055.4 [M$_{Na}$ − Na–C$_7$H$_{12}$O$_5$(MeGlc)]$^-$, 923.4 [M$_{Na}$ − Na–C$_6$H$_{10}$O$_5$(Glc) − C$_6$H$_{10}$O$_4$(Qui)]$^-$, 747.3 [M$_{Na}$ − Na–C$_6$H$_{10}$O$_5$(Glc) − C$_6$H$_{10}$O$_4$(Qui) − C$_7$H$_{12}$O$_5$(MeGlc)]$^-$, 695.1 [M$_{Na}$ − Na − C$_{24}$H$_{37}$O$_3$(Agl) − C$_6$H$_{10}$O$_5$(Glc) − H]$^-$, 565.1 [M$_{Na}$ − Na–C$_{24}$H$_{37}$O$_2$(Agl) − C$_6$H$_{10}$O$_5$(Glc) − C$_6$H$_{10}$O$_4$(Qui) − H]$^-$, 549.1 [M$_{Na}$ − Na–C$_{24}$H$_{37}$O$_3$(Agl) − C$_6$H$_{10}$O$_5$(Glc) − C$_6$H$_{10}$O$_4$(Qui) − H]$^-$, 417.1 [M$_{Na}$ − Na–C$_{24}$H$_{37}$O$_3$(Agl) − C$_6$H$_{10}$O$_5$(Glc) − C$_6$H$_{10}$O$_4$(Qui) − C$_5$H$_8$O$_4$(Xyl) − H]$^-$, 241.0 [M$_{Na}$ − Na–C$_{24}$H$_{37}$O$_3$(Agl) − C$_6$H$_{10}$O$_5$(Glc) − C$_6$H$_{10}$O$_4$(Qui) − C$_5$H$_8$O$_4$(Xyl) − C$_7$H$_{12}$O$_5$(MeGlc) − H]$^-$.

3.3.2. Kuriloside D$_1$ (2)

Colorless powder; $[\alpha]_D^{20}$ −39° (c 0.1, 50% MeOH). NMR: See Table 1 and Table S3, Figures S7–S13. (−)HR-ESI-MS m/z: 1507.6291 (calc. 1507.6268) [M$_{Na}$ − Na]$^-$; (−)ESI-MS/MS m/z: 1349.5 [M$_{Na}$ − Na − C$_8$H$_{15}$O$_3$ + H]$^-$, 1187.5 [M$_{Na}$ − Na − C$_8$H$_{15}$O$_3$ −C$_6$H$_{10}$O$_5$ (Glc) + H]$^-$, 1025.4 [M$_{Na}$ − Na − C$_8$H$_{15}$O$_3$ − C$_6$H$_{10}$O$_5$(Glc) − C$_6$H$_{10}$O$_5$(Glc) + H]$^-$, 879.4 [M$_{Na}$ − Na − C$_8$H$_{15}$O$_3$ −C$_6$H$_{10}$O$_5$(Glc) − C$_6$H$_{10}$O$_5$(Glc) − C$_6$H$_{10}$O$_4$(Qui) + H]$^-$, 565.1 [M$_{Na}$ − Na − C$_{30}$H$_{47}$O$_4$(Agl) − C$_6$H$_{10}$O$_5$(Glc) − C$_6$H$_{10}$O$_5$(Glc) −C$_6$H$_{10}$O$_4$(Qui) − H]$^-$, 417.1 [M$_{Na}$ − Na − C$_{30}$H$_{47}$O$_5$(Agl) − C$_6$H$_{10}$O$_5$(Glc) − C$_6$H$_{10}$O$_5$(Glc) − C$_6$H$_{10}$O$_4$(Qui) − C$_5$H$_8$O$_4$(Xyl) − H]$^-$, 241.0 [M$_{Na}$ − Na − C$_{30}$H$_{47}$O$_5$(Agl) − C$_6$H$_{10}$O$_5$(Glc) − C$_6$H$_{10}$O$_5$(Glc) − C$_6$H$_{10}$O$_4$(Qui) − C$_5$H$_8$O$_4$(Xyl) − C$_7$H$_{12}$O$_5$(MeGlc) − H]$^-$.

3.3.3. Kuriloside G (3)

Colorless powder; $[\alpha]_D^{20}$ −2° (c 0.1, 50% MeOH). NMR: See Table 2 and Table S2, Figures S14–S22. (−)HR-ESI-MS m/z: 1509.5102 (calc. 1509.5132) [M$_{2Na}$ − Na]$^-$; 743.2624 (calc. 743.2626) [M$_{2Na}$ − 2Na]$^{2-}$, (−)ESI-MS/MS m/z: 1389.6 [M$_{2Na}$ − Na − NaHSO$_4$]$^-$, 1333.5 [M$_{2Na}$ − Na − C$_7$H$_{12}$O$_5$(MeGlc)]$^-$, 1231.5 [M$_{2Na}$ − Na − C$_7$H$_{11}$O$_8$SNa(MeGlcSO$_3$Na)]$^-$, 1069.4 [M$_{2Na}$ − Na − C$_7$H$_{11}$O$_8$SNa(MeGlcSO$_3$Na) − C$_6$H$_{10}$O$_5$(Glc)]$^-$, 923.4 [M$_{2Na}$ −Na − C$_7$H$_{11}$O$_8$SNa(MeGlcSO$_3$Na) − C$_6$H$_{10}$O$_5$(Glc)] − C$_6$H$_{10}$O$_4$(Qui)]$^-$.

3.3.4. Kuriloside H (4)

Colorless powder; $[\alpha]_D^{20}$ −3° (c 0.1, 50% MeOH). NMR: See Table 3 and Table S4, Figures S23–S31. (−)HR-ESI-MS m/z: 1683.4701 (calc. 1683.4730) [M$_{3Na}$ − Na]$^-$, 830.2425 (calc. 830.2419) [M$_{3Na}$ − 2Na]$^{2-}$, 545.8332 (calc. 545.8315) [M$_{3Na}$ − 3Na]$^{3-}$; (−)ESI-MS/MS m/z: 1503.5 [M$_{3Na}$ − Na − CH$_3$COOH − NaHSO$_4$]$^-$, 1443.5 [M$_{3Na}$ − Na − 2CH$_3$COOH − NaHSO$_4$]$^-$, 1281.4 [M$_{3Na}$ − Na − 2CH$_3$COOH − NaHSO$_4$ − C$_6$H$_{10}$O$_5$(Glc)]$^-$, 1165.4 [M$_{3Na}$ − Na − 2CH$_3$COOH − NaHSO$_4$ − C$_7$H$_{11}$O$_8$SNa(MeGlcOSO$_3$)]$^-$, 1003.4 [M$_{3Na}$ − Na − 2CH$_3$COOH − NaHSO$_4$ − C$_7$H$_{11}$O$_8$SNa(MeGlcOSO$_3$) − C$_6$H$_{10}$O$_5$ (Glc)]$^-$.

3.3.5. Kuriloside I (5)

Colorless powder; $[\alpha]_D^{20}$ −9° (c 0.1, 50% MeOH). NMR: See Tables 4 and 5, Figures S32–S40. (−)HR-ESI-MS m/z: 1437.3952 (calc. 1437.3991) [M$_{3Na}$ − Na]$^-$, 707.2049 (calc. 707.2049) [M$_{3Na}$ − 2Na]$^{2-}$, 463.8076 (calc. 463.8069) [M$_{3Na}$ − 3Na]$^{3-}$; (−)ESI-MS/MS m/z: 1317.4 [M$_{3Na}$ − Na − NaHSO$_4$]$^-$, 1197.4 [M$_{3Na}$ − Na − 2NaHSO$_4$]$^-$, 1173.4 [M$_{3Na}$ − Na − C$_6$H$_9$O$_8$SNa(GlcOSO$_3$)]$^-$, 1039.4 [M$_{3Na}$ − Na − NaHSO$_4$ − C$_7$H$_{11}$O$_8$SNa(MeGlcOSO$_3$)]$^-$, 1027.3 [M$_{3Na}$ − Na − C$_6$H$_9$O$_8$SNa(GlcOSO$_3$) − C$_6$H$_{10}$O$_4$(Qui)]$^-$, 907.3 [M$_{3Na}$ − Na − NaHSO$_4$ − C$_6$H$_9$O$_8$SNa(GlcOSO$_3$) − C$_6$H$_{10}$O$_4$(Qui)]$^-$, 895.4 [M$_{3Na}$ − Na − C$_6$H$_9$O$_8$SNa (GlcOSO$_3$) − C$_7$H$_{11}$O$_8$SNa (MeGlcOSO$_3$)]$^-$, 667.4 [M$_{3Na}$ − Na − C$_{24}$H$_{39}$O$_2$(Agl) − C$_6$H$_9$O$_8$ SNa(GlcOSO$_3$) − C$_6$H$_{10}$O$_4$(Qui) − H]$^-$, 519.0 [M$_{3Na}$ − Na − C$_{24}$H$_{39}$O$_3$(Agl) − C$_6$H$_9$O$_8$SNa (GlcOSO$_3$) − C$_6$H$_{10}$O$_4$(Qui) − C$_5$H$_8$O$_4$(Xyl) − H]$^-$, 417.1 [M$_{3Na}$ − Na − C$_{24}$H$_{39}$O$_3$(Agl) − C$_6$H$_9$O$_8$SNa(GlcOSO$_3$) − C$_6$H$_{10}$O$_4$(Qui) − C$_5$H$_8$O$_4$(Xyl) − NaHSO$_3$]$^-$.

3.3.6. Kuriloside I$_1$ (6)

Colorless powder; $[\alpha]_D^{20}$ −5° (c 0.1, 50% MeOH). NMR: See Table 4 and Table S4, Figures S41–S47. (−)HR-ESI-MS m/z: 1749.2148 (calc. 747.2155) [M$_{3Na}$ − 2Na]$^{2-}$, 491.8146 (calc. 491.8139) [M$_{3Na}$ − 3Na]$^{3-}$; (−)ESI-MS/MS m/z: 1281.4 [M$_{3Na}$ − Na − 2CH$_3$COOH − NaHSO$_4$]$^-$, 1197.4 [M$_{3Na}$ − Na − CH$_3$COOH − C$_6$H$_9$O$_8$SNa(GlcOSO$_3$)]$^-$, 1137.4 [M$_{3Na}$ − Na − 2CH$_3$COOH − C$_6$H$_9$O$_8$SNa (GlcOSO$_3$)]$^-$, 859.4 [M$_{3Na}$ − Na − 2CH$_3$COOH − C$_6$H$_9$O$_8$SNa(GlcOSO$_3$) − C$_7$H$_{11}$O$_8$SNa(MeGlcOSO$_3$)]$^-$, 719.2 [M$_{3Na}$ − 2Na − CH$_3$COOH]$^{2-}$, 629.2 [M$_{3Na}$ − 2Na − NaHSO$_4$]$^{2-}$, 557.2 [M$_{3Na}$ − 2Na − 2CH$_3$COOH − C$_6$H$_9$O$_8$SNa (GlcOSO$_3$)]$^{2-}$.

3.3.7. Kuriloside J (7)

Colorless powder; $[\alpha]_D^{20}$ −10° (c 0.1, 50% MeOH). NMR: See Tables 6 and 7, Figures S48–S56. (−)HR-ESI-MS m/z: 1377.4687 (calc. 1377.4709) [M$_{2Na}$ − Na]$^-$, 677.2413 (calc. 677.2408) [M$_{2Na}$ − 2Na]$^{2-}$; (−)ESI-MS/MS m/z: 1317.4 [M$_{2Na}$ − Na − CH$_3$COOH]$^-$, 1257.4 [M$_{2Na}$ − Na − NaHSO$_4$]$^-$, 1197.5 [M$_{2Na}$ − Na − CH$_3$COOH − NaHSO$_4$]$^-$, 1155.4 [M$_{2Na}$ − Na − CH$_3$COOH − C$_6$H$_{10}$O$_5$(Glc)]$^-$, 1039.4 [M$_{2Na}$ − Na − CH$_3$COOH − C$_7$H$_{11}$O$_8$SNa(MeGlcOSO$_3$)]$^-$, 1009.4 [M$_{2Na}$ − Na − CH$_3$COOH − C$_6$H$_{10}$O$_5$(Glc) − C$_6$H$_{10}$O$_4$(Qui)]$^-$, 889.4 [M$_{2Na}$ − Na − NaHSO$_4$ − CH$_3$COOH − C$_6$H$_{10}$O$_5$(Glc) − C$_6$H$_{10}$O$_4$(Qui)]$^-$, 667.4 [M$_{2Na}$ − Na − C$_{26}$H$_{41}$O$_3$(Agl) − C$_6$H$_{10}$O$_5$(Glc) − C$_6$H$_{10}$O$_4$(Qui) − H]$^-$, 519.0 [M$_{2Na}$ − Na − C$_{26}$H$_{41}$O$_3$(Agl) − C$_6$H$_{10}$O$_5$(Glc) − C$_6$H$_{10}$O$_4$(Qui) − C$_5$H$_8$O$_4$(Xyl) − H]$^-$, 417.1 [M$_{2Na}$ − Na − C$_{26}$H$_{41}$O$_3$(Agl) − C$_6$H$_{10}$O$_5$ (Glc) − C$_6$H$_{10}$O$_4$ (Qui) − C$_5$H$_8$O$_4$ (Xyl) − NaHSO$_3$]$^-$.

3.3.8. Kuriloside K (8)

Colorless powder; $[\alpha]_D^{20}$ −7° (c 0.1, 50% MeOH). NMR: See Tables 5 and 8, Figures S57–S65. (−)HR-ESI-MS m/z: 1335.4573 (calc. 1335.4603) [M$_{2Na}$ − Na]$^-$, 656.2357 (calc. 656.2356) [M$_{2Na}$ − 2Na]$^{2-}$; (−)ESI-MS/MS m/z: 1215.4 [M$_{2Na}$ − Na − NaHSO$_4$]$^-$, 1159.4 [M$_{2Na}$ − Na − C$_7$H$_{12}$O$_5$(MeGlc)]$^-$, 1071.4 [M$_{2Na}$ − Na − C$_6$H$_9$O$_8$SNa(GlcOSO$_3$)]$^-$, 925.4 [M$_{2Na}$ − Na − C$_6$H$_9$O$_8$SNa (GlcOSO$_3$) − C$_6$H$_{10}$O$_4$ (Qui)]$^-$, 895.4 [M$_{2Na}$ − Na − C$_6$H$_9$O$_8$SNa(GlcOSO$_3$) − C$_7$H$_{12}$O$_5$(MeGlc)]$^-$, 713.3 [M$_{2Na}$ − Na − C$_{24}$H$_{39}$O$_2$(Agl) − C$_6$H$_9$O$_8$SNa(GlcOSO$_3$) − H]$^-$, 417.1 [M$_{2Na}$ − Na − C$_{24}$H$_{39}$O$_3$(Agl) − C$_6$H$_9$O$_8$SNa(GlcOSO$_3$) − C$_6$H$_{10}$O$_4$(Qui) − C$_5$H$_8$O$_4$(Xyl) − H]$^-$, 241.0 [M$_{Na}$ − Na − C$_{24}$H$_{39}$O$_3$(Agl) − C$_6$H$_9$O$_8$SNa(GlcOSO$_3$) − C$_6$H$_{10}$O$_4$(Qui) − C$_5$H$_8$O$_4$(Xyl) − C$_7$H$_{12}$O$_5$(MeGlc) − H]$^-$.

3.3.9. Kuriloside K$_1$ (9)

Colorless powder; $[\alpha]_D^{20}$ −4° (c 0.1, 50% MeOH). NMR: See Tables 7 and 8, Figures S66–S68. (−)HR-ESI-MS m/z: 1377.4723 (calc. 1377.4709) [M$_{2Na}$ − Na]$^-$, 677.2426 (calc. 677.2408) [M$_{2Na}$ − 2Na]$^{2-}$; (−)ESI-MS/MS m/z: 1317.4 [M$_{2Na}$ − Na − CH$_3$COOH]$^-$, 1197.5 [M$_{2Na}$ − Na − CH$_3$COOH − NaHSO$_4$]$^-$, 1069.5 [M$_{2Na}$ − Na − C$_6$H$_{10}$O$_5$ (Glc)]$^-$, 1053.4 [M$_{2Na}$ − Na − CH$_3$COOH − C$_6$H$_9$O$_8$SNa(GlcOSO$_3$)]$^-$, 877.4 [M$_{2Na}$ − Na − CH$_3$COOH − C$_6$H$_9$O$_8$SNa(GlcOSO$_3$) − C$_7$H$_{12}$O$_5$(MeGlc)]$^-$, 731.3 [M$_{2Na}$ − Na − CH$_3$COOH − C$_6$H$_9$O$_8$SNa(GlcOSO$_3$) − C$_7$H$_{12}$O$_5$(MeGlc) − C$_6$H$_{10}$O$_4$(Qui)]$^-$, 565.1 [M$_{2Na}$ − Na − C$_{26}$H$_{41}$O$_3$(Agl) − C$_6$H$_9$O$_8$SNa(GlcOSO$_3$) − C$_6$H$_{10}$O$_4$(Qui) − H]$^-$, 417.1 [M$_{2Na}$ − Na − C$_{26}$H$_{41}$O$_4$(Agl) − C$_6$H$_9$O$_8$SNa(GlcOSO$_3$) − C$_6$H$_{10}$O$_4$(Qui) − C$_5$H$_8$O$_4$(Xyl)]$^-$.

3.4. Cytotoxic Activity (MTT Assay)

All compounds (including cladoloside C used as the positive control) were tested in concentrations from 1.5 µM to 100 µM using two-fold dilution in dH$_2$O. The solutions (20 µL) of tested substances in different concentrations and cell suspension (180 µL) were added in wells of 96-well plates (1 × 10^4 cells/well) and incubated 24 h at 37 °C and 5% CO$_2$. After incubation, the medium with tested substances was replaced by 100 µL of fresh medium. Then, 10 µL of MTT (thiazoyl blue tertrazolium bromide) stock solution (5 mg/mL) was added to each well and the microplate was incubated for 4 h. After that, 100 µL of SDS-HCl solution (1 g SDS/10 mL dH$_2$O/17 µL 6 N HCl) was added to each well followed by incubation for 4–18 h. The absorbance of the converted dye formazan was measured using a Multiskan FC microplate photometer (Thermo Fisher Scientific, Waltham, MA, USA) at a wavelength of 570 nm. Cytotoxic activity of the substances was calculated as the concentration that caused 50% metabolic cell activity inhibition (IC_{50}). All the experiments were made in triplicate, $p < 0.01$.

3.5. Hemolytic Activity

Blood was taken from CD-1 mice (18–20 g). Erythrocytes were isolated from the blood of albino CD-1 mice by centrifugation with phosphate-buffered saline (pH 7.4) for 5 min at 4 °C by $450 \times g$ on a LABOFUGE 400R (Heraeus, Hanau, Germany) centrifuge for three times. Then, the residue of erythrocytes was resuspended in ice cold phosphate saline buffer (pH 7.4) to a final optical density of 1.5 at 700 nm, and kept on ice. For the hemolytic assay, 180 µL of erythrocyte suspension was mixed with 20 µL of test compound solution (including cladoloside C used as the positive control) in V-bottom 96-well plates. After 1 h of incubation at 37 °C, plates were exposed to centrifugation for 10 min at $900 \times g$ on a LMC-3000 (Biosan, Riga, Latvia) laboratory centrifuge. Then, we carefully selected 100 µL of supernatant and transferred it to new flat-plates respectively. Lysis of erythrocytes was determined by measuring the concentration of hemoglobin in the supernatant with a microplate photometer Multiskan FC (Thermo Fisher Scientific, Waltham, MA, USA), $\lambda = 570$ nm. The effective dose causing 50% hemolysis of erythrocytes (ED_{50}) was calculated using the computer program SigmaPlot 10.0. All experiments were made in triplicate, $p < 0.01$.

3.6. Solvolytic Desulfation

A part of the glycosidic sum (350 mg) was dissolved in a mixture of pyridine/dioxane (1/1) and refluxed for 1 h. The obtained mixture was concentrated in vacuo and subsequently purified by using Si gel column chromatography (as depicted in the Section 3.3).

4. Conclusions

Thus, nine unknown earlier triterpene glycosides were isolated from the sea cucumber *Thyonidium* (=*Duasmodactyla*) *kurilensis* in addition to the series of kurilosides found recently [19]. Five new types of the carbohydrate chains (kurilosides of the groups G–K) were discovered. There were trisulfated penta- (kurilosides of the group I (**5**, **6**)) and hexaosides (kuriloside H (**4**)) among them. Kuriloside H (**4**) is the second example of the most polar triterpene glycosides, along with tetrasulfated pentaosides found earlier in the sea cucumber *Psolus fabricii* [20]. The structures of disulfated hexa- and pentasaccharide chains of kurilosides of the groups G (**3**), J (**7**), and K (**8**, **9**) clearly illustrate a combinatorial (mosaic) type of biosynthesis of the glycosides, namely, the positions of the sulfate group attachment. At the same time, the position of one of the sulfate groups (at C(6) Glc, attached to C(4) Xyl1) remained the same in all glycosides found in this species. Three new non-holostane aglycones lacking a lactone ring, two of them being the 22,23,24,25,26,27-hexa-*nor*-lanostane type and one having a normal side chain, were found in glycosides **1–9**. The majority of the aglycones of *T. kurilensis* glycosides differed from each other in the substituents at C-16 (α- and β-oriented hydroxy- or acetoxy groups, or keto-group) and C-20 (hydroxy-, acetoxy-, or keto-groups), representing the biogenetically related rows of the compounds. As mentioned in a previous paper [19], the glycosides with 16α-substituents were isolated from *T. kurilensis* only. The finding of 16β-hydroxylated aglycones is also for the first time. Such compounds can be considered as "hot metabolites", biosynthetic intermediates or precursors of the aglycones with the 16β-acetoxy-group.

Supplementary Materials: The following are available online at https://www.mdpi.com/article/10.3390/md19040187/s1. Table S1. NMR spectrometric data of the carbohydrate moiety of kuriloside A_3 (**1**); Table S2. NMR spectrometric data of the aglycone moiety of kurilosides A_3 (**1**) and G (**3**); Table S3. NMR spectrometric data of the carbohydrate moiety of kuriloside D_1 (**2**); Table S4. NMR spectrometric data of the aglycone moiety of kurilosides H (**4**) and I_1 (**6**); Table S5. NMR spectrometric data of the carbohydrate moiety of DS-kuriloside L (**10**); Table S6. NMR spectrometric data of the aglycone moiety of **10**; Table S7. NMR spectrometric data of the carbohydrate moiety of DS-kuriloside M (**11**); Table S8. NMR spectrometric data of the aglycone moiety of **11**; Figure S1. ^{1}H NMR and ^{13}C NMR spectra of **1**; Figure S2. COSY spectrum of **1**; Figure S3. HSQC spectrum of **1**; Figure S4. ROESY spectrum of **1**; Figure S5. HMBC spectrum of **1**; Figure S6. HR-ESI-MS and ESI-MS/MS spectra of **1**; Figure S7. ^{13}C NMR spectrum of **2**; Figure S8. ^{1}H NMR spectrum of **2**; Figure S9. COSY spectrum of **2**; Figure S10. HSQC spectrum of **2**; Figure S11. HMBC spectrum of **2**; Figure S12. ROESY spectrum of **2**; Figure S13. HR-ESI-MS and ESI-MS/MS spectra of **2**; Figure S14. ^{13}C NMR spectrum of **3**; Figure S15. ^{1}H NMR spectrum of **3**; Figure S16. COSY spectrum of **3**; Figure S17. HSQC spectrum of **3**; Figure S18. HMBC spectrum of **3**; Figure S19. ROESY spectrum of **3**; Figure S20. 1 D TOCSY spectra of Xyl1, Qui2 and Glc3 of **3**; Figure S21. 1 D TOCSY spectra of the MeGlc4, Glc5 and MeGlc6 of **3**; Figure S22. HR-ESI-MS and ESI-MS/MS spectra of **3**; Figure S23. ^{13}C NMR spectrum of **4**; Figure S24. ^{1}H NMR spectrum of **4**; Figure S25. COSY spectrum of **4**; Figure S26. HSQC spectrum of **4**; Figure S27. ROESY spectrum of **4**; Figure S28. HMBC spectrum of **4**; Figure S29. 1 D TOCSY spectra of Xyl1, Qui2 and Glc3 of **4**; Figure S30. 1 D TOCSY spectra of Glc4 and MeGlc6 of **4**; Figure S31. HR-ESI-MS and ESI-MS/MS spectra of **4**; Figure S32. ^{13}C NMR spectrum of kuriloside I (**5**); Figure S33. ^{1}H NMR spectrum of **5**; Figure S34. COSY spectrum of **5**; Figure S35. HSQC spectrum of **5**; Figure S36. HMBC spectrum of **5**; Figure S37. ROESY spectrum of **5**; Figure S38. 1D TOCSY spectra of Xyl1, Qui2 and Glc3 of **5**; Figure S39. 1D TOCSY spectra of Glc4 and MeGlc5 of **5**; Figure S40. HR-ESI-MS and ESI-MS/MS spectra of **5**; Figure S41. ^{13}C NMR spectrum of **6**; Figure S42. ^{1}H NMR spectrum of **6**; Figure S43. COSY spectrum of **6**; Figure S44. HSQC spectrum of **6**; Figure S45. ROESY spectrum of **6**; Figure S46. HMBC spectrum of **6**; Figure S47. HR-ESI-MS and ESI-MS/MS spectra of **6**; Figure S48. ^{13}C NMR spectrum of kuriloside J (**7**); Figure S49. ^{1}H NMR spectrum of **7**; Figure S50. COSY spectrum of **7**; Figure S51. HSQC spectrum of **7**; Figure S52. HMBC spectrum of **7**; Figure S53. ROESY spectrum of **7**; Figure S54. 1 D TOCSY spectra of Xyl1, Qui2 and Glc3 of **7**; Figure S55. 1 D TOCSY spectra of Glc4 and MeGlc5 of **7**; Figure S56. HR-ESI-MS and ESI-MS/MS spectra of **7**; Figure S57. ^{13}C NMR spectrum of kuriloside K (**8**); Figure S58. ^{1}H NMR spectrum of **8**; Figure S59. COSY spectrum of **8**; Figure S60. HSQC spectrum of **8**; Figure S61. HMBC spectrum of **8**; Figure S62. ROESY spectrum of **8**; Figure S63. 1 D TOCSY spectra of Xyl1, Qui2 and Glc3 of **8**; Figure S64. 1 D TOCSY spectra of Glc4 and MeGlc5 of **8**; Figure S65. HR-ESI-MS and ESI-MS/MS spectra of **8**; Figure S66. ^{13}C NMR spectrum of **9**; Figure S67. ^{1}H NMR spectrum of **9** in; Figure S68. HR-ESI-MS and ESI-MS/MS spectra of **9**; Figure S69. ^{13}C NMR spectrum of DS-kuriloside L (**10**); Figure S70. ^{1}H NMR spectrum of **10**; Figure S71. COSY spectrum of **10**; Figure S72. HSQC spectrum of **10**; Figure S73. HMBC spectrum of **10**; Figure S74. ROESY spectrum of **10**; Figure S75. 1 D TOCSY spectra of Xyl1, Qui2 and Glc3 of **10**; Figure S76. HR-ESI-MS (−) and ESI-MS/MS spectra of **10**; Figure S77. ^{13}C NMR spectrum of DS-kuriloside M (**11**); Figure S78. ^{1}H NMR spectrum of **11**; Figure S79. COSY spectrum of **11**; Figure S80. HSQC spectrum of **11**; Figure S81. HMBC spectrum of **11**; Figure S82. ROESY spectrum of **11**; Figure S83. 1 D TOCSY spectra of Xyl1, Qui2 and Glc3 of **11**; Figure S84. 1 D TOCSY spectra of Glc4 and MeGlc5 of **11**; Figure S85. HR-ESI-MS (−), ESI-MS/MS spectra of **11**.

Author Contributions: Conceptualization, A.S.S. and V.I.K.; Methodology, A.S.S. and S.A.A.; Investigation, A.S.S., A.I.K., S.A.A., R.S.P., P.S.D., E.A.C. and P.V.A.; Writing—original draft preparation, A.S.S. and V.I.K.; Writing—review and editing, A.S.S. and V.I.K. All authors have read and agreed to the published version of the manuscript.

Funding: The investigation was carried out with the financial support of a grant from the Ministry of Science and Education, Russian Federation 13.1902.21.0012 (075-15-2020-796) (isolation of individual triterpene glycosides) and a grant from the Russian Foundation for Basic Research No. 19-04-000-14 (elucidation of structures of the glycosides and their biotesting).

Institutional Review Board Statement: The study was conducted according to the guidelines of the Declaration of Helsinki, and approved by the Ethics Committee of the Pacific Institute of Bioorganic Chemistry (Protocol No. 0085.19.10.2020).

Acknowledgments: The study was carried out on the equipment of the Collective Facilities Center "The Far Eastern Center for Structural Molecular Research (NMR/MS) PIBOC FEB RAS". The authors are very appreciative to Professor Valentin A. Stonik (PIBOC FEB RAS, Vladivostok, Russia) for reading and discussion of the manuscript.

Conflicts of Interest: The authors declare no conflict of interest.

References

1. Aminin, D.L.; Menchinskaya, E.S.; Pislyagin, E.A.; Silchenko, A.S.; Avilov, S.A.; Kalinin, V.I. Sea cucumber triterpene glyco-sides as anticancer agents. In *Studies in Natural Product Chemistry*; Atta-ur-Rahman, Ed.; Elsevier B.V.: Amsterdam, The Netherlands, 2016; Volume 49, pp. 55–105.
2. Khotimchenko, Y. Pharmacological Potential of Sea Cucumbers. *Int. J. Mol. Sci.* **2018**, *19*, 1342. [CrossRef]
3. Menchinskaya, E.; Gorpenchenko, T.; Silchenko, A.; Avilov, S.; Aminin, D. Modulation of Doxorubicin Intracellular Accumulation and Anticancer Activity by Triterpene Glycoside Cucumarioside A2-2. *Mar. Drugs* **2019**, *17*, 597. [CrossRef]
4. Pislyagin, E.A.; Menchinskaya, E.S.; Aminin, D.L.; Avilov, S.A.; Silchenko, A.S. Sulfated Glycosides from the Sea Cucumbers Block Ca2+ Flow in Murine Neuroblastoma Cells. *Nat. Prod. Commun.* **2018**, *13*, 953–956. [CrossRef]
5. Zhao, Y.-C.; Xue, C.-H.; Zhang, T.-T.; Wang, Y.-M. Saponins from Sea Cucumber and Their Biological Activities. *J. Agric. Food Chem.* **2018**, *66*, 7222–7237. [CrossRef] [PubMed]
6. Gomes, A.R.; Freitas, A.C.; Duarte, A.C.; Rocha-Santos, T.A.P. Echinoderms: A review of bioactive compounds with poten-tial health effects. In *Studies in Natural Products Chemistry*; Atta-ur-Rachman, Ed.; Esevier Science B.V.: Amsterdam, The Netherlands, 2016; Volume 49, pp. 1–54.
7. Omran, N.E.; Salem, H.K.; Eissa, S.H.; Kabbash, A.M.; Kandeil, M.A.; Salem, M.A. Chemotaxonomic study of the most abundant Egyptian sea-cucumbers using ultra-performance liquid chromatography (UPLC) coupled to high-resolution mass spectrometry (HRMS). *Chemoecology* **2020**, *30*, 35–48. [CrossRef]
8. Kalinin, V.I.; Silchenko, A.S.; Avilov, S.A. Taxonomic significance and ecological role of triterpene glycosides from holothu-rians. *Biol. Bull.* **2016**, *43*, 532–540. [CrossRef]
9. Silchenko, A.S.; Kalinovsky, A.I.; Avilov, S.A.; Adnryjaschenko, P.V.; Dmitrenok, P.S.; Kalinin, V.I.; Martyyas, E.A.; Minin, K.V. Fallaxosides C1, C2, D1 and D2, unusual oligosulfated triterpene glycosides from the sea cucumber Cucumaria fallax (Cu-cumariidae, Dendrochirotida, Holothurioidea) and a taxonomic stratus of this animal. *Nat. Prod. Commun.* **2016**, *11*, 939–945.
10. Kalinin, V.I.; Avilov, S.A.; Silchenko, A.S.; Stonik, V.A. Triterpene Glycosides of Sea Cucumbers (Holothuroidea, Echinodermata) as Taxonomic Markers. *Nat. Prod. Commun.* **2015**, *10*, 21–26. [CrossRef]
11. Kamyab, E.; Rohde, S.; Kellermann, M.Y.; Schupp, P.J. Chemical Defense Mechanisms and Ecological Implications of Indo-Pacific Holothurians. *Molecules* **2020**, *25*, 4808. [CrossRef]
12. Kamyab, E.; Goebeler, N.; Kellermann, M.Y.; Rohde, S.; Reverter, M.; Striebel, M.; Schupp, P.J. Anti-Fouling Effects of Saponin-Containing Crude Extracts from Tropical Indo-Pacific Sea Cucumbers. *Mar. Drugs* **2020**, *18*, 181. [CrossRef]
13. Popov, R.S.; Ivanchina, N.V.; Silchenko, A.S.; Avilov, S.A.; Kalinin, V.I.; Dolmatov, I.Y.; Stonik, V.A.; Dmitrenok, P.S. Me-tabolite profiling of triterpene glycosides of the Far Eastern sea cucumber Eupentacta fraudatrix and their distribution in va-rious body components using LC-ESI QTOF-MS. *Mar. Drugs* **2017**, *14*, 302.
14. Park, J.-I.; Bae, H.-R.; Kim, C.G.; Stonik, V.A.; Kwak, J.Y. Relationships between chemical structures and functions of triter-pene glycosides isolated from sea cucumbers. *Front. Chem.* **2014**, *2*, 77. [CrossRef]
15. Caulier, G.; Flammang, P.; Gerbaux, P.; Eeckhaut, I. When a repellent became an attractant: Harmful saponins are kairo-mones attracting the symbiotic Harlequin crab. *Sci. Rep.* **2013**, *3*, 2639. [CrossRef]
16. Claereboudt, E.J.S.; Caulier, G.; DeCroo, C.; Colson, E.; Gerbaux, P.; Claereboudt, M.R.; Schaller, H.; Flammang, P.; Deleu, M.; Eeckhaut, I. Triterpenoids in Echinoderms: Fundamental Differences in Diversity and Biosynthetic Pathways. *Mar. Drugs* **2019**, *17*, 352. [CrossRef]
17. Kalinin, V.I.; Silchenko, A.S.; Avilov, S.A.; Stonik, V.A. Non-holostane aglycones of sea cucumber triterpene glycosides. Structure, biosynthesis, evolution. *Steroids* **2019**, *147*, 42–51. [CrossRef]
18. Silchenko, A.S.; Kalinovsky, A.I.; Avilov, S.A.; Andryjashchenko, P.V.; Dmitrenok, P.S.; Kalinin, V.I.; Stonik, V.A. 3β-O-Glycosylated 16β-acetoxy-9β-H-lanosta-7,24-diene-3β,18,20β-triol, an intermediate metabolite from the sea cucumber Eupentacta fraudatrix and its biosynthetic significance. *Biochem. Syst. Ecol.* **2012**, *44*, 53–60. [CrossRef]
19. Silchenko, A.S.; Kalinovsky, A.I.; Avilov, S.A.; Andrijaschenko, P.V.; Popov, R.S.; Dmitrenok, P.S.; Chingizova, E.A.; Kali-nin, V.I. Kurilosides A1, A2, C1, D, E and F—triterpene glycosides from the Far Eastern sea cucumber Thyonidium (=Duasmodactyla) kurilensis (Levin): Structures with unusual non-holostane aglycones and cytotoxicities. *Mar. Drugs* **2020**, *18*, 551. [CrossRef]
20. Silchenko, A.S.; Kalinovsky, A.I.; Avilov, S.A.; Kalinin, V.I.; Andrijaschenko, P.V.; Dmitrenok, P.S.; Popov, R.S.; Chingizova, E.A. Structures and Bioactivities of Psolusosides B1, B2, J, K, L, M, N, O, P, and Q from the Sea Cucumber Psolus fabricii. The First Finding of Tetrasulfated Marine Low Molecular Weight Metabolites. *Mar. Drugs* **2019**, *17*, 631. [CrossRef]
21. Avilov, S.A.; Kalinovskii, A.I. New triterpene aglycone from the holothurian Duasmodactyla kurilensis. *Chem. Nat. Compd.* **1989**, *25*, 309–311. [CrossRef]
22. Avilov, S.A.; Kalinovskii, A.I.; Stonik, V.A. Two new triterpene glycosides from the holothurian Duasmodactyla kurilensis. *Chem. Nat. Compd.* **1991**, *27*, 188–192. [CrossRef]
23. Silchenko, A.S.; Kalinovsky, A.I.; Avilov, S.A.; Andryjaschenko, P.V.; Dmitrenok, P.S.; Yurchenko, E.A.; Dolmatov, I.Y.; Kalinin, V.I.; Stonik, V.A. Structure and Biological Action of Cladolosides B1, B2, C, C1, C2 and D, Six New Triterpene Glycosides from the Sea Cucumber Cladolabes schmeltzii. *Nat. Prod. Commun.* **2013**, *8*, 1527–1534. [CrossRef]
24. Aminin, D.; Pislyagin, E.; Astashev, M.; Es'Kov, A.; Kozhemyako, V.; Avilov, S.; Zelepuga, E.; Yurchenko, E.; Kaluzhskiy, L.; Kozlovskaya, E.; et al. Glycosides from edible sea cucumbers stimulate macrophages via purinergic receptors. *Sci. Rep.* **2016**, *6*, 39683. [CrossRef]

25. Isaeva, M.P.; Likhatskaya, G.N.; Guzev, K.V.; Baldaev, S.N.; Bystritskaya, E.P.; Stonik, V.A. Molecular cloning of sea cu-cumber oxidosqualene cyclases. Вестник Дальневосточного отделения Российскойакадемии наук **2018**, *6*, 84–85.
26. Liu, H.; Kong, X.; Chen, J.; Zhang, H. De novo sequencing and transcriptome analysis of Stichpous horrens to reveal genes related to biosynthesis of triterpenoids. *Aquaculture* **2018**, *491*, 358–367. [CrossRef]
27. Li, Y.; Wang, R.; Xun, X.; Wang, J.; Bao, L.; Thimmappa, R.; Ding, J.; Jiang, J.; Zhang, L.; Li, T.; et al. Sea cucumber genome provides insights into saponin biosynthesis and aestivation regulation. *Cell Discov.* **2018**, *4*, 85–86. [CrossRef]
28. Cuong, N.X.; Vien, L.T.; Hoang, L.; Hanh, T.T.H.; Thao, D.T.; Thann, N.V.; Nam, N.H.; Thung, D.C.; Kiem, P.V.; Minh, C.V. Cytotoxic triterpene glycosides from the sea cucumber Stichopus horrens. *Bioorganic Med. Chem. Lett.* **2017**, *27*, 2939–2942. [CrossRef] [PubMed]
29. Vien, L.T.; Hoang, L.; Hanh, T.T.H.; Van Thanh, N.; Cuong, N.X.; Nam, N.H.; Thung, D.C.; Van Kiem, P.; Van Minh, C. Triterpene tetraglycosides from the sea cucumber Stichopus horrens. *Nat. Prod. Res.* **2017**, *32*, 1039–1043. [CrossRef]
30. Maltsev, I.; Stonik, V.; Kalinovsky, A.; Elyakov, G. Triterpene glycosides from sea cucumber Stichopus japonicus Selenka. *Comp. Biochem. Physiol. Part B Comp. Biochem.* **1984**, *78*, 421–426. [CrossRef]
31. Zhang, X.-M.; Li, X.-B.; Zhang, S.-S.; He, Q.-X.; Hou, H.-R.; Dang, L.; Guo, J.-L.; Chen, Y.-F.; Yu, T.; Peng, D.-J.; et al. LC-MS/MS Identification of Novel Saponins from the Viscera of Sea Cucumber Apostichopus japonicus. *Chem. Nat. Compd.* **2018**, *54*, 721–725. [CrossRef]

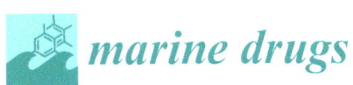

Review

Application of MS-Based Metabolomic Approaches in Analysis of Starfish and Sea Cucumber Bioactive Compounds

Roman S. Popov *, Natalia V. Ivanchina and Pavel S. Dmitrenok *

G.B. Elyakov Pacific Institute of Bioorganic Chemistry, Far Eastern Branch of Russian Academy of Sciences, 159 Prospect 100-let Vladivostoku, Vladivostok 690022, Russia; ivanchina@piboc.dvo.ru
* Correspondence: popov_rs@piboc.dvo.ru (R.S.P.); paveldmt@piboc.dvo.ru (P.S.D.); Tel.: +7-423-231-1132 (P.S.D.)

Abstract: Today, marine natural products are considered one of the main sources of compounds for drug development. Starfish and sea cucumbers are potential sources of natural products of pharmaceutical interest. Among their metabolites, polar steroids, triterpene glycosides, and polar lipids have attracted a great deal of attention; however, studying these compounds by conventional methods is challenging. The application of modern MS-based approaches can help to obtain valuable information about such compounds. This review provides an up-to-date overview of MS-based applications for starfish and sea cucumber bioactive compounds analysis. While describing most characteristic features of MS-based approaches in the context of starfish and sea cucumber metabolites, including sample preparation and MS analysis steps, the present paper mainly focuses on the application of MS-based metabolic profiling of polar steroid compounds, triterpene glycosides, and lipids. The application of MS in metabolomics studies is also outlined.

Keywords: starfish; sea cucumber; polyhydroxysteroids; triterpene glycosides; steroid glycosides; lipids; mass spectrometry; metabolomics; metabolomic profiling

Citation: Popov, R.S.; Ivanchina, N.V.; Dmitrenok, P.S. Application of MS-Based Metabolomic Approaches in Analysis of Starfish and Sea Cucumber Bioactive Compounds. *Mar. Drugs* 2022, 20, 320. https://doi.org/10.3390/md20050320

Academic Editor: Espen Hansen

Received: 19 April 2022
Accepted: 11 May 2022
Published: 12 May 2022

Publisher's Note: MDPI stays neutral with regard to jurisdictional claims in published maps and institutional affiliations.

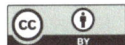

Copyright: © 2022 by the authors. Licensee MDPI, Basel, Switzerland. This article is an open access article distributed under the terms and conditions of the Creative Commons Attribution (CC BY) license (https://creativecommons.org/licenses/by/4.0/).

1. Introduction

The emergence of novel diseases and resistant forms of known diseases in recent years and the emergence of multidrug-resistant pathogens has led to a renewed interest in the exploration of new sources of bioactive compounds. The sea environment possesses extraordinary ecological variety, and its inhabitants exhibit enormous biochemical diversity. At present, over 29,000 marine natural products have been discovered [1–4]. To date, several dozen marine natural products or their derivatives have been approved as therapeutic agents or are undergoing Phase III, II, or I drug development [5]. As the biodiversity of marine organisms is higher than that of terrestrial plants and animals, and as only a minor portion of metabolites present in marine species has been studied, it can be assumed that the number of new marine compounds will continue to increase, providing new therapeutic alternatives.

Marine invertebrates have long been considered an inexhaustible source of novel natural products. Although Porifera and Cnidaria are the two major sources of new marine natural products, Echinodermata is viewed as another abundant source of new bioactive compounds. Over the past five years, just over two hundred new compounds have been isolated from echinoderms [1–4,6]. The phylum Echinodermata includes about 7500 species found in all seas at every depth, from intertidal to abyssal, and in all ecosystems, from coral reefs to shallow shores. Echinoderms are divided into five different taxonomic classes, including Asteroidea (starfish) and Holothuroidea (sea cucumbers).

Starfish and sea cucumbers are extensively employed in traditional medicine, being a rich source of bioactive compounds. Several starfish species are used to treat rheumatism or as tonics in traditional Chinese medicine [7,8]. Sea cucumbers are one of the most valuable aquaculture species in China, Korea, and Japan, as well as other countries, where they are used as functional foods. Traditional medicine in China and other countries in Asia and the Middle East uses sea cucumbers widely to treat a broad range of diseases, including asthma, arthritis, hypertension, and kidney disease [9,10].

Unique pharmacological properties, including anticancer, antioxidant, antithrombotic, and immunostimulating activities, among others, are associated with bioactive starfish and sea cucumber compounds [11–15]. Moreover, the secondary metabolites of sea cucumbers affect the biological clock and circadian rhythm of lipid metabolism [16], reduce fat accumulation [17], and protect against high fat diet-induced metabolic disorders in mice [18]. Extracts of certain specimens may accelerate wound healing and tissue regeneration [19].

The distinctive chemical composition of starfish and sea cucumbers seems to be the main reason for these beneficial properties. Starfish and sea cucumbers are high in valuable nutrients such as vitamins, minerals, and metabolites such as peptides, sterols, phenolics, sphingolipids, glycosaminoglycans, sulfated polysaccharides, and lectins [10]. Among these compounds the most exciting are unique polar steroid compounds and triterpene glycosides, which are characteristic of starfish and sea cucumbers. These compounds have unusual chemical structures and demonstrate a variety of biological effects, such as cytotoxic, antifungal, antiviral, antibacterial, anti-inflammatory, analgesic, ichthyotoxic, hemolytic, anti-biofouling, anticancer, immunomodulating, and neuritogenic actions [12,20–33].

Secondary metabolites are usually present in the extracts of starfish and sea cucumbers as complex mixtures of very similar compounds. Conventional methods for the structural study of bioactive compounds are usually time-consuming and labor-intensive procedures that include the isolation of individual compounds by a combination of chromatographic techniques and structure elucidation through a combination of different methods [20]. The final structure confirmation of a new compound is always performed with a set of independent methods, such as nuclear magnetic resonance (NMR) spectroscopy, mass spectrometry (MS), or other analytical methods and chemical transformation. Despite the instrumentation developments of recent years, the analysis of bioactive natural compounds using conventional approaches remains a challenging task due to the difficulty of isolating individual compounds from fractions consisting of many components and with high chemical diversity covering a broad concentration range. As a result, only certain compounds can be described; overall, the entire metabolite pool remains poorly studied.

At present, modern mass spectrometry techniques are widely employed for the identification and structural analysis of novel natural compounds [34–36]. Hyphenated techniques combining various separation methods with mass spectrometry are applied for metabolomic and target profiling and allow for the characterization of compounds in complex mixtures extracted from biological material. Different MS-imaging techniques precisely localize and quantify the metabolites in tissues [37]. Recently developed ion mobility (IM) methods add dimension to conventional chromatography separation, allowing the stereoisomers that cannot be separated by liquid chromatography (LC) to be identified [38].

Mass spectrometry is used in various fields of marine sciences today, including marine proteomics [39], metabolomics [40,41], lipidomics [42], marine toxicology [43], ecology studies [44], and others. The introduction of modern mass-spectrometric approaches has greatly contributed to the development of metabolomics as a transdisciplinary science that aims at the qualitative and quantitative determination of the whole metabolite pool of organisms. Although no single analytical method exists that can determine all members of the metabolome simultaneously, MS-based metabolomics has been successfully applied to analyze a wide range of compounds from various sources. In recent years, MS-based metabolomics has emerged as a useful tool in natural product research. In addition to metabolic fingerprinting, two approaches used in metabolomics studies can be distinguished [45]. The first, metabolic profiling, focuses on the analysis of structure-related metabolites or metabolites related to a specific metabolic pathway. Such an approach provides information on the chemical composition of extracts or fractions and allows for the dereplication of known bioactive compounds and detection of new compounds as well as the evaluation of the their isolation possibility [34]. The metabolome-oriented approach aims to detect differences in metabolic profiles that occur in response to stress, disease, changing environmental conditions, or other influences in comparative experiments.

Metabolomic studies of marine organisms is a field that uses a variety of modern approaches, including MS, NMR methods, and hyphenated techniques [40,41,44]. This review focuses on the use of MS-based metabolomics techniques applied in studies of extracts and fractions of starfish and sea cucumber bioactive compounds. The following section provides a general overview of the characteristic features in workflows, including sample preparation and analytical approaches. Section 3 includes illustrative examples of MS-based applications in the analysis of bioactive compounds such as polar steroids, triterpene glycosides, cerebroside, and ganglioside, as well as examples of the multi-class approach application. Instrumental and methodological details are highlighted and summarized in tables (Table 1, Table 2, Tables S1 and S2). Section 4 reviews the recently published advances in the field of metabolome-oriented studies of starfish and sea cucumbers.

2. Overview of MS-Based Metabolomic Workflows in the Analysis of Starfish and Sea Cucumber Bioactive Compounds

In terms of workflow, a typical MS-based metabolomic study involves the stages of sample collection, extraction, fractionation and/or purification, measurement, identification, and analysis of the results (Figure 1). The analytical protocols used in MS-based marine metabolomics have several important differences from those used to analyze the metabolites of terrestrial animals and plants [41]. This section discusses the characteristic features of MS-based metabolomic approaches in the context of starfish and sea cucumber bioactive compounds, including steps of sample preparation, acquisition, and analysis.

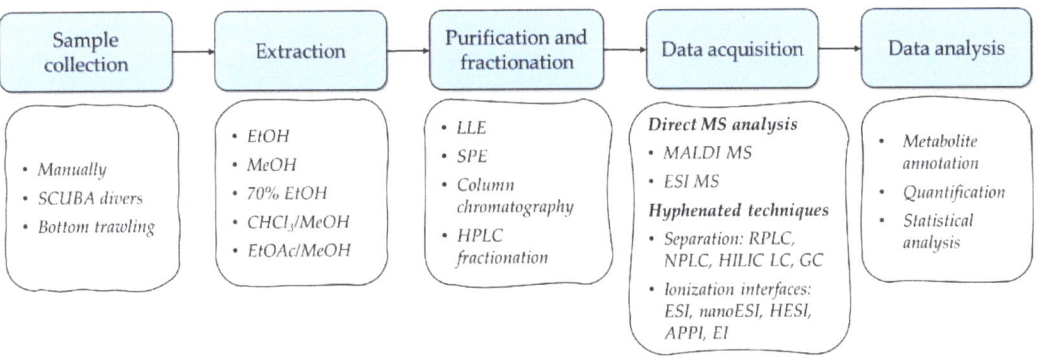

Figure 1. Main research stages in MS-based metabolomics studies of starfish and sea cucumber bioactive compounds.

2.1. Sample Preparation

The sample preparation stage, which comprises sample collection and extraction, is the most important in metabolomics research. Most of the studied starfish and sea cucumbers are collected from the coastal area manually or by SCUBA divers, or, if the depth exceeds 30 m, by bottom trawling. The main difficulties encountered in the collection of echinoderms are related to accessibility and their limited quantity. Many starfish and sea cucumbers are common species found in coastal areas where collection is unproblematic, while others occur in restricted or inaccessible geographic areas or in limited populations. Certain sea cucumber species, such as *Apostichopus japonicus* and *Holothuria scabra*, are aquaculture species, making their collection much simpler than the collection of wild specimens. In contrast to terrestrial ecosystems, when collecting marine samples the depth, salinity, and oxygen concentration of the water must be considered in addition to general factors such as temperature and light. A specimen's location, physiological state, sex, and season can have a great metabolic influence. Difficulties are often caused by significant distances between the collection site and the laboratory, which requires more complicated logistics and specific sample preparation protocols.

Stress caused by handling induces responses in animals at the biochemical level [46] and can cause sea cucumber evisceration, the expulsion of the internal organs from the body [47]. To avoid such changes, as well as metabolomic changes resulting from enzymatic turnover during transportation or sample processing, it is highly recommended to quench the metabolism rapidly [48]. There are protocols designed for quenching, including flash-freezing using liquid nitrogen or dry ice, lyophilization, and freeze-drying; however, some of these are difficult to implement when animals are collected in the wild. Therefore, in most cases researchers use alternative protocols such as freezing or direct extraction with organic solvents [41].

The collected sample material must be processed to extract the metabolites of interest and remove salts and impurities. Extractions with organic solvents are commonly used for this purpose. Due to the high chemical diversity of metabolites, there is no single solvent capable of capturing all the required compounds without related impurities and contaminants. Generally, polar and semi-polar metabolites such as triterpene glycosides, asterosaponins, and gangliosides are preferentially extracted with hydro-alcoholic solutions, while lipid, sterol, terpene, and other non-polar compound extraction can be achieved with hydrophobic solvents (chloroform, hexane) or liquid–liquid extraction (LLE) by Folch's [49] and Bligh and Dyer's [50] methods. Extraction with methyl tert-butyl ether (MTBE) [51] can be used for the recovery of both polar and non-polar metabolites into separate fractions. In addition, the selected extraction protocols and solvents must be related to the analytical methods used.

It should be noted that most starfish and sea cucumber extracts contain significant amounts of salts, even if a non-polar solvent is used for extraction. Such samples are incompatible with analytical techniques such as mass spectrometry and NMR because of the effect of salts on analytical performance. For example, the presence of a small concentration of NaCl can cause the appearance of unexpected adducts at ESI MS, while larger concentrations can suppress analyte ionization and lead to salt crystal deposits in the ion source and the capillary, which can cause the instrument malfunction. MALDI MS is more tolerant to salt impurities and can be used for preliminary screening of extracts without additional purification. Desalting of marine extracts typically involves column chromatography (CC), liquid–liquid extraction, and solid-phase extraction (SPE).

Another problem can be the presence of lipid impurities and/or proteins in samples of polar secondary metabolites. For example, when extracting starfish polar steroid compounds or sea cucumber triterpene glycosides the crude hydro-alcoholic extracts may contain a large concentration of phospholipids, which can complicate chromatographic separations and suppress the ionization of the target analytes. If lipid compounds are not included in the target pool, additional purification of the extract can improve both LC separation and MS identification of target analytes. In order to remove such interfering compounds, column chromatography with Amberlite XAD-4, Sephadex LH-60, or other sorbents, LLE or SPE is usually used. In order to simplify the analysis of extremely complex extracts and obtain a mixture containing only structure-related metabolites of interest, fractionation using column chromatography, flash chromatography, or HPLC is used.

The choice of extraction solvent and purification methods affects the efficiency of the sample preparation stage. The use of unsuitable solvents and extraction methods can result in quantitatively and qualitatively incomplete extraction, while the use of suboptimal purification or fractionation procedures can lead to loss of the target metabolites. To the best of our knowledge, there are no published studies comparing the effectiveness of the most commonly used sample preparation protocols for the analysis of starfish and sea cucumber bioactive compounds.

2.2. Data Acquisition

Structural elucidation of starfish and sea cucumber bioactive compounds remains a difficult task due to the great diversity of these compounds and the complexity of the analyzed mixtures. Usually, these compounds form very complicated mixtures which are difficult to separate into pure compounds by chromatography. In the past, the application of chemical methods was required in order to identify the structure of such compounds. In particular, acid hydrolysis was used to recognize steroid and triterpene glycoside structures. While this approach allowed the partial characterization of aglycon structures and the determination of qualitative and quantitative monosaccharide composition, the destruction of native aglycon was frequent.

For a long time, electron ionization (EI) was the only possible mass spectrometry technique. Rashkes et al. carried out mass spectrometry research on six polyhydroxysteroid compounds and glycosides isolated from the Far Eastern starfish *Patiria pectinifera* and determined the characteristic fragmentation pattern of starfish polyhydroxysteroid under EI conditions [52]. EI and GC-EI MS were widely used for the determination of structures of aglycones and oligosaccharide chains of asterosaponins and triterpene glycosides after hydrolysis of glycosides and chemical derivatization of monosaccharides [20]. GC coupled with EI MS remains one of the most suitable metabolomic techniques for analyzing the wide range of volatile, semi-volatile non-polar compounds and derivatized polar metabolites. Electron impact ionization results in highly reproducible fragmentation patterns that can be used for identification by database search along with retention times indexes.

The application of fast atom bombardment (FAB) MS allows for analysis of the more polar and unstable compounds. Introduced in 1983, FAB has been successfully used for the determination of the structures of starfish steroid glycosides and sea cucumber triterpene glycosides as well as cerebrosides and gangliosides, which could not be analyzed by EI MS [53]. FAB mass spectra of starfish and sea cucumber glycosides can show molecular ions as well as fragmentation products, providing information about molecular formulae, the presence and location of sulfate groups, the structures of carbohydrate chains, and aglycon. Collision-induced dissociation (CID) experiments can provide additional structural information on the structural features of aglycon, the quantity and type of monosaccharides attached to aglycon, and their location.

Electrospray ionization (ESI) and Matrix-Assisted Laser Desorption/Ionization (MALDI) have significantly expanded the possibilities of mass spectrometry for the analysis of natural products. ESI has had an enormous impact on the analysis of polar and non-volatile molecules as well as large biomolecules. In contrast to electron ionization, in-source fragmentation under ESI conditions is practically unrealized; tandem MS methods are used to initiate the fragmentation of these ions. ESI mass spectrometry is currently the most common ionization technique; it has been widely used for the characterization of natural compounds, including steroid and triterpene glycosides, polar lipids, and other compounds from purified starfish and sea cucumber extracts. MALDI MS is another efficient method for the analysis of natural compounds. The necessity of using matrices and the presence of matrix ion peaks at spectra in the low mass range are drawbacks; however, due to its high sensitivity, high speed of analysis, and tolerance to inorganic salts impurities, MALDI MS is widely used for rapid screening and chemical characterization of complex mixtures. Recent advances in analytical techniques, including high-resolution time-of-flight (TOF), Fourier transform (FT), and Orbitrap mass analyzers have high scan speeds along with extended dynamic range and sensitivity, allowing for the development of hybrid instruments and new ionization interfaces such as nanoelectrospray (nanoESI) and heated electrospray ionization (HESI) and leading to the establishment of high-throughput protocols for the analysis of the most complex mixtures of natural compounds. The development of hyphenated techniques combining liquid chromatography or gas chromatography with mass spectrometry (LC-MS or GC-MS) makes allows for straightforward analysis of the compounds present in complicated extracts.

2.3. Data Analysis

Data analysis is the next important stage of MS-based research. Generally, the processing of data obtained using chromatography-MS methods has included the steps of identifying *m/z* signals, chromatographic peak detection, filtering, alignment, and identification [54]. Many freely available (XCMS [55], MZmine 2 [56], OpenMS [57], and MS-DIAL [58]) and commercial software tools are currently available for the processing of LC-MS and GC-MS data. While the processing of GC-MS data is well-established and relatively simple, the results are usually limited to known compounds presented in databases. LC-MS is a more versatile method, covering broad chemistries and sensitivity ranges, although it produces more complex data. Due to the lower resolution and reproducibility of LC separation and the presence of adduct, isotope, fragment, and contamination peaks in ESI spectra, LC-MS data processing is much more difficult.

In certain cases, special approaches are useful for data processing. In order to process MS profiling data, methods based on scanning neutral losses, characteristic fragments, and an in-house library for rapid screening of the compounds of interest are often used. For example, the construction of ion chromatograms for negative fragment ions at m/z 96.96 can be used for detecting sulfated compounds like asterosaponins and sulfated triterpene glycosides, and cerebrosides can be detected according to the neutral loss fragments of 180 Da [59].

Similar to common metabolomic studies, metabolite identification is a current bottleneck in the analysis of starfish and sea cucumber metabolites. Chromatography-MS-based analysis can result in a huge number of peaks that are extremely difficult to identify. Even when analyzing well-studied organisms, only small percentages of the data collected in a typical LC-MS experiment can be matched to known molecules [60]. The chemical composition of starfish and sea cucumbers remains poorly investigated and the percentage of identified compounds can be extremely low. According to Metabolomics Standards Initiative recommendations, high identification confidence can be obtained by comparing an accurate high-resolution monoisotopic mass, MS/MS spectra, and retention times with data from an authentic chemical standard [61]. However, the available libraries of certified standards do not cover the entire scope of biochemical diversity, especially in the area of marine bioactive compounds. Although only putative annotation is possible without matching experimental data to data for authentic chemical standards [61], the availability of comprehensive open-access databases is extremely important for the successful application of mass spectrometry to the analysis of complex mixtures of natural compounds. Existing databases cover various natural compounds [62], and several databases, such as the GNPS database [63], MassBank [64], Metlin [65], the Human Metabolome Database [66], and MassBank of North America (https://mona.fiehnlab.ucdavis.edu, accessed on 1 April 2022) include MS/MS spectra of natural compounds from different sources. Databases such as the Dictionary of Marine Natural Products (https://dmnp.chemnetbase.com, accessed on 1 April 2022) and MarinLit (https://marinlit.rsc.org, accessed on 1 April 2022) include structural information, and the NMR and UV spectra of marine-derived compounds, although MS and MS/MS data on marine natural compounds in all existing databases is extremely limited. There are currently no databases covering taxonomic, structural, and experimental mass spectrometry data on bioactive metabolites of marine echinoderms.

Moreover, unlike peptides, oligosaccharides, and lipids, the MS fragmentation of most secondary metabolites is less studied due to the vast structural variability, and the de novo identification of metabolites by MS/MS spectra is very difficult. Several computational approaches based on machine learning or quantum chemistry calculations have been proposed for the in silico generation of MS/MS spectra or the prediction of structural features of compounds based on the experimental MS/MS spectra [67,68]. The molecular networking approach is based on the clustering of detected compounds by the similarity of their MS/MS spectra and allows for the annotation of related metabolites [63]. Using models for the in silico prediction of LC retention times can help to improve the reliability of identification in metabolomics analysis [69]. However, despite the recent advances in computational approaches, the currently used algorithms need to be significantly improved before effective identification and structural elucidation of marine bioactive compounds is possible. Along with the huge degree of structural variability, these issues limit the application of MS for annotation, dereplication, and structural elucidation in studies of metabolites from marine organisms.

In the case of research aimed at discovering metabolomic alterations between distinct biological groups of organisms, the statistical analysis is applied to the peak lists obtained after the processing of MS data. The choice of statistical methods is often determined by the study design, and can be divided into univariate (*t*-test, analysis of variance (ANOVA), fold-change analysis) and multivariate (unsupervised Principal Component Analysis (PCA) and supervised Partial Least Squares Discriminant Analysis (PLS-DA)) methods of analysis. Generally, the statistical methods used in the analysis of starfish and sea cucumber metabolites are the same as those used for conventional metabolomics studies, which are thoroughly discussed in [70]. Tables S1–S3 provide a general overview of the statistical approaches used for the treatment of analytical data in research on starfish and sea cucumber bioactive compounds.

3. MS-Based Metabolomic Profiling Approaches to the Study of Starfish and Sea Cucumber Bioactive Compounds

3.1. Starfish Polar Steroid Compounds

Unlike other echinoderms, starfish are characterized by a wide variety of steroid compounds, both non-polar sterols and polar steroid compounds. The latter form a large group of biologically active compounds, including polyhydroxysteroids, related glycosides, and steroid oligoglycosides (asterosaponins) (Figure 2). Starfish polyhydroxysteroids are steroid compounds, and usually contain from four to nine hydroxy groups in a steroidal nucleus and side chain. Polyhydroxylated glycosides have one, two, or rarely three monosaccharides attached to a steroid moiety, either to side chains or to the steroid nucleus and side chain simultaneously. The most common sugar residues in these compounds are xylose or its derivatives and arabinose. Polyhydroxylated glycosides have been found in both sulfated and non-sulfated forms. A characteristic feature of the asterosaponins is the 3β,6α-dihydroxysteroid aglycon with a 9(11)-double bond and a sulfate group at C-3. The asterosaponin carbohydrate chain consists of four to six sugars and is attached to C-6. The oligosaccharide chain of pentaosides contains one branching at the second monosaccharide, while hexaosides can have one or two branches at the second and third monosaccharide residues of the chain. Hexoses (glucose, galactose), pentoses (arabinose, xylose), and deoxyhexoses (fucose, quinovose) are the most common sugar residues in asterosaponins. Monosaccharides in asterosaponins are always in pyranose forms and are connected, as a rule, by β-glycosidic bonds (Figure 2).

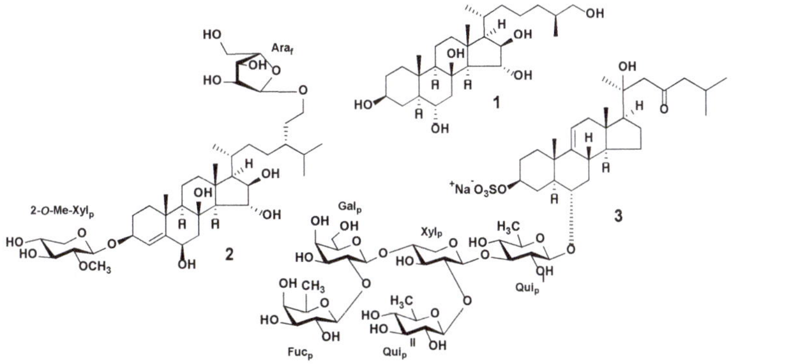

Figure 2. The structures of typical starfish polyhydroxysteroid (5α-cholestane-3β,6α,8,15α,16β,26-hexaol (**1**) from the starfish *Protoreaster nodosus* [71]), a glycoside of polyhydroxysteroid (linckoside

A (**2**) from the starfish *Linckia laevigata* [72]), and asterosaponin (thornasteroside A (**3**) from the starfish *Acanthaster planci* [73]).

Demonstrating significant structural diversity, individual representatives of starfish polar steroids show a variety of biological effects including cytotoxic, neuritogenic hemolytic, antibacterial, antiviral, and anti-inflammatory effects [12,20,27–31]. Several starfish polar steroids are promising antitumor and cancer-preventing agents [14]. A recent study has reported that starfish polar steroids in combination with X-ray radiation affect colony formation and apoptosis induction in human colorectal carcinoma cells [74]. Starfish polar steroids have shown a combined anticancer effect with alga polysaccharides on human cell lines in models of 2D and 3D cultures [75,76].

ESI and MALDI are currently the most suitable and widely used ionization techniques for analyzing starfish polar steroids (Table 1). Typically, starfish sulfated steroid glycosides are detected as $[M + Na]^+$ and $[M - Na]^-$ ions in the positive and negative ion modes of ESI MS, respectively. Non-sulfated polyhydroxysteroids and related glycosides are usually revealed as $[M - H]^-$ and $[M + Cl]^-$ ions in the negative ion mode and as $[M + Na]^+$ ions in the positive ion mode. Although both positive and negative ion mass spectra are good enough to characterize all types of glycosides, the negative ion mode contains peaks of higher intensities and is more suitable for the analysis of sulfated compounds, while non-sulfated glycosides are analyzed by the positive ion mode [77–79].

Preliminary asterosaponin structures can be predicted from experimental tandem MS data because typical fragment ions and neutral losses provides valuable information about aglycon structures and sequences of monosaccharide units in carbohydrate chains. Tandem mass spectra show intensive characteristic fragment peaks for all asterosaponins and sulfated glycosides, indicating the sulfate group (peak at m/z 96.9 in negative ion mode and neutral loss of 120 Da and peak at m/z 142.9 in positive ion mode) (Figure 3). In the negative product ion spectra, an intense Y-type ion series (nomenclature by Domon and Costello [80]) associated with the cleavages of glycosidic bonds and corresponding sequential losses of sugar units has been observed. The analogous Y-type product ion series corresponding to losses of monosaccharide units as well as B- and C-type product ion series can be observed in the positive ion spectra of asterosaponins. The fragmentation of certain asterosaponins under CID conditions produces a very intense characteristic product ion series corresponding to the loss of side chain neutral fragments. For example, the spectra of many asterosaponins display neutral loss of a fragment of 100 Da as well as the Y–100 product ion series. This fragmentation corresponds to the loss of the $C_6H_{12}O$ molecule associated with the C-20–C-22 bond cleavage and 1H transfer, which is characteristic of asterosaponins containing an aglycon with a 20-hydroxy-cholestan-23-one side chain (Figure 3) [20]. The similar product ion series Y–114 and Y–128 indicate aglycons with 20-hydroxy-24-methyl-cholestan-23-one and 20-hydroxy-24-ethyl-cholestan-23-one side chains.

The structural characterization of polyhydroxysteroids and glycosides of polyhydroxysteroids is challenging due to the great diversity of compounds in this class. Spectra of polyhydroxysteroid compounds and related glycosides contain fragmentation patterns indicate a number of hydroxy groups and structures of the side chains and steroid nuclei. Tandem spectra of polyhydroxysteroid glycosides with sulfated monosaccharide unit usually show diagnostic ion B_0 at m/z 241.0 $[C_6H_9O_8S]^-$, 225.0 $[C_6H_9O_7S]^-$ or 210.9 $[C_5H_7O_7S]^-$, which are characteristic of sulfated hexose, methylated pentose, or pentose units, respectively, whereas the presence of intense Y-type ions is associated with non-sulfated compounds or sulfated aglycon. In certain cases the A- and X-type product ions formed by cross-ring cleavages of sulfated monosaccharides can be detected, potentially allowing isomeric monosaccharides with different positions of the sulfate group to be distinguished [81,82]. In other cases, the structure of the polyhydroxysteroidal aglycon can be proposed from both obtained MS data and from biosynthetic considerations [77,83].

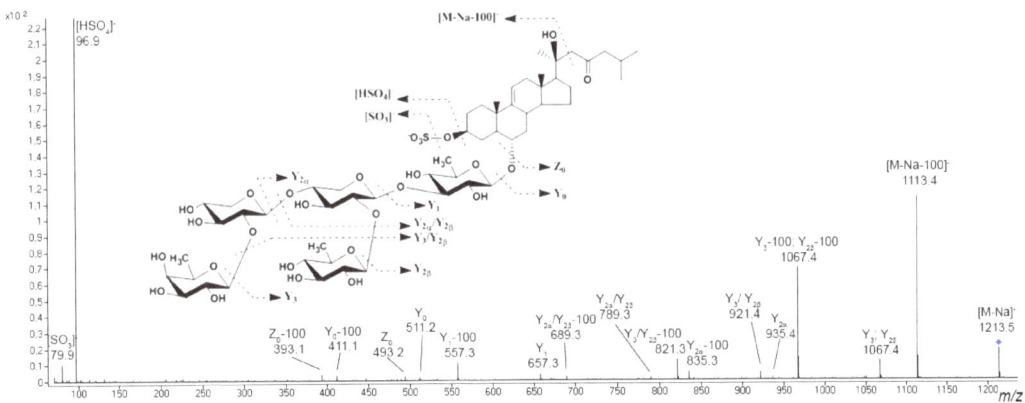

Figure 3. ESI MS/MS spectrum of $[M - Na]^-$ precursor ion at m/z 1213 identified as ophidianoside F (modified from [77]).

Table 1 provides a general overview of the approaches used for metabolomic profiling of starfish polar steroids and triterpene glycosides of sea cucumbers, including extractions, purification methods, and analytical techniques. Table S1 provides more expansive technical details of these particular approaches, including sample preparation protocols and the instrumental setups of the ESI MS, MALDI MS, and hyphenated techniques.

Table 1. Selected examples illustrating MS-based approaches for the analysis of starfish polar steroids and sea cucumber triterpene glycosides *.

Species Name	Extraction	Purification Methods	MS Approach	Research Results	Number of Detected Analytes	Ref.
Asteroidea						
Asterias rubens	MSPD extraction		RPLC-NMR-ESI-IT MS	A combination of MSPD extraction with on-flow LC–NMR–MS for rapid chemical screening and structural elucidation was applied; a series of new asterosaponins were found and their structures were established	17 asterosaponins	[84]
A. rubens	90% MeOH	LLE, CC	MALDI-QTOF MS; MALDI-TOF/TOF MSI; RPLC-ESI-QQQ MS	A series of known and new asterosaponins were detected and characterized; localization, inter- and intra-organ variability of asterosaponin were described	26 asterosaponins	[85,86]
Aphelasterias japonica	EtOH	SPE	RPLC-ESI-QTOF MS	A series of new polar steroid compounds were detected and characterized; a theoretical scheme of biogenesis of several polar steroids was proposed	33 asterosaponins, 28 polyhydroxylated glycosides, 7 polyhydroxysteroids	[77]

Table 1. Cont.

Species Name	Extraction	Purification Methods	MS Approach	Research Results	Number of Detected Analytes	Ref.
Patiria pectinifera	EtOH	SPE	RPLC-ESI-QTOF MS	A series of new polar steroid compounds were detected and characterized; peculiarities of the biosynthesis of the starfish polar steroids were discussed. Changes in steroid metabolome induced by environmental factors were studied	35 asterosaponins, 22 polyhydroxysteroids, and 15 polyhydroxylated glycosides	[78,87]
Luidia senegalensis	70% EtOH	SPE	RPLC-ESI-IT MS	New asterosaponins were detected and annotated	5 asterosaponins, 2 polyhydroxysteroids	[88]
Lethasterias fusca	EtOH	LLE, SPE	nanoRPLC-CSI-QTOF MS	A series of new polar steroids compounds were detected and their fragmentation behaviors were extensively investigated; variations in the distribution of individual representatives in different organs were found	106 asterosaponins, 81 polyhydroxylated glycosides, 14 polyhydroxysteroids	[79,89]
Echinaster sepositus	60% MeOH	LLE	ESI-QOrbitrap MS	New asterosaponins were detected and annotated; significant inter-organ variability in asterosaponins was demonstrated	11 asterosaponins	[90]
Heliaster helianthus	EtOH	LLE, CC	ESI-QTOF MS	The presence of sulfated steroidal glycosides in the fractions studied was confirmed and their structures were established	1 asterosaponin, 2 polyhydroxylated glycosides	[91]
Holothuroidea						
Holothuria forskali	70% EtOH	LLE, CC	MALDI-QTOF MS; RPLC-ESI-QTOF MS	A series of triterpene glycosides were detected and characterized; variations in triterpene glycoside composition in Cuvierian tubules and body walls were demonstrated	26 triterpene glycosides	[92]
H. forskali	70% EtOH	LLE, CC	MALDI-TOF/TOF MS; MALDI-TOF/TOF MSI	Statistical differences in triterpene glycoside distribution between control and stressed groups were described	8 triterpene glycosides	[93]
H. atra, H. leucospilota, Pearsonothuria graeffei, Actinopyga echinites, Bohadschia subrubra	70% EtOH	LLE, CC	MALDI-QTOF MS; RPLC-ESI-QTOF MS	A series of new and known glycosides were detected and characterized; variations between species and between body compartments were established	H. atra—4, H. leucospilota—6, P. graeffei—8, A. echinites—10, B. subrubra—19 triterpene glycosides	[94]

Table 1. Cont.

Species Name	Extraction	Purification Methods	MS Approach	Research Results	Number of Detected Analytes	Ref.
H. forskali	70% EtOH	LLE, CC	MALDI-QTOF MS; RPLC-ESI-QTOF MS	Localization of triterpene glycosides in the body wall tissues was described; variations of secreted glycosides were found in the seawater surroundings of non-stressed and stressed animals	8 triterpene glycosides	[95]
H. scabra, H. impatiens, H. fuscocinerea	70% EtOH	LLE, HPLC	nanoRPLC-ESI-QTOF MS; MALDI-FTICR MS	Triterpene glycoside compositions of three sea cucumber species were described; variations and sample-specific compounds were found	H. scabra—32, H. impatiens—32, H. fuscocinerea—33 triterpene glycosides	[96]
H. scabra	MeOH	LLE, CC	MALDI-QTOF MS	The triterpene glycoside composition of the H. scabra body wall was characterized, as was processed holothurian,	6 triterpene glycosides	[97]
H. sanctori	MeOH	LLE, CC	MALDI-QTOF MS	Qualitative and quantitative differences in the body wall and Cuvierian tubules of composition were described	18 triterpene glycosides	[98]
Eupentacta fraudatrix	EtOH	SPE	RPLC-ESI-QTOF MS	A series of triterpene glycosides were discovered and characterized; qualitative and quantitative variations in the body wall and viscera were found	54 triterpene glycosides	[99]
H. scabra		SPE	RPLC-multimode source-QTOF MS	Several known and new triterpene glycosides were identified in conditioned water of H. scabra	16 triterpene glycosides	[100]
H. forskali	MeOH	LLE	MALDI-QTOF MS; RPLC-ESI-QQQ MS; RPLC-ESI-IM-QTOF MS	The triterpene glycoside compositions of the body wall, gonads, and Cuvierian tubules of H. forskali were described	26 triterpene glycosides	[101]
H. leucospilota	70% EtOH; H_2O or n-BuOH	LLE	MALDI-TOF/TOF MS; MALDI-TOF/TOF MSI	The presence of triterpene glycosides was confirmed in the body wall and epidermis extracts; epidermal pigmented cells were reported to involve in the accumulation and release of the triterpene glycosides to the surrounding seawater	12 triterpene glycosides	[102]

Table 1. Cont.

Species Name	Extraction	Purification Methods	MS Approach	Research Results	Number of Detected Analytes	Ref.
H. atra	EtOAc/MeOH	LLE	RPLC-ESI-QOrbitrap MS	A combination of LC-MS profiling and molecular networking followed by target compound isolation was applied; variations in triterpene glycoside composition between H. atra from the Persian Gulf and previously reported results were described	15 triterpene glycosides (4—isolated as pure compounds)	[103]
Apostichopus japonicus	70% EtOH	LLE	RPLC-ESI-QOrbitrap MS	Variability in triterpene glycoside composition among different types of A. japonicus was described	5 triterpene glycosides	[104]
H. polii, H. leucospilota, H. atra, H. edulis, Bohadschia marmorata, Actinopyga mauritiana	96% EtOH	LLE	RPLC-ESI-QOrbitrap MS	MS-based profiling results were applied for chemotaxonomy of sea cucumber species	4 triterpene glycosides; 15 fatty acids, 45 triacylglycerols	[105]
H. whitmaei, H. hilla, H. atra, H. edulis, Bohadschia argus, B. vittiensis, Bohadschia sp., Actinopyga echinites, A. mauritiana	MeOH:EtOAc, MeOH	LLE, SPE, HPLC	RPLC-ESI-QTOF MS	A series of triterpene glycosides were detected in crude extracts; anti-fouling activity of sea cucumber extracts was found to be species-specific and related to total concentration of triterpene glycosides.	102 triterpene glycosides in crude extracts (including 23 triterpene glycosides in B. argus fractions)	[106]
H. scabra	MeOH	flash chromatography, LLE	MALDI-QTOF MS; RPLC-ESI-IM-QTOF MS	The qualitative and quantitative composition of triterpene glycosides in dried viscera and its desulfation by microwave activation products were described	26 triterpene glycosides	[107]

* Abbreviations: CC, column chromatography; CSI, captive spray ionization; ESI, electrospray ionization; FTICR, Fourier-transform ion cyclotron resonance; HPLC, high-performance liquid chromatography; IM, ion mobility; IT, ion trap; LC, liquid chromatography; LLE, liquid-liquid extraction; NMR, nuclear magnetic resonance; MALDI, matrix-assisted laser desorption/ionization; MS, mass spectrometry; MSI, mass spectrometry imaging; MSPD, matrix solid-phase dispersion; nanoESI, nanoelectrospray; QOrbitrap, quadrupole-Orbitrap; QTOF, quadrupole time-of-flight; QQQ, triple-quadrupole; RPLC, reverse-phase liquid chromatography; SPE, solid-phase extraction; TOF, time-of-flight.

Polar steroid compounds are usually extracted from animal materials using methanol, ethanol, or hydro-alcoholic solutions. As crude extracts contain a large concentration of impurities and inorganic salt, there is a need for additional purification procedures before analysis. SPE with reverse-phase (RP) sorbents is the most fast and versatile way of obtaining the purified total fraction of polar steroids [77,78]. Regarding asterosaponin fraction extraction, LLE is preferred. The most commonly used protocol is adapted from that in [108], and includes the dilution of the dry extract in 90% methanol followed by successive partitioning against n-hexane, dichloromethane, and chloroform. After column chromatography with an Amberlite XAD-4 column, the eluate is extracted against isobutanol. The resulting fraction contained purified asterosaponins [85,90].

Although LC coupled to MS through electrospray ionization interface is the most popular combination for profiling due to its efficiency, versatility, and capability in analyzing isomeric compounds, MALDI is commonly used as the primary technique for the rapid screening of extracts [85]. All of the researchers reviewed here used columns with RP C18 sorbents for analytical separation; however, it should be noted that the high complexity of the extracts and fractions places high demands on both chromatography and detection. The use of high-resolution MS analyzers (TOF and Orbitrap) enables calculation of the elemental composition of the analytes via high accuracy measurements and true isotopic patterns, while using tandem techniques allows for structural characterization of the detected compound.

LC-NMR-MS was used for the profiling and characterization of *Asterias rubens* asterosaponins [84,109]. The on-flow LC-NMR-MS screening showed novel asterosaponins in *A. rubens*, and their tentative structures were proposed by MS and NMR data [109]. Using a similar experimental setup, the authors replaced time-consuming classical extraction with matrix solid-phase dispersion (MSPD) extraction, which combines both sample homogenization and extraction in a single step starting from the intact sample material. The structures of seventeen asterosaponins were established based on complementary structural information from both MS and NMR detection, including 1H-NMR spectra obtained in on-flow mode, 2D WET-TOCSY spectra from the MS-triggered stopped-flow mode, information about molecular mass before and after H-D exchange, and fragmentation patterns and characteristic neutral losses [84].

Further studies on *A. rubens* using a combination of MALDI MS, MALDI imaging (MALDI MSI), and LC-MS have focused on the diversity, body distribution, and localization of asterosaponins [85,86]. Asterosaponins from the body walls, stomach, pyloric caeca, and gonads were extracted and analyzed by MALDI-TOF MS and LC-ESI MS [85]. As a result, seventeen known and nine novel asterosaponins were detected. It was found that each organ was characterized by a specific mixture of asterosaponins, and that their concentration varies considerably among individuals. MALDI MSI was used to clarify the inter- and intraorgan distribution of asterosaponins [86]. Sample preparation is a particularly important step in MALDI imaging. Because the starfish body wall contains calcareous ossicles, the researchers used carboxymethyl cellulose as an embedding medium to facilitate the cryosectioning procedure. The results confirmed that asterosaponin distributions are not homogeneous, and revealed that certain asterosaponins are located both inside the body wall and within the outer mucus layer, where they probably protect the animal.

As a part of starfish polar steroid exploration, metabolite profiling of polar steroids in the Far Eastern starfishes *Aphelasterias japonica* and *Patiria pectinifera* was performed [77,78]. A detailed LC-MS analysis of the complicated mixture of polar steroids from *A. japonica* revealed 68 polar steroid metabolites, including 33 asterosaponins, 28 polyhydroxysteroid glycosides, and seven polyhydroxysteroids [77]. Fragmentation analysis indicated asterosaponins with rare and atypical units in their oligosaccharide chains that have thus far not been identified from marine sources. The profiling of polar steroid compounds of *P. pectinifera* using the LC-MS allowed many different polar steroid compounds to be discovered [78]. LC-ESI MS analysis revealed 72 components (35 asterosaponins, 15 sulfated glycosides of polyhydroxysteroids, and 22 polyhydroxylated steroids). Annotation was based on MS data obtained in both negative and positive ion modes. Liquid chromatography coupled with atmospheric pressure photoionization (LC-APPI) MS was applied for non-sulfated polyhydroxysteroid compounds. APPI MS/MS exhibited extensive fragmentation, with sequential neutral losses of H_2O molecules and cleavages in side chains and tetracyclic nucleus. The comparison of the steroid constituents of *P. pectinifera* and *A. japonica* revealed significant differences associated with details of the biosynthesis of starfish polar steroids.

A combination of SPE and ultra-high performance liquid chromatography (UPLC) coupled with ion trap (IT) mass spectrometry was used to profile asterosaponins from the Brazilian starfish *Luidia senegalensis* [88]. Seven components were detected as a result, and five of which were characterized as asterosaponins. ESI MS was used together with NMR to detect and characterize asterosaponins and sulfated polyhydroxysteroid glycosides in bioactive fractions obtained by LLE and chromatography purification of the ethanolic extract from the starfish *Heliaster helianthus* [91].

The profiling of polar steroids from the starfish *Lethasterias fusca* was carried out by nanoflow liquid chromatography coupled with captive spray ionization (CSI) mass spectrometry [79]. As a result, the structure of the largest number of polar steroid metabolites was discovered, and the MS fragmentation of a large series of starfish polar steroids was studied. A total of 207 compounds, including 106 asterosaponins, 81 glycosides of polyhydroxysteroids, and 14 polyhydroxylated steroids, were detected and characterized. Further study of the distribution of the detected compounds in *L. fusca* body components showed that the polar steroid compositions in the body walls, coelomic fluid, gonads, stomach, and pyloric caeca were qualitatively and quantitatively different [89]. Research on the distribution of asterosaponins from *Echinaster sepositus* revealed eleven compounds, and found significant variability in asterosaponin composition depending on the organ, sex, and season [90].

In summarizing the aforementioned results it is necessary to note the huge variety of starfish polar steroids. Each studied species contained dozens, and in several cases, hundreds of polar steroids, most of which had not been previously described [77–79]. Additional studies of the polar steroids in the studied species often lead to the identification of both known compounds and new previously-undescribed metabolites. For example, the study of asterosaponins of *A. rubens* by LC-NMR-MS revealed seventeen asterosaponins [84]. Subsequent studies led to the detection of both previously discovered compounds as well as the discovery of new asterosaponins [85,86]. This is related both to the instrumental advancements involving increasing sensitivity and selectivity of analysis and to the great variability in the polar steroid composition of starfish, even among representatives of the same species. The observed large structural variability together with the huge number of structures in each species studied and the small number of species studied (a total of six species have been studied using metabolomic methods) may indicate a potentially huge chemical space for starfish polar steroids.

Most studies have focused on both the description of the structural diversity and on the study of the localization of the discovered compounds. It has been determined that each organ is characterized by a certain composition of polar steroids. The comparison of the content of individual steroids in different starfish organs probably suggests the different biological roles of these metabolites in the starfish. Asterosaponins, which are the most toxic starfish compounds, have been found in all organs of the starfish [85,86,89]. However, the body walls often show the highest content of asterosaponins. In addition, these compounds have been found in the outer layer of mucus [86]. This may be due to the toxic, protective, or antimicrobial properties of these compounds. The main potion of polyhydroxysteroid glycosides is located in the pyloric caeca, which confirms the digestive function of these steroids in starfish [89,110]. At the same time, the levels of polar steroids can vary greatly depending on the individual, season, and sex [85,90,111]. This high interindividual variability may be associated with different physiological statuses of the animals, and partly with the biogenesis of certain compounds from dietary steroids.

3.2. Sea Cucumber Triterpene Glycosides

Triterpene glycosides are the characteristic secondary metabolites of sea cucumbers. Their chemical structures are characterized by the large variability of certain structural features, although the general structure of these compounds is rather conservative. Most sea cucumber triterpene glycosides have a lanostane-type aglycon with an 18(20)-lactone. Usually, aglycon has a polycyclic nucleus with a 7(8)- or 9(11)-double bond and oxygen-containing substituents, which may be bonded to C-12, C-17, or C-16. Structures of the side chains of aglycons demonstrate significant natural diversity and may have one or more double bonds, hydroxyl or acetate groups, and other substituents. Certain glycosides have aglycons with shortened side chains. The carbohydrate chains of sea cucumber glycosides may include up to six sugar units and be attached to C-3 of the aglycon. Xylose, glucose, quinovose, 3-O-methylglucose, and rarely 3-O-methylxylose are the most common sugar residues in triterpene glycosides. The first monosaccharide unit is always xylose, and monosaccharides with the 3-O-methyl group are always terminal ones. Many glycosides have up to four sulfate groups in the first xylose, glucose, and 3-O-methylglucose units. The oligosaccharide chains that have up to four monosaccharide units usually represent a linear structure, while the penta- and hexaosides contain a branching at the first or second monosaccharide unit (Figure 4) [21,23,24,32,33].

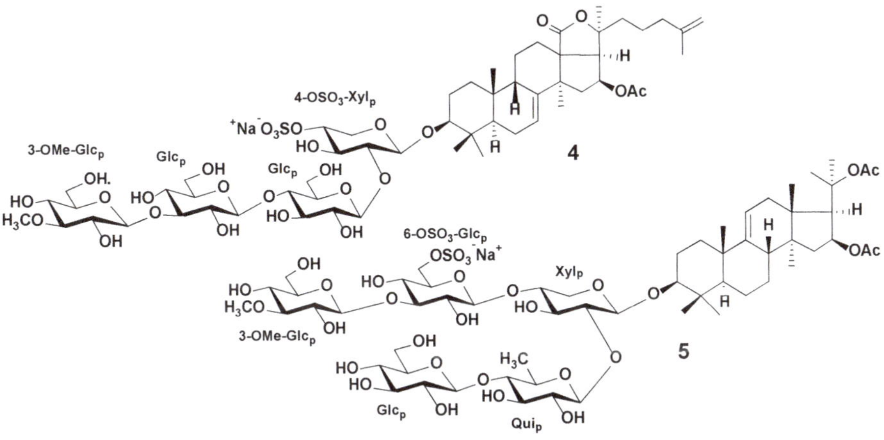

Figure 4. The structures of typical holothurian triterpene glycosides with holostane aglycon (okhotoside B$_1$ (**4**) from the sea cucumber *Cucumaria okhotensis* [112]) and rare non-holostane aglycon (kurilosides A$_1$ (**5**) from the sea cucumber *Thyonidium* (=*Duasmodactyla*) *kurilensis* [113]), demonstrating different carbohydrate chain architecture.

Triterpene glycosides demonstrate both biological and pharmacological effects, including cytotoxic, antifungal, bactericidal, antiviral, and antiparasitic effects [21,22,32,33]. The most interesting of these is the ability of certain glycosides to induce apoptosis and inhibit tumor cell growth; thus, sea cucumbers have become a promising source for the discovery of new drugs [114]. Additionally, certain triterpene glycosides have been reported to exhibit immunomodulatory properties [115]. Several species of sea cucumber are an important aquaculture resource and are used as functional foods [116]. It has been suggested that dietary triterpene glycoside supplements can improve lipid metabolism, significantly suppress adipose accumulation, and reduce serum and hepatic lipids [117].

Most triterpene glycosides have been detected within m/z range from 1000 to 1600 as [M + Na]$^+$ ions. In most cases, sulfated and disulfated triterpene glycosides are detected in negative ion mode as [M − Na]$^−$ and [M − 2Na]$^{2-}$ ions, respectively, whereas non-sulfated compounds are detected as [M − H]$^−$ ions. The tandem mass spectra of triterpene glycosides usually reveal B- and C-type product ion series arising from the cleavage of glycosidic bonds. These product ion series are characteristic, and they provide information about the sequence of monosaccharide residues in carbohydrate chains (Figure 5).

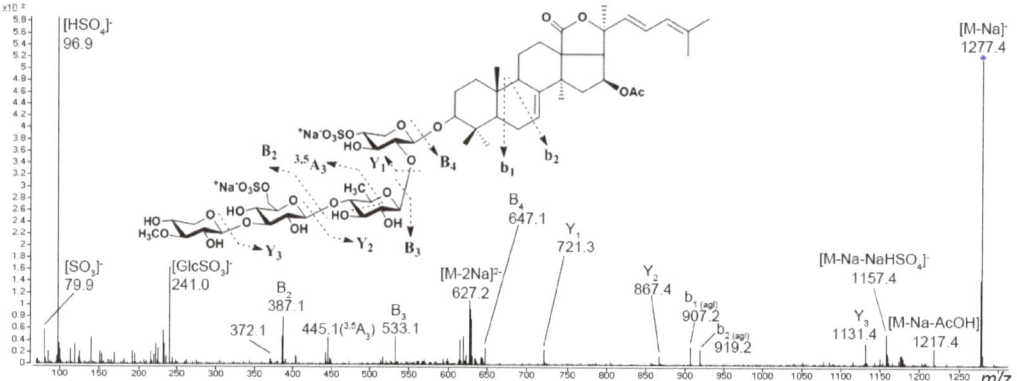

Figure 5. ESI MS/MS spectrum of [M − Na]⁻ precursor ion at m/z 1277, identified as cucumarioside F_2 (modified from [118]).

Tandem mass spectra of many triterpene glycosides show typical mass losses related to aglycon fragmentation, and can provide information about the structure of the nucleus and the side chain. In the MS/MS spectra of certain glycosides a mass loss of 60 Da between the precursor and the intense fragment ion has been detected, which corresponds to the loss of the $C_2H_4O_2$ molecule and is a characteristic of glycosides containing an acetoxy group. An intense fragment ion with a mass loss of 104 Da from the precursor is related to the loss of a $[C_2H_4O_2 + CO_2]$ fragment, which is characteristic of compounds with an acetoxy group and an 18(20)-lactone cycle. Certain triterpene glycosides tend to lose the neutral fragments of the side chain under CID conditions.

Regarding the extraction of triterpene glycosides from animal tissue, the most preferred solvents are 70% ethanol and methanol, although ethanol and ethyl acetate:methanol mixtures have been used (Tables 1 and S1). Crude extracts must be purified before analysis to remove inorganic salts, lipid, and protein contaminants. For these purposes, most researchers use successive liquid–liquid partitioning against n-hexane, dichloromethane, and chloroform, followed by column chromatography with an Amberlite XAD-4 column and extraction against butanol or similar LLE-based protocols. Another purification approach includes SPE with C18 cartridges [99,100]. Omran et al. used LLE with a solvent combination of MTBE/MeOH/H_2O for the purification of crude ethanol extract to obtain the polar fraction of the triterpene glycosides and non-polar fraction of lipids in a single extraction step [105]. The purified extracts can be fractionated using HPLC [96,106] or flash chromatography [107].

MALDI MS is often used as the primary technique for rapid screening of triterpene glycoside mixtures. As sea cucumber triterpene glycosides are characterized by the presence of isomeric compounds, the LC-MS technique can be used as a tool for discriminating different isomers and structure confirmation. In order to separate glycosides, most LC-MS applications use analytical columns with C18 sorbents. Ion mobility technology provides additional orthogonal separation for the discrimination and structural characterization of isomeric compounds [119].

A combination of MALDI MS and ESI MS was used to annotate the triterpene glycosides in purified fractions of the Australian sea cucumber *Holothuria lessoni* [120–123]. As a result, a series of known and novel triterpene glycosides were annotated by extensive MS fragmentation. It should be noted that the authors determined the structures of novel glycosides based only on MS data. However, it is known that different epimeric monosaccharides as well as types of bonds between sugars and absolute configuration of asymmetric atoms cannot be strictly distinguished by MS [124]. The proposed structures are therefore tentative, and must be verified by additional approaches such as NMR spectroscopy.

MS-based approaches were used for screening, characterization, and study of the bodily distribution of the triterpene glycosides of the sea cucumber *Holothuria forskali* [92,93,95]. Triterpene glycosides were extracted from two different body components, the body wall and the Cuvierian tubules (a defensive organ that can be ejected in response to predator attacks), and analyzed by a combination of MALDI MS, MALDI MSI, and LC-ESI MS. The analysis revealed at least 26 triterpene glycosides, including twelve glycosides in the body wall and twenty-six in the Cuvierian tubules. The glycosides detected in the body wall were found in the Cuvierian tubules, with the latter containing fourteen other specific glycosides as well. A more detailed study of triterpene glycoside localization in the body wall revealed that the glycosides were mainly localized in the epidermis and mesothelium [95]. A combination of MALDI, LC-ESI MS, and LC-ESI-IM MS was used in order to better tackle the structural complexity of *H. forskali* glycosides [101]. As a result, at least 10, 16, and 22 different triterpene glycosides within the body wall, gonads, and Cuvierian tubules, respectively, were detected. Glycosides with pentasaccharide chains were dominant within the extracts from the gonads and the Cuvierian tubules, whereas the body wall extract exhibited equally abundant tetra-, penta- and hexaosides. In addition, the authors described the interaction of branched triterpene glycosides with sodium ions, and proposed a new schematic for data representation using sector diagrams constructed from MS data.

The diversity of triterpene glycosides was studied in five tropical sea cucumber species [94]. Triterpene glycosides from the body wall and the Cuvierian tubules were extracted and analyzed with a combination of MALDI MS, ESI MS, and LC-MS. The researchers indicated that the smallest number of glycosides was observed in *Holothuria atra*, which contained a total of four compounds, followed by *Holothuria leucospilota*, *Pearsonothuria graeffei*, and *Actinopyga echinites* with six, eight, and ten compounds, respectively. *Bohadschia subrubra* showed the highest triterpene glycoside diversity. Differences between the glycoside composition in the body walls and the Cuvierian tubules were highlighted.

The profiles of three tropical sea cucumber species were determined and compared to examine their chemical diversity with phylogenetic data [96]. Semi-purified extracts from the body wall of *Holothuria scabra*, *H. impatiens*, and *H. fuscocinerea* were first analyzed by MALDI-FT MS and chip-HPLC-ESI MS. The obtained data showed holothurines common for three species (for example, holothurin A) as well as glycosides specific for certain species (for example, impatienside A in *H. impatiens*). Glycosidic fractions of three species contained approximately the same number of compounds (32 glycosides in *H. scabra* and *H. impatiens* and 33 glycosides in *H. fuscocinerea*); however, the glycoside profiles were both quantitatively and qualitatively different from each other. Moreover, the authors demonstrated a relationship between metabolomic and phylogenetic data. Their obtained results show the possibility of effectively using MS-based metabolomic profiling for chemotaxonomy purposes in sea cucumbers.

The MALDI MS analysis of triterpene glycosides of *Holothuria scabra* revealed six major compounds saved during the processing of the body wall [97]. Mitu et al. showed that *H. scabra* releases triterpene glycosides into the surrounding seawater [100]. The characterization of these compounds by LC-multimode source MS led to the annotation of sixteen new and known compounds. A recent study used MALDI MS and LC-IM MS to characterize the triterpene glycoside composition of the viscera of *H. scabra* [107]. A combined analysis revealed 26 sulfated triterpene glycosides.

MALDI MS was used for the rapid structural characterization of triterpene glycosides in the body wall and Cuvierian tubules of the sea cucumber *Holothuria sanctori* [98]. Mass spectrometry analysis revealed eighteen triterpene glycosides, including eight novel compounds. Body wall triterpene glycosides showed higher diversity than those from the Cuvierian tubules.

LC-MS profiling of the sea cucumber *Eupentacta fraudatrix* revealed 26 sulfated, 18 nonsulfated, and 10 disulfated triterpene glycosides [99]. Many novel compounds were characterized by tandem MS, including those with previously unknown oligosaccharide chain types. Two new glycosides were isolated and their tentative structures were confirmed by NMR. Based on the literature data and obtained results, a biosynthetic pathway for oligosaccharide fragments of *E. fraudatrix* glycosides was proposed. LC-MS analysis of extracts from the respiratory trees, body walls, gonad tubules, guts, and aquapharyngeal bulbs indicated triterpene glycosides in all body components, although quantitative variability for certain triterpene glycosides was observed.

A combined technique involving microscopic analysis, MALDI MS, and MALDI MSI was used to study triterpene glycoside localization in the body wall of *Holothuria leucospilota* [102]. MALDI MS analysis of the body wall and the epidermal tissue extracts revealed twelve triterpene glycosides. The following MALDI MSI analysis showed the presence of detected glycosides in the epidermis of *H. leucospilota*, whereas in the dermis the circular and longitudinal muscle bands had no glycosides.

The composition of triterpene glycoside in the sea cucumber *Holothuria atra*, collected in the Persian Gulf, was studied using a modern analytical approach combining LC-MS, molecular networking, pure compound isolation, and NMR spectroscopy. In order to evaluate the entire pool of triterpene glycosides, the purified extract was subjected to LC-MS analysis using a column with pentafluorophenyl phase. The obtained MS data were used to create a molecular network using the GNPS Molecular Networking website. As a result, twelve triterpene glycosides were found, including three novel glycosides. Four major triterpene glycosides were isolated by HPLC, and their structures were confirmed by NMR [103].

The metabolic profiling of the polar fractions obtained from MTBE-based LLE of six sea cucumbers allowed for the identification of two sulfated glycosides found in all species and two species-specific nonsulfated glycosides [105]. Metabolic profiling was used for the screening of crude extracts of nine tropical sea cucumber species related to anti-fouling activities [106]. LC-MS analysis detected glycosides in all extracts; in total 102 triterpene glycosides were detected. The extract of *Bohadschia argus* represents one of the most active anti-fouling extracts, and includes 23 glycosides. The obtained results demonstrate that anti-fouling activities in sea cucumber extracts are species-specific and related to both triterpene glycoside total concentration and structures of presented triterpene glycosides. In another study, the relation between anti-fouling activities and the presence of triterpene glycosides was observed [125]. The UPLC-MS approach was used to evaluate the glycoside composition of *Apostichopus japonicus* [104]. As a result, five triterpene glycosides were detected and the variability of content of identified triterpene glycosides among the different types of *A. japonicus* was described.

The results of the aforementioned metabolomics studies indicate a huge structural variability of triterpene glycosides, as in the case of starfish polar steroids. Interestingly, certain species contain only a few triterpene glycosides, while dozens of glycosides have been found in the extracts of others. The maximum number of triterpene glycosides was detected in the extract of *E. fraudatrix*, with 54 compounds [99]. It should be noted that certain researchers used only MALDI MS methods, which do not distinguish between isomeric compounds in mixtures; thus, the real number of structures may be somewhat higher. Several studies have demonstrated the strict taxonomic specificity of the chemical composition of studied systematic groups of sea cucumbers [96,105]. Thus, MS-based metabolomic profiling can easily be used for chemotaxonomy purposes, both to clarify the species identity of unknown specimens and to confirm or revise the status of taxa.

The application of MALDI MSI and LC-MS profiling of extracts from various organs provides a better understanding of the distribution and localization of triterpene glycosides in animal tissues. Although glycosides are present in all organs, their distribution is heterogeneous [99]. Maximum total concentrations and number of structures can be found for the body walls and Cuvierian tubules [94,98,101]. By using MS-based methods, it has been found that sea cucumbers secrete toxic triterpene glycosides into the surrounding water [95]. These facts confirm the suggestion that triterpene glycosides have multiple defensive roles, including defense against predators and protection from parasites and microorganisms.

3.3. Starfish and Sea Cucumber Lipids

Marine invertebrates are known to be a valuable source of bioactive and dietary lipids, which are connected to the prevention of diseases and have applications in nutrition, cosmetics, pharmacy, and other fields. In this respect, an essential part of modern lipidomic studies is focused on fatty acids, glycerophospholipids, and sphingolipids in marine organisms such as sponges, cnidarians, worms, molluscs, and arthropods. Regarding starfish and sea cucumbers, research interest is largely linked to studying fatty acid composition and bioactive sphingolipids, including unique cerebrosides and gangliosides [126].

Sea cucumbers and starfish contain fatty acids in relatively small amounts [127]. Sea cucumber fatty acids usually account for less than 8% of their total weight, enriched in unsaturated fatty acids that may account for up to 70% [128]. The main fatty acids of sea cucumbers are 20:4 (n-6), 20:1, 20:5 (n-3), 16:0 and 18:0 [129]. Starfish are characterized by a high level of polyunsaturated acids, among which 20:5 (n-3) and 20:4 (n-6) are dominant [130]. MS-based analysis of fatty acids can be considered a well-established approach in view of both sample preparation and analysis protocols. Nowadays, GC-MS with chemical derivatization is routinely used to obtain an exhaustive view of the composition and metabolism of fatty acids. Analytical approaches and scientific results on fatty acid composition in marine invertebrates, including sea cucumbers and starfish, are discussed in detail in [13,131–133]. Fatty acid and sterol compositions of numerous sea cucumber [134] and starfish species [135] have been analyzed using GS-MS-based approaches. In addition, the variability in fatty acid content studied by GC-MS is used to analyze the effects of diet [136] and geographical origin [137,138] and to distinguish between wild and cultured animals [139].

The major phospholipids in Echinodermata include phosphatidylcholine, phosphatidylethanolamine, and phosphatidylserine. Sea cucumbers are characterized by high phosphatidylinositol content, while their lysophosphatidylcholine, lysophosphatidylethanolamine, diphosphatidylglycerol, phosphatidic acid, and phosphatidylinositol-4-phosphate contents are low [140].

Sample preparation for phospholipid determination in sea cucumbers and starfish is commonly based on extractions from the fresh whole body, body walls, or viscera via the classic Folch method [141], the Bligh and Dyer method [142], or extraction using a solvent combination of MTBE/MeOH/H$_2$O [105] (Table 2 and Table S2). Different phospholipid headgroups and alterations in chain length, amount and position of double bonds in fatty acids, and ester bond types lead to an extremely complex composition of phospholipid mixtures. Traditionally, protocols that use deacylation and derivatization followed by GC or GC-MS identification were used to establish the fatty acid composition of phospholipids. However, such approaches are associated with the destruction of the original structures. In contrast, LC-MS methods allow for the detailed investigation of complex lipid mixtures in a high-throughput manner without prior purification and chemical modification. However, good chromatographic separation is critical for the accurate identification of lipids in such complex mixtures. Most frequently used reverse-phase sorbents, such as C8 or C18, allow for the separation of the molecules of phospholipids according to chain length and degree of saturation of acyl fatty acids. The use of HILIC or normal-phase (NP) columns, on the other hand, allows for the separation of molecules based on the structure of the polar head groups.

Table 2. Selected examples illustrating MS-based approaches for the analysis of starfish and sea cucumber lipids *.

Species Name	Extraction	Purification Method	MS Approach	Research Findings	Number of Analytes	Ref.
Acaudina molpadioides, Cucumaria frondosa, Apostichopus japonicus	CHCl$_3$/MeOH	LLE, CC	RPLC-ESI-ITTOF MS	Cerebroside compositions of three sea cucumber species were characterized; many novel glucocerebroside structures were described	Cerebroside molecular species: *A. japonicus*—26, *C. frondosa*—40, *A. molpadioides*—12	[143]

Table 2. Cont.

Species Name	Extraction	Purification Method	MS Approach	Research Findings	Number of Analytes	Ref.
A. japonicus, Thelenota ananas, A. molpadioides, Bohadschia marmorata	CHCl$_3$/MeOH	LLE, SPE	RPLC-ESI-QTOF MS	A series of cerebrosides from four sea cucumber species were detected and annotated; the relation of long-chain base structures and fatty acids to sea cucumber genera were described	Cerebroside molecular species: A. japonicus—55, T. ananas—107, A. molpadioides—87, B. marmorata—75	[59]
Pearsonothria graeffei	CHCl$_3$/MeOH	LLE, SPE	RPLC-ESI-QTOF MS	A series of cerebrosides of the sea cucumber P. graeffei were detected and annotated; characteristic structural features of sea cucumber cerebrosides were described	89 cerebroside molecular species	[144]
C. frondosa	CHCl$_3$/MeOH/H$_2$O	LLE, CC	RPLC-HESI-QOrbitrap MS	The sphingolipid composition of the sea cucumber C. frondosa was investigated; the relationship between sea cucumber sphingolipid structures and pro-apoptotic activities was discussed	35 cerebroside molecular species, 8 ceramide molecular species, 2 sphingosines	[145]
Asterias amurensis	Bligh and Dyer protocol	CC	RPLC-ESI-ITTOF MS	Cerebroside composition and distribution in viscera of the starfish A. amurensis were investigated; the potential usefulness of starfish as a source of raw material for cerebrosides was discussed	23 cerebrosides molecular species	[146]
Parastichopus californicus, C. frondosa, Isostichopus fuscus, Holothuria mexicana, H. polli, Bohadschia marmorata	Bligh and Dyer protocol		NPLC-ESI-TripleTOF MS	A series of phospholipids, including rare representatives, were detected and annotated; qualitative and quantitative variations between sea cucumber species were established; the possibility of using phospholipid data for classification was shown	From 295 to 445 molecular species from 7 phospholipid classes (PG, PE, PI, PS, LPE, PC, LPC)	[142]
B. marmorata, I. fuscus, H. polli, H. mexicana, C. frondosa P. californicus	H$_2$O	LLE, SPE	HILIC LC-HESI-QOrbitrap MS	Seventeen ganglioside subclasses, including rare and new ganglioside structures, were discovered in six sea cucumber species; variations and characteristic features of the ganglioside composition of sea cucumbers were described	17 ganglioside subclasses	[147]

* Abbreviations: CC, column chromatography; ESI, electrospray ionization; HESI, heated electrospray ionization; HILIC, hydrophilic interaction chromatography; IT, ion trap; LC, liquid chromatography; LLE, liquid-liquid extraction; LPC, lysophosphatidylcholine; LPE, lysophosphatidylethanolamine; NPLC, normal-phase liquid chromatography; MS, mass spectrometry; PC, phosphatidylcholine; PE, phosphatidylethanolamine; PG, phosphatidylglycerol; PI, phosphatidylinositol; PS, phosphatidylserine; QOrbitrap, quadrupole-Orbitrap; QTOF, quadrupole time-of-flight; RPLC, reverse-phase liquid chromatography; SPE, solid-phase extraction; TOF, time-of-flight.

Although phospholipids have drawn intense interest in recent years as substances with the potential for human health benefits, and although modern LC-MS lipidomic methods have been used extensively, only limited studies are available on the phospholipid content of starfish and sea cucumbers [148]. The investigation of the composition of phospholipids in several echinoderm species by LC-ESI MS revealed the predomination of alkylacyl-PC and alkenylacyl-PE forms in starfish and sea cucumbers [141]. Structural characterization was achieved by comparing the retention times and in-source fragmentation patterns obtained in negative and positive ion modes with single-stage MS. The NPLC-ESI TripleTOF MS was employed to study the phospholipid composition of the dried body walls of six sea cucumber species [142]. The application of normal-phase liquid chromatography as a separation technique allowed for the division of complex mixtures into subclasses with reproducible retention times as well as the separation of isobaric molecules in the same subclass. As a result, between 295 to 445 molecular species belonging to eleven phospholipid subclasses (phosphatidylcholines, phosphatidylserines, phosphatidylethanolamines, phosphatidylinositol, phosphatidic acids, phosphatidylglycerols, lysophosphatidylcholines, lysophosphatidylethanolamine, lysophosphatidylserine, lysophosphatidylinositol, and rare phosphonoethanolamine) were detected in each species. Identification and structure elucidation were based on retention times, ion forms, and specific fragmentation patterns obtained in negative ion mode using the LIPIDMAPS database. Semiquantitation followed by statistical analysis demonstrated differences in the phospholipid profiles of the studied species. Analysis of the nonpolar fraction obtained by extraction of six Egyptian sea cucumber species was performed using UPLC-Orbitrap MS in positive and negative ion modes [105]. For metabolite identification, the obtained data (m/z, retention time, isotope and fragmentation patterns) were searched against public databases. A total of fifteen free fatty acids and 45 triacyl glycerols were detected. Statistical analysis showed that quantitative variations in lipid content between the studied species were associated with habitat or food changes, not with taxonomical relationships.

Sphingolipids constitute an extremely diverse class of bioactive polar lipids. As components of cell membranes and intracellular mediators, sphingolipids are involved in cell recognition and signal transduction processes [149,150]. Sphingolipids from marine organisms exhibit various activities, including antitumor, immunomodulatory, antiviral, neuritogenic, and other activities [126,151].

Sphingolipids, particularly cerebrosides and gangliosides, are important components of echinoderm lipids that have drawn attention because of their structure and bioactivity. Compared to those present in mammals and plants, the sphingolipids present in echinoderms have notable structural differences. Variations in chain length and in the degree of saturation and/or hydroxylation of the sphingoid backbone and fatty acids lead to the extensive variety of cerebrosides structures. Starfish and sea cucumber gangliosides remain little studied. These compounds have a specific sugar core, including sialic acids within carbohydrate chains, as well as additional monosaccharide residues and unusual types of glycosidic bonds between them (Figure 6) [126]. The determination of their diverse structures and variety of sphingoid backbones are very important for understanding the functional and nutritional significance of dietary sphingolipids. To date, about 150 sphingolipids from fifteen starfishes and nine sea cucumbers have been studied, several of which have demonstrated biological activity [126]. Cerebrosides from sea cucumbers and starfish show activity against nonalcoholic fatty liver disease [152] and an inhibitory effect on cell proliferation through the induction of apoptosis in cancer cells [153]. Sea cucumber sphingosine has strong cytotoxicity against colon cancer cells [154]. Gangliosides of starfish and sea cucumbers show slight neuritogenic activity. However, the bioactivity of these compounds remains poorly investigated [126].

Regarding cerebroside extraction from starfish and sea cucumbers, LLE with methanol: chloroform mixtures is preferred, although extraction following the Bligh and Dyer method or modifications of it is applicable. Subsequent purification of crude extracts by LLE, SPE, or silica gel column chromatography provides pure fractions containing cerebrosides. High-speed counter-current chromatography (HSCCC) has recently been pointed out as a way to improve the resulting cerebroside fractions without requiring extraction procedures or additional purification [145]. Gangliosides, as the more polar compounds, can be extracted from sea cucumber body walls by homogenization in water followed by purification using LLE with a solvent combination of $CHCl_3/MeOH/H_2O$ followed by SPE purification using C8 sorbent [147] (Tables 2 and S2).

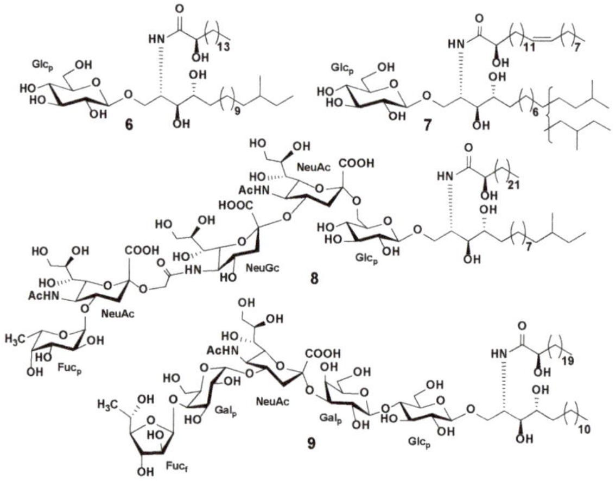

Figure 6. The structures of typical echinoderm cerebrosides (luidiacerebroside A (**6**) from the starfish *Luidia maculata* [155] and glucocerebroside HPC-3-A (**7**) from the sea cucumber *Holothuria pervicax* [156]) and gangliosides (ganglioside molecular species from the sea cucumber *H. pervicax* (**8**) [157] and acanthaganglioside I (**9**) from the starfish *Acanthaster planci* [158]).

Because of their structural complexity, sphingolipids are difficult to analyze using one method. Formerly, sphingolipids were quantified by thin-layer chromatography (TLC); structure elucidation comprised many stages of chemical decomposition and derivatization followed by GC, GC-MS, HPLC, MS, and NMR analyses [159]. Today, LC-MS with electrospray ionization is the main tool for the detection and annotation of sphingolipids, including both known and novel molecular species. RPLC with isocratic elution with 95% MeOH with 5 mM ammonium acetate and 0.05% acetic acid or elution with 95% ACN is commonly used to separate sphingolipids. HILIC-LC on the GOLD-amino column has been used in the separation of gangliosides from sea cucumbers [147]. In this approach, the ganglioside subclasses are eluted in a specific time range based on their amounts of sialic acid residues.

The ESI in positive ion mode is the most extensively used ionization technique for the analysis of cerebrosides (Table 2). Although the locations of the double bonds in the fatty acyl chain often cannot be unequivocally identified by CID, the specific fragment ions from fatty acid, sphingosine, and sugar units allow putative structures to be proposed [59,143–145]. Gangliosides detected in the negative ion mode mainly form deprotonated or double deprotonated ions. Characteristic fragment ions and neutral losses formed by oligosaccharide chain fragmentation reveal a monosaccharide composition and different sialic acid types [147].

The investigation of cerebrosides from various sources by LC-MS showed that the cerebroside composition of sea cucumbers differs from those of plants (maize, rice) and mushrooms (maitake). [160]. Research into the cerebroside composition of the sea cucumbers *Apostichopus japonicus, Thelenota ananas, Acaudina molpadioides, Bohadschia marmorata, Cucumaria frondosa*, and *Pearsonothria graeffei* using LC-MS led to the discovery of a large series of compounds and showed that sea cucumber sphingolipids are much more diverse than was conventionally thought [59,143–145] (Table 2). Each studied species contained several dozen cerebroside molecular species, with the most complicated composition belonging to *T. ananas*. Several sea cucumber species were found to have similar sphingolipid compositions, while the profiles of others were dramatically distinctive. The analysis of many structures allowed identification of the characteristic structural features of sea cucumber cerebrosides. A sphingoid base (d17:1) is typically predominant in sea cucumber cerebrosides and is not widely found in plants, mammals, or fungi. In addition, the occurrence of C23:1h is characteristic of sea cucumber cerebrosides and is rarely found in plants, mammals, or fungi. The FA contained in cerebrosides from sea cucumbers is similar to those of common mammals, although it has more double bonds and hydroxylation. The study of the cerebroside composition of the gonads, viscera, and whole body of the starfish *Asterias amurensis* revealed a characteristic structure distribution that can be divided into three major structural groups [146].

HILIC-ESI MS was used to identify gangliosides in six sea cucumber species. Seventeen ganglioside subclasses were detected, and their oligosaccharide chains were characterized by tandem MS [147]. The results indicated that sea cucumber gangliosides differ from mammalian gangliosides in monosaccharide composition, number, and types of sialic acids. Moreover, gangliosides with phosphoinositidyled sialic acid and tetrasialogangliosides were identified in sea cucumbers for the first time.

3.4. Multi-Class Profiling Studies

In contrast to the single-class approach, the multi-class approach attempts to simultaneously detect the qualitative and quantitative characterization of various metabolites of different chemical groups in a single analysis run. Essentially, research that uses a multi-class approach aims to investigate crude extracts or study the composition of bioactive fractions. Due to the complicated composition of marine invertebrates, such extracts or fractions contain a wide diversity of compounds. The chemical pool of such extracts depends primarily on the solvent used and/or on the extraction protocol. Methanol, ethanol, dichloromethane, chloroform, ethyl acetate, and their mixtures are often used for extraction. Non-polar solvents extract complex mixtures of fatty acids, lipids, carotenoids, triterpenes, and sterols, while the use of polar solvents leads to extracts containing mixtures of polar steroid compounds or triterpene glycosides, polar lipids, and other compounds. The results depend on the analytical method and platform. The widely used multi-class GC-MS approach is used for analysis and accurate identification via a database search of sterols, triterpenes, and fatty acids such as methyl esters. LC-MS is used to characterize more polar compounds.

The LC-MS metabolic profiling of sea cucumber *Holothuria spinifera* extract indicated secondary metabolites of several classes [161]. Gradient elution on the C18 column with ESI-Orbitrap MS operating in positive and negative ion modes was used for the investigation of methanol:dichloromethane extract. It is worth noting that only 4% of metabolites were detected in either mode. The molecular formula was predicted using the MZmine algorithm and identification was achieved using MarinLit and the Dictionary of Natural Products databases. As a result, thirteen secondary metabolites belonging to the fatty acids, phenolic diterpenes, and triterpenes were identified.

Investigation of antifouling and antibacterial activities of three extracts from different organs of the sea cucumber *Holothuria leucospilota* showed that ethyl acetate extract of the body wall possessed the most pronounced activity [162]. In order to determine its bioactive compounds, GC-MS was used. Using the NIST GC-MS library, seventeen metabolites, including five terpenes and terpenoids and six fatty acids, were identified.

The lipid, fatty acid, and sterol compositions of four sea cucumbers were analyzed to assess their feeding habits [163]. The extracts were obtained using a modified Bligh and Dyer protocol and analyzed using a thin-layer chromatography-flame ionization detector (TLC-FID) analyzer to quantify lipid classes and GC-MS for the identification of individual metabolites. The sea cucumbers were found to be rich in phytosterols and algal-derived fatty acids, suggesting tight trophic coupling to phytodetritus, while the relatively large proportions of stanols were probably the result of enteric bacteria. GC-MS was used for targeted profiling of fatty acids as methyl esters and amino acids after sample derivatization with N-methyl-N-tert-butyldimethylsilyltrifluoroacetamide (BSTFA) and trimethylchlorosilane (TMCS) of three sea cucumber species [127].

Dichloromethane, methanol, and aqueous extracts of *Linckia laevigata*, *Fromia indica*, *Cryptasterina pentagona*, and *Archaster typicus* were tested in order to identify surface-bound metabolites that protect the starfish from fouling; the most biologically active fractions were analyzed by GC-MS [164]. Several fatty acids and sterols were identified using the NIST and Wiley GC-MS databases. GC-MS analyses of the surface-extracted metabolites of each starfish specimen identified hexadecanoic acid, cholesterol, lathosterol, and sitosterol as the compounds responsible for the antifouling effects.

Pereira et al. proposed the GC-MS method for simultaneous analysis of fatty acids, amino acids, sterols, and lupanes in marine animals and applied this method to the characterization of the starfish *Marthasterias glacialis* extract [165]. Using ethanol as the extraction solvent at 40 °C and N-methyl-N-(trimethylsilyl)-trifluoroacetamide (MSTFA) as the derivatization reagent, forty compounds (including fifteen amino acids, sixteen fatty acids, six sterols, and three lupanes were detected and quantified.

The LC-MS approach was used for the profiling and identification of the active compounds of dichloromethane:methanol extract of the holothurian *Pseudocolochirus violaceus*, which exhibited strong antiproliferative effects [166]. The mixture was separated on a C18 column and metabolites were detected using ESI MS in positive and negative ionization modes. Compound identification was performed by accurate mass measurement and comparison of the obtained data with previously reported information. As a result, 24 compounds, belonging mainly to the terpenes, steroids, and fatty acids, were detected using both positive and negative ionization modes, several of which have previously been reported to exhibit antiproliferative capacity in cancer cells.

A combination of the GC-MS and LC-MS methods was applied to obtain a comprehensive view of the composition of ethyl acetate extract of the sea cucumber *Holothuria forskali* [167]. The GC-MS analysis revealed 25 major components identified by the NIST GC-MS library, while LC-MS showed eight molecules, including fat-soluble vitamins, phytosterols, and phenolic acids, identified by comparison of retention times and MS data obtained for pure standards.

Zakharenko et al. proposed an alternative method for the extraction of bioactive compounds from sea cucumbers using a two-step process with carbon dioxide extraction followed by extraction with CO_2 and ethanol as a co-solvent [168]. The obtained extracts were tested by LC-IT MS in negative and positive ion modes and tandem MS. The identification of the metabolites was achieved using the Bruker library database and literature data, and revealed the presence of fifteen triterpene glycosides, eighteen styrene compounds, and fourteen carotenoids.

Variability in the chemical composition of the viscera and body walls of the sea cucumber *A. japonicus* extracted by methanol was investigated by the LC-MS approach, and 85 metabolites were determined [169]. Multivariate data analysis using PCA and PLS-DA revealed significant differences between the viscera and body walls. To identify the main characteristic compounds of viscera, several sphingoid-based nucleoside analogs were isolated and their structures were confirmed by MS/MS and NMR methods.

The investigation of sea cucumber metabolites is not restricted to metabolite profiling of extract, and can be applied to the profiling of volatile compounds as well. Volatile compounds of eight dried sea cucumber species with different geographical origins were analyzed using a combination of headspace solid-phase microextraction and GC-MS [170]. Metabolite identification was achieved by matching data with NIST and Wiley GC-MS databases and confirmed by comparing retention times and mass spectra with standard compounds. As a result, 42 volatile compounds, including aldehydes, alcohols, aromatic compounds, and furans, were identified in the dried sea cucumbers, several of which were determined as odour-active compounds.

4. Applications of Metabolome-Oriented Approaches in Studies of Starfish and Sea Cucumbers

MS-based targeted metabolomics were applied to investigate the influence of different environmental factors on the polar steroids of the starfish *P. pectinifera* [87]. Extracts of control starfishes and starfishes exposed to water heating, oxygen deficiency, feeding, injury, and different water salinity levels were purified by SPE and analyzed using LC-ESI-QTOF

MS. An in-house library of retention times and MS data on previously characterized polar steroid metabolites of *P. pectinifera* were used for metabolite identification. Univariate and multivariate statistical analyses revealed variations in the steroid metabolome between the control and treatment groups. In order to further evaluate stress-induced differences, PCA and PLS-DA analyses were carried out on each group of starfish individually with the control group. The results revealed that differences caused by feeding, injury, and heating were greater than in the other starfish groups. These states had similarities in their effects on the steroid metabolome of starfish. Most asterosaponins were reduced, and most polyhydroxysteroids and related glycosides were increased. These differences in steroid metabolite profiles may relate to the biological multifunctionality of these compounds.

MALDI MSI was applied to study the precise localization of sea cucumber *H. forskali* triterpene glycosides in the Cuvierian tubules of control and stressed sea cucumbers [93]. Stressed animals were mechanically disturbed for 4 h by repetitive hitting using a specific device. Statistical multivariate tests using PCA showed statistical differences in triterpene glycoside composition between the control and stressed groups. Triterpene glycosides with corresponding ions at m/z 1287 and 1303 were mainly localized in the connective tissue of the tubules of both control and stressed sea cucumbers. Glycoside ions at m/z 1125 and 1141 were present in relaxed animals, while ions at m/z 1433, 1449, 1463, and 1479 were observed in the Cuvierian tubules of stressed animals in the outer part of the connective tissue. The authors proposed that the latest glycosides are stress-specific compounds formed by modifications of the glycosides with shortened oligosaccharide chains. Another study revealed that *H. forskali* releases glycosides into the surrounding seawater. Among these secreted glycosides, holothurinoside G was detected in the seawater surrounding relaxed sea cucumbers, while holothurinosides C, F, M, L, and desholothurin A were secreted when the animals were stressed [95].

The most extensive metabolomics research has been performed on the commercially important sea cucumber *Apostichopus japonicus* (Table S3). Most of these studies used a non-targeted UPLC-QTOF MS approach and focused on primary metabolites such as amino acids, sugars, fatty acids, and common metabolites, and did not involve sea cucumber-specific triterpene glycosides and gangliosides.

High temperature and low oxygen concentration are the common environmental stress factors for marine invertebrates, and their impact on *A. japonicus* has been studied using MS-based metabolomics [171]. Changes in the concentrations of 84, 68, and 417 metabolites related to the responses to heat, hypoxia, and combined stress, respectively, were detected by LC-MS and multivariate statistical analysis. Among the detected metabolites, compounds atypical for echinoderms such as the plant glycoside tokoronin, the synthetic drug tirofiban, and others were found, which may be due to identification errors (the authors did not provide information on how metabolite identification was performed). Another investigation of acute hypoxia in *A. japonicus* showed that levels of most lipids increased with the elongation of hypoxia. These results imply that the homeostasis of synthesis and degradation of lipids and their derivatives are strongly affected by hypoxic stress [172]. Liu et al., used GC-MS to compare the metabolic profiles of a thermotolerant strain of *A. japonicus* with a control group, and found significant differences in the concentrations of 52 metabolites [173]. Evisceration is a well-known stress response of sea cucumbers, although the biochemistry of this process is unclear. Metabolomic analysis of coelomic fluids ejected during *A. japonicus* evisceration using LC-MS followed by univariate and multivariate analysis revealed five significantly changed signaling pathways [47]. In response to high temperatures, sea cucumbers can enter a state characterized by inactivity, cessation of feeding, gut degeneration, and decreased metabolic rate. This physiological state is called aestivation. Yang et al. used transcriptomic and metabolomic approaches to explore alterations in *A. japonicus* during the aestivation stage [174]. LC-MS analysis revealed that downregulated metabolites were associated with fatty acid metabolism, carbohydrate metabolism, and the TCA cycle. UPLC-QTOF MS was used to describe the metabolic changes induced by skin ulceration syndrome, the main disease affecting the development of *Apostichopus japonicus* in the aquaculture industry [175]. As a result, variations in metabolites mainly related to amino acid metabolism, energy metabolism, immunity, osmoregulation, and neuroactive ligand-receptor interaction has been discovered.

Another research focus has been directed towards the study of metabolomic changes induced by the impact of various factors. LC-MS has been used to highlight metabolomic differences between cage-cultured, pond-cultured, and bottom-sowed *A. japonicus* [176]. Multivariate analysis and enrichment of metabolic pathway analyses revealed differential metabolites participating in lipid, amino acid, carbohydrate, and nucleotide metabolism. The investigation of *A. japonicus* coelomic fluids in different sexes and reproductive states by UPLC-QTOF MS and multivariate statistical analysis revealed variations in phenylalanine metabolism and unsaturated fatty acid synthesis [177]. LC-MS highlighted significant metabolic differences in the muscle tissue of animals between the nonbreeding and growth stages [178]. The metabolite profiles obtained using UPLC-QTOF-MS of four *A. japonicus* varieties (green, white, purple, and spiny) were compared, and differences were identified using multivariate analysis [179]. Differential metabolites included fatty acids, amino acids, phospholipids, and sugars. In another study, a similar approach was applied to reveal the metabolic changes in white, green, and purple *A. japonicus* body walls during the pigmentation process [180]. Statistical analysis differentiated the body wall chemical composition among the three color morphs, and thirteen annotated metabolites showed significant differences in white, green, and purple sea cucumbers. UPLC-QTOF MS metabolomic profiling was applied to distinguish *A. japonicus* from different geographical origins [181]. Data analysis using OPLS-DA showed that differential metabolites mainly included amino acids and lipids.

Melatonin-induced metabolomic changes in the muscle tissues of *A. japonicus* have been tested using UPLC-QTOF MS [182]. Statistical analysis with PCA, PLS-DA, fold-change analysis, and *t*-test showed alterations in the levels of 22 different metabolites, including serotonin, retinoic acids, and fatty acids, which can explain the observed sedative effect of melatonin on this species. The LC-MS metabolomic analysis revealed that pedal peptide-type neuropeptides involved in the regulation of locomotor behavior in *A. japonicus* induce changes in the levels of certain phospholipids [183].

Most of the mentioned metabolomics studies of *A. japonicus* used a similar workflow involving the extraction of tissue samples with methanol, methanol:water, or methanol: acetonitrile mixtures, homogenization, centrifugation, and LC-MS analysis mainly using RP separation and ESI-QTOF mass spectrometers for the detection of metabolites operating in the mass ranges from 50 to 1200 Da in positive and negative ion modes. Although a huge number of metabolites (from several dozen to 4435 metabolites) are found in almost every work, the compounds that are mainly responsible for the bioactive properties of sea cucumbers (triterpene glycosides, cerebrosides, and gangliosides) remain undetected, and their variations under the studied conditions remain unclear. At the same time, the results of the other works [87,93] indicate statistically significant changes in the levels of specific metabolites, namely, starfish polar steroids and sea cucumber triterpene glycosides, in response to stresses and environmental factors. Thus, the influence of many factors and physiological phenomena, such as aestivation and evisceration, on large groups of bioactive metabolites remains unexplored. It is well known that starfish and sea cucumbers have extraordinary regenerative potential, however, the features of this process remain poorly explored at the metabolome level.

5. Conclusions and Perspectives

The unique features of biosynthesis and metabolism and the diversity of their metabolites explain the researchers' interest in these organisms. Starting in the middle of the last century, chemical research on echinoderm metabolites has resulted in hundreds of compounds, many of which have demonstrated biological and pharmacological effects. The structural elucidation of the bioactive compounds of starfish and sea cucumbers is a difficult task, combining isolation of pure compounds with modern MS and NMR techniques to unambiguously determine the structures of new compounds.

MS-based metabolomics approaches have proven to be a powerful research tool in the natural product area. The application of MS-based techniques has made it possible to study chemical compounds without the laborious process of isolating individual compounds. Using modern metabolomics methods in the marine sciences allows evaluation of the biochemical diversity of marine systems and expands our understanding of the chemical space of marine compounds.

To date, only a few dozen species of starfish and sea cucumbers have been studied using MS-based metabolomics approaches, a very small fraction of the more than 3600 known species. Most of the studied species are aquaculture species or readily available and widely distributed species, and most deep-sea and rare species remain almost unexplored.

In summarizing MS-based metabolomics studies on the bioactive secondary metabolites of starfish and sea cucumbers, it was found that this approach allows for the ready detection and annotation of polar steroids, triterpene glycosides, and lipids in producer organisms. Obtained data allow for their exact or preliminary structures to be proposed. The data obtained thus far make it possible to assess the prospects for the search for new bioactive molecules as well as to draw conclusions about their taxonomic distribution, biogenesis, and biological functions. These methods are used to compare metabolomic profiles of different echinoderm species and populations in ecological, dietary, and biosynthesis studies.

The main difficulties of applying MS-based metabolomics approaches are related to the extreme complexity of the mixtures being analyzed. However, the use of modern chromatography and mass spectrometry methods allows these methods to be successfully applied. UPLC with analytical columns packed with sub-2-μm sorbents allows metabolites with closely related structures to be separated. The introduction of cutting-edge mass-spectrometry techniques such as ion mobility, improved ion dissociation techniques, and ultra-high resolution mass analyzers can provide high-performance MS analyses. While identification of detected peaks remain the main problem in MS data analysis, constructing specialized databases of echinoderm metabolites and improving in silico computational algorithms may improve the obtained results considerably.

Supplementary Materials: The following supporting information can be downloaded at: https://www.mdpi.com/article/10.3390/md20050320/s1, Table S1: Instrumental and methodological details of MS-based applications for the analysis of starfish polar steroids and sea cucumber triterpene glycosides; Table S2: Instrumental and methodological details of MS-based applications for the analysis of starfish and sea cucumbers lipids; Table S3: Instrumental and methodological details in metabolomics studies of starfish and sea cucumbers.

Author Contributions: Writing—original draft preparation and writing—review and editing, R.S.P. and N.V.I.; conceptualization and validation, P.S.D. All authors have read and agreed to the published version of the manuscript.

Funding: This work was carried out with the support of the Russian Science Foundation (RSF) Grant Number 21-73-00180.

Conflicts of Interest: The authors declare no conflict of interest.

References

1. Carroll, A.R.; Copp, B.R.; Davis, R.A.; Keyzers, R.A.; Prinsep, M.R. Marine natural products. *Nat. Prod. Rep.* **2019**, *36*, 122–173. [CrossRef] [PubMed]
2. Carroll, A.R.; Copp, B.R.; Davis, R.A.; Keyzers, R.A.; Prinsep, M.R. Marine natural products. *Nat. Prod. Rep.* **2020**, *37*, 175–223. [CrossRef] [PubMed]
3. Carroll, A.R.; Copp, B.R.; Davis, R.A.; Keyzers, R.A.; Prinsep, M.R. Marine natural products. *Nat. Prod. Rep.* **2021**, *23*, 9–10. [CrossRef] [PubMed]
4. Carroll, A.R.; Copp, B.R.; Davis, R.A.; Keyzers, R.A.; Prinsep, M.R. Marine natural products. *Nat. Prod. Rep.* **2022**. [CrossRef] [PubMed]

5. Jiménez, C. Marine natural products in medicinal chemistry. *ACS Med. Chem. Lett.* **2018**, *9*, 959–961. [CrossRef]
6. Blunt, J.W.; Carroll, A.R.; Copp, B.R.; Davis, R.A.; Keyzers, R.A.; Prinsep, M.R. Marine natural products. *Nat. Prod. Rep.* **2018**, *35*, 8–53. [CrossRef]
7. Zhang, L.-X.; Fan, X.; Shi, J.-G. A novel pyrrole oligoglycoside from the starfish *Asterina pectinifera*. *Nat. Prod. Res.* **2006**, *20*, 229–233. [CrossRef]
8. Yang, X.W.; Chen, X.Q.; Dong, G.; Zhou, X.F.; Chai, X.Y.; Li, Y.Q.; Yang, B.; Zhang, W.D.; Liu, Y. Isolation and structural characterisation of five new and 14 known metabolites from the commercial starfish *Archaster typicus*. *Food Chem.* **2011**, *124*, 1634–1638. [CrossRef]
9. Purcell, S.W. Managing sea cucumber fisheries with an ecosystem approach. In *FAO Fisheries and Aquaculture Technical Paper*; No. 520; Lovatelli, A., Vasconcellos, M., Yimin, Y., Eds.; FAO: Rome, Italy, 2010; 157p, ISBN 978-92-5-106489-4.
10. Bordbar, S.; Anwar, F.; Saari, N. High-value components and bioactives from sea cucumbers for functional foods—A review. *Mar. Drugs* **2011**, *9*, 1761–1805. [CrossRef]
11. Li, Y.X.; Himaya, S.W.A.; Kim, S.K. Triterpenoids of marine origin as anti-cancer agents. *Molecules* **2013**, *18*, 7886–7909. [CrossRef]
12. Gomes, A.R.; Freitas, A.C.; Rocha-Santos, T.A.P.; Duarte, A.C. Bioactive compounds derived from echinoderms. *RSC Adv.* **2014**, *4*, 29365–29382. [CrossRef]
13. Khotimchenko, Y. Pharmacological potential of sea cucumbers. *Int. J. Mol. Sci.* **2018**, *19*, 1342. [CrossRef] [PubMed]
14. Lazzara, V.; Arizza, V.; Luparello, C.; Mauro, M.; Vazzana, M. Bright spots in the darkness of cancer: A review of starfishes-derived compounds and their anti-tumor action. *Mar. Drugs* **2019**, *17*, 617. [CrossRef] [PubMed]
15. Zhou, Y.; Farooqi, A.A.; Xu, B. Comprehensive review on signaling pathways of dietary saponins in cancer cells suppression. *Crit. Rev. Food Sci. Nutr.* **2021**, *9*, 1–26. [CrossRef] [PubMed]
16. Wen, M.; Cui, J.; Xu, J.; Xue, Y.; Wang, J.; Xue, C.; Wang, Y. Effects of dietary sea cucumber saponin on the gene expression rhythm involved in circadian clock and lipid metabolism in mice during nighttime-feeding. *J. Physiol. Biochem.* **2014**, *70*, 801–808. [CrossRef]
17. Chumphoochai, K.; Chalorak, P.; Suphamungmee, W.; Sobhon, P.; Meemon, K. Saponin-enriched extracts from body wall and Cuvierian tubule of *Holothuria leucospilota* reduce fat accumulation and suppress lipogenesis in *Caenorhabditis elegans*. *J. Sci. Food Agric.* **2019**, *99*, 4158–4166. [CrossRef]
18. Liu, X.; Xu, J.; Xue, Y.; Gao, Z.; Li, Z.; Leng, K.; Wang, J.; Xue, C.; Wang, Y. Sea cucumber cerebrosides and long-chain bases from *Acaudina molpadioides* protect against high fat diet-induced metabolic disorders in mice. *Food Funct.* **2015**, *6*, 3428–3436. [CrossRef]
19. Luparello, C.; Mauro, M.; Lazzara, V.; Vazzana, M. Collective locomotion of human cells, wound healing and their control by extracts and isolated compounds from marine invertebrates. *Molecules* **2020**, *25*, 2471. [CrossRef]
20. Minale, L.; Riccio, R.; Zollo, F. Steroidal Oligoglycosides and polyhydroxysteroids from echinoderms. *Prog. Chem. Org. Nat. Prod.* **1993**, *62*, 75–308.
21. Chludil, H.D.; Murray, A.P.; Seldes, A.M.; Maier, M.S. Biologically active triterpene glycosides from sea cucumbers (Holothuroidea, Echinodermata). In *Studies in Natural Products Chemistry*; Atta-ur-Rahman, Ed.; Elsevier Science Publisher: Amsterdam, The Netherlands, 2003; Volume 28, pp. 587–615.
22. Kim, S.; Himaya, S.W.A. Triterpene glycosides from sea cucumbers and their biological activities. *Adv. Food Nutr. Res.* **2012**, *65*, 297–319.
23. Kalinin, V.I.; Silchenko, A.S.; Avilov, S.A.; Stonik, V.A. Progress in the studies of triterpene glycosides from sea cucumbers (Holothuroidea, Echinodermata) Between 2017 and 2021. *Nat. Prod. Commun.* **2021**, *16*, 1934578X211053934. [CrossRef]
24. Kalinin, V.I.; Avilov, S.A.; Silchenko, A.S.; Stonik, V.A.; Elyakov, G.B. Triterpene glycosides of sea cucumbers (Holothuroidea, Echinodermata) as taxonomic markers. *Nat. Prod. Commun.* **2015**, *10*, 21–26. [CrossRef] [PubMed]
25. Kalinin, V.I.; Silchenko, A.S.; Avilov, S.A.; Stonik, V.A. Non-holostane aglycones of sea cucumber triterpene glycosides. Structure, biosynthesis, evolution. *Steroids* **2019**, *147*, 42–51. [CrossRef] [PubMed]
26. Stonik, V.A.; Ivanchina, N.V.; Kicha, A.A. New polar steroids from starfish. *Nat. Prod. Commun.* **2008**, *3*, 1587–1610. [CrossRef]
27. Ivanchina, N.V.; Kicha, A.A.; Stonik, V.A. Steroid glycosides from marine organisms. *Steroids* **2011**, *76*, 425–454. [CrossRef]
28. Dong, G.; Xu, T.; Yang, B.; Lin, X.; Zhou, X.; Yang, X.; Liu, Y. Chemical constituents and bioactivities of starfish. *Chem. Biodivers.* **2011**, *8*, 740–791. [CrossRef]
29. Ivanchina, N.; Kicha, A.; Malyarenko, T.; Stonik, V. Recent studies of polar steroids from starfish: Structures, biological activities and biosynthesis. In *Advances in Natural Products Discovery*; Nova Science Publishers: New York, NY, USA, 2017; pp. 191–224.
30. Xia, J.M.; Miao, Z.; Xie, C.L.; Zhang, J.W.; Yang, X.W. Chemical constituents and bioactivities of starfishes: An update. *Chem. Biodivers.* **2020**, *17*, e1900638. [CrossRef]
31. Stonik, V.A.; Kicha, A.A.; Malyarenko, T.V.; Ivanchina, N.V. Asterosaponins: Structures, taxonomic distribution, biogenesis and biological activities. *Mar. Drugs* **2020**, *18*, 584. [CrossRef]
32. Kalinin, V.I.; Aminin, D.L.; Avilov, S.A.; Silchenko, A.S.; Stonik, V.A. Triterpene glycosides from sea cucucmbers (Holothurioidea, Echinodermata). Biological activities and functions. In *Studies in Natural Products Chemistry (Bioactive Natural Products)*; Atta-ur-Rahman, Ed.; Elsevier Science Publisher: Amsterdam, The Netherlands, 2008; Volume 35, pp. 135–196, ISBN 1572-5995.
33. Careaga, V.P.; Maier, M.S. Cytotoxic triterpene glycosides from sea cucumbers. In *Handbook of Anticancer Drugs from Marine Origin*; Kim, S.-K., Ed.; Springer International Publishing: Cham, Switzerland, 2015; pp. 515–528, ISBN 978-3-319-07145-9.

34. Wolfender, J.L.; Litaudon, M.; Touboul, D.; Queiroz, E.F. Innovative omics-based approaches for prioritisation and targeted isolation of natural products-new strategies for drug discovery. *Nat. Prod. Rep.* **2019**, *36*, 855–868. [CrossRef]
35. Alvarez-Rivera, G.; Ballesteros-Vivas, D.; Parada-Alfonso, F.; Ibañez, E.; Cifuentes, A. Recent applications of high resolution mass spectrometry for the characterization of plant natural products. *TrAC Trends Anal. Chem.* **2019**, *112*, 87–101. [CrossRef]
36. Aydoğan, C. Recent advances and applications in LC-HRMS for food and plant natural products: A critical review. *Anal. Bioanal. Chem.* **2020**, *412*, 1973–1991. [CrossRef] [PubMed]
37. Boughton, B.A.; Thinagaran, D.; Sarabia, D.; Bacic, A.; Roessner, U. Mass spectrometry imaging for plant biology: A review. *Phytochem. Rev.* **2016**, *15*, 445–488. [CrossRef] [PubMed]
38. Zhang, X.; Quinn, K.; Cruickshank-Quinn, C.; Reisdorph, R.; Reisdorph, N. The application of ion mobility mass spectrometry to metabolomics. *Curr. Opin. Chem. Biol.* **2018**, *42*, 60–66. [CrossRef] [PubMed]
39. Chandramouli, K. Marine proteomics: Challenges and opportunities. *J. Data Min. Genom. Proteom.* **2016**, *7*, 3–4. [CrossRef]
40. Stuart, K.A.; Welsh, K.; Walker, M.C.; Edrada-Ebel, R.A. Metabolomic tools used in marine natural product drug discovery. *Expert Opin. Drug Discov.* **2020**, *15*, 499–522. [CrossRef]
41. Bayona, L.M.; de Voogd, N.J.; Choi, Y.H. Metabolomics on the study of marine organisms. *Metabolomics* **2022**, *18*, 17. [CrossRef]
42. Yeo, J.D.; Parrish, C.C. Mass spectrometry-based lipidomics in the characterization of individual triacylglycerol (TAG) and phospholipid (PL) species from marine sources and their beneficial health effects. *Rev. Fish. Sci. Aquac.* **2022**, *30*, 81–100. [CrossRef]
43. Christian, B.; Luckas, B. Determination of marine biotoxins relevant for regulations: From the mouse bioassay to coupled LC-MS methods. *Anal. Bioanal. Chem.* **2008**, *391*, 117–134. [CrossRef]
44. Goulitquer, S.; Potin, P.; Tonon, T. Mass spectrometry-based metabolomics to elucidate functions in marine organisms and ecosystems. *Mar. Drugs* **2012**, *10*, 849. [CrossRef]
45. Fiehn, O. Metabolomics—The link between genotypes and phenotypes. *Plant Mol. Biol.* **2002**, *48*, 155–171. [CrossRef]
46. Tonn, N.; Novais, S.C.; Silva, C.S.E.; Morais, H.A.; Correia, J.P.S.; Lemos, M.F.L. Stress responses of the sea cucumber *Holothuria forskali* during aquaculture handling and transportation. *Mar. Biol. Res.* **2016**, *12*, 948–957. [CrossRef]
47. Ding, K.; Zhang, L.; Huo, D.; Guo, X.; Liu, X.; Zhang, S. Metabolomic analysis of coelomic fluids reveals the physiological mechanisms underlying evisceration behavior in the sea cucumber *Apostichopus Jpn. Aquac.* **2021**, *543*, 736960. [CrossRef]
48. Vuckovic, D. Current trends and challenges in sample preparation for global metabolomics using liquid chromatography-mass spectrometry. *Anal. Bioanal. Chem.* **2012**, *403*, 1523–1548. [CrossRef] [PubMed]
49. Folch, J.; Lees, M.; Stanley, G.H.S. A simple method for the isolation and purification of total lipides from animal tissues. *J. Biol. Chem.* **1957**, *226*, 497–509. [CrossRef]
50. Bligh, E.G.; Dyer, W.J. A rapid method of total lipid extraction and purification. *Can. J. Biochem. Physiol.* **1959**, *37*, 911–917. [CrossRef] [PubMed]
51. Matyash, V.; Liebisch, G.; Kurzchalia, T.V.; Shevchenko, A.; Schwudke, D. Lipid extraction by methyl-tert-butyl ether for high-throughput lipidomics. *J. Lipid Res.* **2008**, *49*, 1137–1146. [CrossRef]
52. Rashkes, Y.V.; Kicha, A.; Levina, E.V.; Stonik, V.A. Mass spectra of polyhydrosysteroids of the starfish *Patiria pectinifera*. *Chem. Nat. Compd.* **1985**, *21*, 337–342. [CrossRef]
53. Komori, T.; Nanri, H.; Itakura, Y.; Sakamoto, K.; Taguchi, S.; Higuchi, R.; Kawasaki, T.; Higuchi, T. Biologically active glycosides from Asteroidea, III. Steroid oligoglycosides from the starfish *Acanthaster planci* L., 2. Structures of two newly characterized genuine sapogenins and an oligoglycoside sulfate. *Liebigs Ann. Der Chem.* **1983**, *1983*, 37–55. [CrossRef]
54. Alonso, A.; Marsal, S.; JuliÃ, A. Analytical methods in untargeted metabolomics: State of the art in 2015. *Front. Bioeng. Biotechnol.* **2015**, *3*, 23. [CrossRef]
55. Smith, C.A.; Want, E.J.; O'Maille, G.; Abagyan, R.; Siuzdak, G. XCMS: Processing Mass Spectrometry Data for metabolite profiling using nonlinear peak alignment, matching, and identification. *Anal. Chem.* **2006**, *78*, 779–787. [CrossRef]
56. Pluskal, T.; Castillo, S.; Villar-Briones, A.; Orešič, M. MZmine 2: Modular framework for processing, visualizing, and analyzing mass spectrometry-based molecular profile data. *BMC Bioinform.* **2010**, *11*, 395. [CrossRef] [PubMed]
57. Röst, H.L.; Sachsenberg, T.; Aiche, S.; Bielow, C.; Weisser, H.; Aicheler, F.; Andreotti, S.; Ehrlich, H.C.; Gutenbrunner, P.; Kenar, E.; et al. OpenMS: A flexible open-source software platform for mass spectrometry data analysis. *Nat. Methods* **2016**, *13*, 741–748. [CrossRef] [PubMed]
58. Tsugawa, H.; Ikeda, K.; Takahashi, M.; Satoh, A.; Mori, Y.; Uchino, H.; Okahashi, N.; Yamada, Y.; Tada, I.; Bonini, P.; et al. A lipidome atlas in MS-DIAL 4. *Nat. Biotechnol.* **2020**, *38*, 1159–1163. [CrossRef] [PubMed]
59. Jia, Z.; Cong, P.; Zhang, H.; Song, Y.; Li, Z.; Xu, J.; Xue, C. Reversed-phase liquid chromatography–quadrupole-time-of-flight mass spectrometry for high-throughput molecular profiling of sea cucumber cerebrosides. *Lipids* **2015**, *50*, 667–679. [CrossRef]
60. Aksenov, A.A.; Da Silva, R.; Knight, R.; Lopes, N.P.; Dorrestein, P.C. Global chemical analysis of biology by mass spectrometry. *Nat. Rev. Chem.* **2017**, *1*, 0054. [CrossRef]
61. Sumner, L.W.; Amberg, A.; Barrett, D.; Beale, M.H.; Beger, R.; Daykin, C.A.; Fan, T.W.M.; Fiehn, O.; Goodacre, R.; Griffin, J.L.; et al. Proposed minimum reporting standards for chemical analysis: Chemical Analysis Working Group (CAWG) Metabolomics Standards Initiative (MSI). *Metabolomics* **2007**, *3*, 211–221. [CrossRef]

62. Wolfender, J.L.; Nuzillard, J.M.; Van Der Hooft, J.J.J.; Renault, J.H.; Bertrand, S. Accelerating metabolite identification in natural product research: Toward an ideal combination of liquid chromatography-high-resolution tandem mass spectrometry and nmr profiling, in silico databases, and chemometrics. *Anal. Chem.* **2019**, *91*, 704–742. [CrossRef]
63. Wang, M.; Carver, J.J.; Phelan, V.V.; Sanchez, L.M.; Garg, N.; Peng, Y.; Nguyen, D.D.; Watrous, J.; Kapono, C.A.; Luzzatto-Knaan, T.; et al. Sharing and community curation of mass spectrometry data with Global Natural Products Social Molecular Networking. *Nat. Biotechnol.* **2016**, *34*, 828–837. [CrossRef]
64. Horai, H.; Arita, M.; Kanaya, S.; Nihei, Y.; Ikeda, T.; Suwa, K.; Ojima, Y.; Tanaka, K.; Tanaka, S.; Aoshima, K.; et al. MassBank: A public repository for sharing mass spectral data for life sciences. *J. Mass Spectrom.* **2010**, *45*, 703–714. [CrossRef]
65. Smith, C.A.; Maille, G.O.; Want, E.J.; Qin, C.; Trauger, S.A.; Brandon, T.R.; Custodio, D.E.; Abagyan, R.; Siuzdak, G. METLIN a metabolite mass spectral database. *Ther. Drug Monit.* **2005**, *27*, 747–751. [CrossRef]
66. Wishart, D.S.; Feunang, Y.D.; Marcu, A.; Guo, A.C.; Liang, K.; Vázquez-Fresno, R.; Sajed, T.; Johnson, D.; Li, C.; Karu, N.; et al. HMDB 4.0: The human metabolome database for 2018. *Nucleic Acids Res.* **2018**, *46*, D608–D617. [CrossRef] [PubMed]
67. Krettler, C.A.; Thallinger, G.G. A map of mass spectrometry-based in silico fragmentation prediction and compound identification in metabolomics. *Brief. Bioinform.* **2021**, *22*, bbab073. [CrossRef] [PubMed]
68. Böcker, S. Searching molecular structure databases using tandem MS data: Are we there yet? *Curr. Opin. Chem. Biol.* **2017**, *36*, 1–6. [CrossRef] [PubMed]
69. Stanstrup, J.; Neumann, S.; Vrhovšek, U. PredRet: Prediction of retention time by direct mapping between multiple chromatographic systems. *Anal. Chem.* **2015**, *87*, 9421–9428. [CrossRef]
70. Ren, S.; Hinzman, A.A.; Kang, E.L.; Szczesniak, R.D.; Lu, L.J. Computational and statistical analysis of metabolomics data. *Metabolomics* **2015**, *11*, 1492–1513. [CrossRef]
71. Riccio, R.; Minale, L.; Pagonis, S.; Pizza, C.; Zollo, F.; Pusset, J. A novel group of highly hydroxylated steroids from the starfish *Protoreaster nodosus*. *Tetrahedron* **1982**, *38*, 3615–3622. [CrossRef]
72. Qi, J.; Ojika, M.; Sakagami, Y. Linckosides A and B, two new neuritogenic steroid glycosides from the Okinawan starfish *Linckia laevigata*. *Bioorg. Med. Chem.* **2002**, *10*, 1961–1966. [CrossRef]
73. Kitagawa, I.; Kobayashi, M. Saponin and sapogenol. XXVI. Steroidal saponins from the starfish *Acanthaster planci* L. (crown of thorns). 2. Structure of the major saponin thornasteroside A. *Chem. Pharm. Bull.* **1978**, *26*, 1864–1873. [CrossRef]
74. Malyarenko, O.S.; Malyarenko, T.V.; Kicha, A.A.; Ivanchina, N.V.; Ermakova, S.P. Effects of polar steroids from the starfish *Patiria* (=*asterina*) *pectinifera* in combination with x-ray radiation on colony formation and apoptosis induction of human colorectal carcinoma cells. *Molecules* **2019**, *24*, 3154. [CrossRef]
75. Malyarenko, O.S.; Malyarenko, T.V.; Usoltseva, R.V.; Silchenko, A.S.; Kicha, A.A.; Ivanchina, N.V.; Ermakova, S.P. Fucoidan from brown algae *Fucus evanescens* potentiates the anti-proliferative efficacy of asterosaponins from starfish *Asteropsis carinifera* in 2D and 3D models of melanoma cells. *Int. J. Biol. Macromol.* **2021**, *185*, 31–39. [CrossRef]
76. Malyarenko, O.S.; Malyarenko, T.V.; Usoltseva, R.V.; Surits, V.V.; Kicha, A.A.; Ivanchina, N.V.; Ermakova, S.P. Combined anticancer effect of sulfated laminaran from the brown alga *Alaria angusta* and polyhydroxysteroid glycosides from the starfish *Protoreaster lincki* on 3D colorectal carcinoma HCT 116 cell line. *Mar. Drugs* **2021**, *19*, 540. [CrossRef] [PubMed]
77. Popov, R.S.; Ivanchina, N.V.; Kicha, A.A.; Malyarenko, T.V.; Dmitrenok, P.S.; Stonik, V.A. Metabolite profiling of polar steroid constituents in the far eastern starfish *Aphelasterias japonica* using LC-ESI MS/MS. *Metabolomics* **2014**, *10*, 1152–1168. [CrossRef]
78. Popov, R.S.; Ivanchina, N.V.; Kicha, A.A.; Malyarenko, T.V.; Dmitrenok, P.S.; Stonik, V.A. LC-ESI MS/MS profiling of polar steroid metabolites of the Far Eastern starfish *Patiria* (=*Asterina*) *Pectinifera*. *Metabolomics* **2016**, *12*, 21. [CrossRef]
79. Popov, R.S.; Ivanchina, N.V.; Kicha, A.A.; Malyarenko, T.V.; Dmitrenok, P.S. Structural characterization of polar steroid compounds of the Far Eastern starfish *Lethasterias fusca* by nanoflow liquid chromatography coupled to quadrupole time-of-flight tandem mass spectrometry. *J. Am. Soc. Mass Spectrom.* **2019**, *30*, 743–764. [CrossRef]
80. Domon, B.; Costello, C.E. A systematic nomenclature for carbohydrate fragmentations in FAB-MS/MS spectra of glycoconjugates. *Glycoconj. J.* **1988**, *5*, 397–409. [CrossRef]
81. Minamisawa, T.; Hirabayashi, J. Fragmentations of isomeric sulfated monosaccharides using electrospray ion trap mass spectrometry. *Rapid Commun. Mass Spectrom.* **2005**, *19*, 1788–1796. [CrossRef]
82. Gonçalves, A.G.; Ducatti, D.R.B.; Grindley, T.B.; Duarte, M.E.R.; Noseda, M.D. ESI-MS differential fragmentation of positional isomers of sulfated oligosaccharides derived from carrageenans and agarans. *J. Am. Soc. Mass Spectrom.* **2010**, *21*, 1404–1416. [CrossRef]
83. Popov, R.S.; Dmitrenok, P.S. Stereospecific fragmentation of starfish polyhydroxysteroids in electrospray ionization mass spectrometry. *J. Anal. Chem.* **2016**, *71*, 1368–1376. [CrossRef]
84. Sandvoss, M.; Weltring, A.; Preiss, A.; Levsen, K.; Wuensch, G. Combination of matrix solid-phase dispersion extraction and direct on-line liquid chromatography-nuclear magnetic resonance spectroscopy-tandem mass spectrometry as a new efficient approach for the rapid screening of natural products: Application to the t. *J. Chromatogr. A* **2001**, *917*, 75–86. [CrossRef]
85. Demeyer, M.; De Winter, J.; Caulier, G.; Eeckhaut, I.; Flammang, P.; Gerbaux, P. Molecular diversity and body distribution of saponins in the sea star *Asterias rubens* by mass spectrometry. *Comp. Biochem. Physiol. Part B Biochem. Mol. Biol.* **2014**, *168*, 1–11. [CrossRef]

86. Demeyer, M.; Wisztorski, M.; Decroo, C.; De Winter, J.; Caulier, G.; Hennebert, E.; Eeckhaut, I.; Fournier, I.; Flammang, P.; Gerbaux, P. Inter- and intra-organ spatial distributions of sea star saponins by MALDI imaging. *Anal. Bioanal. Chem.* **2015**, *407*, 8813–8824. [CrossRef] [PubMed]
87. Popov, R.S.; Ivanchina, N.V.; Kicha, A.A.; Malyarenko, T.V.; Grebnev, B.B.; Dmitrenok, P.S.; Stonik, V.A. LC–MS-based metabolome analysis on steroid metabolites from the starfish *Patiria* (=*Asterina*) *pectinifera* in conditions of active feeding and stresses. *Metabolomics* **2016**, *12*, 106. [CrossRef]
88. Tangerina, M.M.P.; Cesário, J.P.; Pereira, G.R.R.; Costa, T.M.; Valenti, W.C.; Vilegas, W. Chemical profile of the sulphated saponins from the starfish *Luidia senegalensis* collected as by-catch fauna in Brazilian coast. *Nat. Prod. Bioprospect.* **2018**, *8*, 83–89. [CrossRef] [PubMed]
89. Popov, R.S.; Ivanchina, N.V.; Kicha, A.A.; Malyarenko, T.V.; Grebnev, B.B.; Stonik, V.A.; Dmitrenok, P.S. The distribution of asterosaponins, polyhydroxysteroids and related glycosides in different body components of the Far Eastern starfish *Lethasterias fusca*. *Mar. Drugs* **2019**, *17*, 523. [CrossRef]
90. Dahmoune, B.; Bachari-Houma, F.; Chibane, M.; Jéhan, P.; Guegan, J.P.; Dahmoune, F.; Aissou-Akrour, C.; Mouni, L.; Ferrières, V.; Hauchard, D. Saponin contents in the starfish *Echinaster sepositus*: Chemical characterization, qualitative and quantitative distribution. *Biochem. Syst. Ecol.* **2021**, *96*, 104262. [CrossRef]
91. Maier, M.S.; Centurión, R.; Muniain, C.; Haddad, R.; Eberlin, M.N. Identification of sulfated steroidal glycosides from the starfish *Heliaster helianthus* by electrospray ionization mass spectrometry. *Arkivoc* **2006**, *2007*, 301. [CrossRef]
92. Van Dyck, S.; Gerbaux, P.; Flammang, P. Elucidation of molecular diversity and body distribution of saponins in the sea cucumber *Holothuria forskali* (Echinodermata) by mass spectrometry. *Comp. Biochem. Physiol. B Biochem. Mol. Biol.* **2009**, *152*, 124–134. [CrossRef]
93. van Dyck, S.; Flammang, P.; Meriaux, C.; Bonnel, D.; Salzet, M.; Fournier, I.; Wisztorski, M. Localization of secondary metabolites in marine invertebrates: Contribution of MALDI MSI for the study of saponins in Cuvierian tubules of *H. forskali*. *PLoS ONE* **2010**, *5*, e13923. [CrossRef]
94. Van Dyck, S.; Gerbaux, P.; Flammang, P. Qualitative and quantitative saponin contents in five sea cucumbers from the Indian ocean. *Mar. Drugs* **2010**, *8*, 173–189. [CrossRef]
95. Van Dyck, S.; Caulier, G.; Todesco, M.; Gerbaux, P.; Fournier, I.; Wisztorski, M.; Flammang, P. The triterpene glycosides of *Holothuria forskali*: Usefulness and efficiency as a chemical defense mechanism against predatory fish. *J. Exp. Biol.* **2011**, *214*, 1347–1356. [CrossRef]
96. Bondoc, K.G.V.; Lee, H.; Cruz, L.J.; Lebrilla, C.B.; Juinio-Meñez, M.A. Chemical fingerprinting and phylogenetic mapping of saponin congeners from three tropical holothurian sea cucumbers. *Comp. Biochem. Physiol. B Biochem. Mol. Biol.* **2013**, *166*, 182–193. [CrossRef] [PubMed]
97. Caulier, G.; Flammang, P.; Rakotorisoa, P.; Gerbaux, P.; Demeyer, M.; Eeckhaut, I. Preservation of the bioactive saponins of *Holothuria scabra* through the processing of trepang. *Cah. Biol. Mar.* **2013**, *54*, 685–690.
98. Caulier, G.; Mezali, K.; Soualili, D.L.; Decroo, C.; Demeyer, M.; Eeckhaut, I.; Gerbaux, P.; Flammang, P. Chemical characterization of saponins contained in the body wall and the Cuvierian tubules of the sea cucumber *Holothuria* (*Platyperona*) *sanctori* (Delle Chiaje, 1823). *Biochem. Syst. Ecol.* **2016**, *68*, 119–127. [CrossRef]
99. Popov, R.S.; Ivanchina, N.V.; Silchenko, A.S.; Avilov, S.A.; Kalinin, V.I.; Dolmatov, I.Y.; Stonik, V.A.; Dmitrenok, P.S. Metabolite profiling of triterpene glycosides of the far eastern sea cucumber *Eupentacta fraudatrix* and their distribution in various body components using LC-ESI QTOF-MS. *Mar. Drugs* **2017**, *15*, 302. [CrossRef]
100. Mitu, S.A.; Bose, U.; Suwansa-ard, S.; Turner, L.H.; Zhao, M.; Elizur, A.; Ogbourne, S.M.; Shaw, P.N.; Cummins, S.F. Evidence for a saponin biosynthesis pathway in the body wall of the commercially significant sea cucumber *Holothuria scabra*. *Mar. Drugs* **2017**, *15*, 349. [CrossRef]
101. Decroo, C.; Colson, E.; Demeyer, M.; Lemaur, V.; Caulier, G.; Eeckhaut, I.; Cornil, J.; Flammang, P.; Gerbaux, P. Tackling saponin diversity in marine animals by mass spectrometry: Data acquisition and integration. *Anal. Bioanal. Chem.* **2017**, *409*, 3115–3126. [CrossRef]
102. Sroyraya, M.; Kaewphalug, W.; Anantachoke, N.; Poomtong, T.; Sobhon, P.; Srimongkol, A.; Suphamungmee, W. Saponins enriched in the epidermal layer of *Holothuria leucospilota* body wall. *Microsc. Res. Tech.* **2018**, *81*, 1182–1190. [CrossRef]
103. Grauso, L.; Yegdaneh, A.; Sharifi, M.; Mangoni, A.; Zolfaghari, B.; Lanzotti, V. Molecular networking-based analysis of cytotoxic saponins from sea cucumber *Holothuria atra*. *Mar. Drugs* **2019**, *17*, 86. [CrossRef]
104. Dai, Y.L.; Kim, E.A.; Luo, H.M.; Jiang, Y.F.; Oh, J.Y.; Heo, S.J.; Jeon, Y.J. Characterization and anti-tumor activity of saponin-rich fractions of South Korean sea cucumbers (*Apostichopus japonicus*). *J. Food Sci. Technol.* **2020**, *57*, 2283–2292. [CrossRef]
105. Omran, N.E.; Salem, H.K.; Eissa, S.H.; Kabbash, A.M.; Kandeil, M.A.; Salem, M.A. Chemotaxonomic study of the most abundant Egyptian sea-cucumbers using ultra-performance liquid chromatography (UPLC) coupled to high-resolution mass spectrometry (HRMS). *Chemoecology* **2020**, *30*, 35–48. [CrossRef]
106. Kamyab, E.; Goebeler, N.; Kellermann, M.Y.; Rohde, S.; Reverter, M.; Striebel, M.; Schupp, P.J. Anti-fouling effects of saponin-containing crude extracts from tropical Indo-Pacific sea cucumbers. *Mar. Drugs* **2020**, *18*, 181. [CrossRef] [PubMed]
107. Savarino, P.; Colson, E.; Caulier, G.; Eeckhaut, I.; Flammang, P.; Gerbaux, P. Microwave-assisted desulfation of the hemolytic saponins extracted from *Holothuria scabra* viscera. *Molecules* **2022**, *27*, 537. [CrossRef] [PubMed]

108. Campagnuolo, C.; Fattorusso, E.; Taglialatela-Scafati, O. Feroxosides A-B, two norlanostane tetraglycosides from the Caribbean sponge *Ectyoplasia ferox*. *Tetrahedron* **2001**, *57*, 4049–4055. [CrossRef]
109. Sandvoss, M.; Pham, L.H.; Levsen, K.; Preiss, A.; Mügge, C.; Wünsch, G. Isolation and structural elucidation of steroid oligoglycosides from the starfish *Asterias rubens* by means of direct online LC-NMR-MS hyphenation and one- and two-dimensional NMR investigations. *Eur. J. Org. Chem.* **2000**, *2000*, 1253–1262. [CrossRef]
110. Kicha, A.A.; Ivanchina, N.V.; Gorshkova, I.A.; Ponomarenko, L.P.; Likhatskaya, G.N.; Stonik, V.A. The distribution of free sterols, polyhydroxysteroids and steroid glycosides in various body components of the starfish *Patiria* (=*Asterina*) *pectinifera*. *Comp. Biochem. Physiol. Part B Biochem. Mol. Biol.* **2001**, *128*, 43–52. [CrossRef]
111. Kicha, A.A.; Ivanchina, N.V.; Stonik, V.A. Seasonal variations in the levels of polyhydroxysteroids and related glycosides in the digestive tissues of the starfish *Patiria* (*Asterina*) *pectinifera*. *Comp. Biochem. Physiol. Part B Biochem. Mol. Biol.* **2003**, *136*, 897–903. [CrossRef]
112. Silchenko, A.S.; Avilov, S.A.; Kalinin, V.I.; Kalinovsky, A.I.; Dmitrenok, P.S.; Fedorov, S.N.; Stepanov, V.G.; Dong, Z.; Stonik, V.A. Constituents of the sea cucumber *Cucumaria okhotensis*. Structures of okhotosides B1-B3 and cytotoxic activities of some glycosides from this species. *J. Nat. Prod.* **2008**, *71*, 351–356. [CrossRef]
113. Silchenko, A.S.; Kalinovsky, A.I.; Avilov, S.A.; Andrijaschenko, P.V.; Popov, R.S.; Dmitrenok, P.S.; Chingizova, E.A.; Kalinin, V.I. Kurilosides A1, A2, C1, D, E and F—triterpene glycosides from the far eastern sea cucumber *Thyonidium* (=*Duasmodactyla*) *kurilensis* (Levin): Structures with unusual non-holostane aglycones and cytotoxicities. *Mar. Drugs* **2020**, *18*, 551. [CrossRef]
114. Aminin, D.; Menchinskaya, E.; Pisliagin, E.; Silchenko, A.; Avilov, S.; Kalinin, V. Anticancer activity of sea cucumber triterpene glycosides. *Mar. Drugs* **2015**, *13*, 1202–1223. [CrossRef]
115. Aminin, D.L.; Pislyagin, E.A.; Menchinskaya, E.S.; Silchenko, A.S.; Avilov, S.A.; Kalinin, V.I. Immunomodulatory and anticancer activity of sea cucumber triterpene glycosides. In *Studies in Natural Products Chemistry*; Atta-ur-Rahman, Ed.; Elsevier: Amsterdam, The Netherlands, 2014; pp. 75–94, ISBN 9780444632944.
116. Han, Q.; Keesing, J.K.; Liu, D. A Review of sea cucumber aquaculture, ranching, and stock enhancement in China. *Rev. Fish. Sci. Aquac.* **2016**, *24*, 326–341. [CrossRef]
117. Hu, X.Q.; Xu, J.; Xue, Y.; Li, Z.J.; Wang, J.F.; Wang, J.H.; Xue, C.H.; Wangy, Y.M. Effects of bioactive components of sea cucumber on the serum, liver lipid profile and lipid absorption. *Biosci. Biotechnol. Biochem.* **2012**, *76*, 2214–2218. [CrossRef] [PubMed]
118. Popov, R.S.; Avilov, S.A.; Silchenko, A.S.; Kalinovsky, A.I.; Dmitrenok, P.S.; Grebnev, B.B.; Ivanchina, N.V.; Kalinin, V.I. Cucumariosides F1 and F2, two new triterpene glycosides from the sea cucumber *Eupentacta fraudatrix* and their LC-ESI MS/MS identification in the starfish *Patiria pectinifera*, a predator of the sea cucumber. *Biochem. Syst. Ecol.* **2014**, *57*, 191–197. [CrossRef]
119. Decroo, C.; Colson, E.; Lemaur, V.; Caulier, G.; De Winter, J.; Cabrera-Barjas, G.; Cornil, J.; Flammang, P.; Gerbaux, P. Ion mobility mass spectrometry of saponin ions. *Rapid Commun. Mass Spectrom.* **2019**, *33*, 22–33. [CrossRef] [PubMed]
120. Bahrami, Y.; Zhang, W.; Franco, C. Discovery of novel saponins from the viscera of the sea cucumber *Holothuria lessoni*. *Mar. Drugs* **2014**, *12*, 2633–2667. [CrossRef]
121. Bahrami, Y.; Zhang, W.; Chataway, T.; Franco, C. Structural elucidation of novel saponins in the sea cucumber *Holothuria lessoni*. *Mar. Drugs* **2014**, *12*, 4439–4473. [CrossRef] [PubMed]
122. Bahrami, Y.; Franco, C.M.M. Structure elucidation of new acetylated saponins, Lessoniosides A, B, C, D, and E, and non-acetylated saponins, Lessoniosides F and G, from the viscera of the sea cucumber *Holothuria lessoni*. *Mar. Drugs* **2015**, *13*, 597–617. [CrossRef] [PubMed]
123. Bahrami, Y.; Zhang, W.; Franco, C.M.M.; Franco, C.M.M. Distribution of saponins in the sea cucumber *Holothuria lessoni*; the body wall versus the viscera, and their biological activities. *Mar. Drugs* **2018**, *16*, 423. [CrossRef]
124. Shajahan, A.; Heiss, C.; Ishihara, M.; Azadi, P. Glycomic and glycoproteomic analysis of glycoproteins—a tutorial. *Anal. Bioanal. Chem.* **2017**, *409*, 4483–4505. [CrossRef]
125. Mert Ozupek, N.; Cavas, L. Triterpene glycosides associated antifouling activity from *Holothuria tubulosa* and *H. polii*. *Reg. Stud. Mar. Sci.* **2017**, *13*, 32–41. [CrossRef]
126. Malyarenko, T.V.; Kicha, A.A.; Stonik, V.A.; Ivanchina, N.V. Sphingolipids of asteroidea and holothuroidea: Structures and biological activities. *Mar. Drugs* **2021**, *19*, 330. [CrossRef]
127. González-Wangüemert, M.; Roggatz, C.C.; Rodrigues, M.J.; Barreira, L.; da Silva, M.M.; Custódio, L. A new insight into the influence of habitat on the biochemical properties of three commercial sea cucumber species. *Int. Aquat. Res.* **2018**, *10*, 361–373. [CrossRef]
128. Bechtel, P.J.; Oliveira, A.C.M.; Demir, N.; Smiley, S. Chemical composition of the giant red sea cucumber, *Parastichopus californicus*, commercially harvested in Alaska. *Food Sci. Nutr.* **2013**, *1*, 63–73. [CrossRef] [PubMed]
129. Svetashev, V.I.; Levin, V.S.; Lam, C.N.; Nga, D.T. Lipid and fatty acid composition of holothurians from tropical and temperate waters. *Comp. Biochem. Physiol.* **1991**, *98*, 489–494. [CrossRef]
130. Howell, K.L.; Pond, D.W.; Billett, D.S.M.; Tyler, P.A. Feeding ecology of deep-sea seastars (Echinodermata: Asteroidea): A fatty-acid biomarker approach. *Mar. Ecol. Prog. Ser.* **2003**, *255*, 193–206. [CrossRef]
131. Bergé, J.P.; Barnathan, G. Fatty acids from lipids of marine organisms: Molecular biodiversity, roles as biomarkers, biologically active compounds, and economical aspects. *Adv. Biochem. Eng. Biotechnol.* **2005**, *96*, 49–125. [CrossRef]
132. Chiu, H.H.; Kuo, C.H. Gas chromatography-mass spectrometry-based analytical strategies for fatty acid analysis in biological samples. *J. Food Drug Anal.* **2020**, *28*, 60–73. [CrossRef]

133. Tang, B.; Row, K.H. Development of gas chromatography analysis of fatty acids in marine organisms. *J. Chromatogr. Sci.* **2013**, *51*, 599–607. [CrossRef]
134. Ginger, M.L.; Santos, V.L.C.S.; Wolff, G.A. A preliminary investigation of the lipids of abyssal holothurians from the north-east Atlantic Ocean. *J. Mar. Biol. Assoc. U. K.* **2000**, *80*, 139–146. [CrossRef]
135. Svetashev, V.I.; Kharlamenko, V.I. Fatty acids of abyssal echinodermata, the sea star *Eremicaster vicinus* and the sea urchin *Kamptosoma abyssale*: A New Polyunsaturated Fatty Acid Detected, 22:6(n-2). *Lipids* **2020**, *55*, 291–296. [CrossRef]
136. Hasegawa, N.; Sawaguchi, S.; Tokuda, M.; Unuma, T. Fatty acid composition in sea cucumber *Apostichopus japonicus* fed with microbially degraded dietary sources. *Aquac. Res.* **2014**, *45*, 2021–2031. [CrossRef]
137. Zhang, X.; Liu, Y.; Li, Y.; Zhao, X. Identification of the geographical origins of sea cucumber (*Apostichopus japonicus*) in northern China by using stable isotope ratios and fatty acid profiles. *Food Chem.* **2017**, *218*, 269–276. [CrossRef] [PubMed]
138. Zhang, X.; Cheng, J.; Han, D.; Chen, X.; Zhao, X.; Liu, Y. Regional differences in fatty acid composition of sea cucumber (*Apostichopus japonicus*) and scallop (*Patinopecten yesoensis*) in the coastal areas of China. *Reg. Stud. Mar. Sci.* **2019**, *31*, 100782. [CrossRef]
139. Imbs, A.B.; Svetashev, V.I.; Rodkina, S.A. Differences in lipid class and fatty acid composition between wild and cultured sea cucumbers, *Apostichopus japonicus*, explain modification and deposition of lipids. *Aquac. Res.* **2022**, *53*, 810–819. [CrossRef]
140. Kostetsky, E.Y.; Velansky, P.V.; Sanina, N.M. Phospholipids of the organs and tissues of echinoderms and tunicates from Peter the great bay (Sea of Japan). *Russ. J. Mar. Biol.* **2012**, *38*, 64–71. [CrossRef]
141. Kostetsky, E.Y.; Sanina, N.M.; Velansky, P.V. The thermotropic behavior and major molecular species composition of the phospholipids of echinoderms. *Russ. J. Mar. Biol.* **2014**, *40*, 131–139. [CrossRef]
142. Wang, X.; Cong, P.; Chen, Q.; Li, Z.; Xu, J.; Xue, C. Characterizing the phospholipid composition of six edible sea cucumbers by NPLC-Triple TOF-MS/MS. *J. Food Compos. Anal.* **2020**, *94*, 103626. [CrossRef]
143. Xu, J.; Duan, J.; Xue, C.; Feng, T.; Dong, P.; Sugawara, T.; Hirata, T. Analysis and comparison of glucocerebroside species from three edible sea cucumbers using liquid chromatography ion trap time-of-flight mass spectrometry. *J. Agric. Food Chem.* **2011**, *59*, 12246–12253. [CrossRef]
144. Jia, Z.; Li, S.; Cong, P.; Wang, Y.; Sugawara, T.; Xue, C.; Xu, J. High throughput analysis of cerebrosides from the sea cucumber *Pearsonothria graeffei* by liquid chromatography—Quadrupole-time-of-flight mass spectrometry. *J. Oleo Sci.* **2015**, *64*, 51–60. [CrossRef]
145. Jia, Z.; Song, Y.; Tao, S.; Cong, P.; Wang, X.; Xue, C.; Xu, J. Structure of sphingolipids from sea cucumber *Cucumaria frondosa* and structure-specific cytotoxicity against human HepG2 cells. *Lipids* **2016**, *51*, 321–334. [CrossRef]
146. Yamaguchi, R.; Kanie, Y.; Kanie, O.; Shimizu, Y. A unique structural distribution pattern discovered for the cerebrosides from starfish *Asterias amurensis*. *Carbohydr. Res.* **2019**, *473*, 115–122. [CrossRef]
147. Wang, X.; Wang, X.; Cong, P.; Zhang, X.; Zhang, H.; Xue, C.; Xu, J. Characterizing gangliosides in six sea cucumber species by HILIC–ESI-MS/MS. *Food Chem.* **2021**, *352*, 129379. [CrossRef] [PubMed]
148. Imbs, A.B.; Ermolenko, E.V.; Grigorchuk, V.P.; Sikorskaya, T.V.; Velansky, P.V. Current progress in lipidomics of marine invertebrates. *Mar. Drugs* **2021**, *19*, 660. [CrossRef] [PubMed]
149. Degroote, S.; Wolthoorn, J.; Vanmeer, G. The cell biology of glycosphingolipids. *Semin. Cell Dev. Biol.* **2004**, *15*, 375–387. [CrossRef] [PubMed]
150. Wennekes, T.; Van Den Berg, R.J.B.H.N.; Boot, R.G.; Van Der Marel, G.A.; Overkleeft, H.S.; Aerts, J.M.F.G. Glycosphingolipids-Nature, function, and pharmacological modulation. *Angew. Chem. Int. Ed.* **2009**, *48*, 8848–8869. [CrossRef]
151. Muralidhar, P.; Radhika, P.; Krishna, N.; Rao, D.V.; Rao, C.B. Sphingolipids from marine organisms: A review. *Nat. Prod. Sci.* **2003**, *9*, 117–142.
152. Xu, J.; Wang, Y.M.; Feng, T.Y.; Zhang, B.; Sugawara, T.; Xue, C.H. Isolation and anti-fatty liver activity of a novel cerebroside from the sea cucumber *Acaudina molpadioides*. *Biosci. Biotechnol. Biochem.* **2011**, *75*, 1466–1471. [CrossRef]
153. Du, L.; Li, Z.J.; Xu, J.; Wang, J.F.; Xue, Y.; Xue, C.H.; Takahashi, K.; Wang, Y.M. The anti-tumor activities of cerebrosides derived from sea cucumber *Acaudina molpadioides* and starfish *Asterias amurensis* in vitro and in vivo. *J. Oleo Sci.* **2012**, *61*, 321–330. [CrossRef]
154. Sugawara, T.; Zaima, N.; Yamamoto, A.; Sakai, S.; Noguchi, R.; Hirata, T. Isolation of sphingoid bases of sea cucumber cerebrosides and their cytotoxicity against human colon cancer cells. *Biosci. Biotechnol. Biochem.* **2006**, *70*, 2906–2912. [CrossRef]
155. Kawatake, S.; Nakamura, K.; Inagaki, M.; Higuchi, R. Isolation and structure determination of six glucocerebrosides from the starfish *Luidia maculata*. *Chem. Pharm. Bull.* **2002**, *50*, 1091–1096. [CrossRef]
156. Yamada, K.; Sasaki, K.; Harada, Y.; Isobe, R.; Higuchi, R. Constituents of Holothuroidea, 12. Isolation and structure of glucocerebrosides from the sea cucumber *Holothuria pervicax*. *Chem. Pharm. Bull.* **2002**, *50*, 1467–1470. [CrossRef]
157. Yamada, K.; Hara, E.; Miyamoto, T.; Higuchi, R.; Isobe, R.; Honda, S. Isolation and structure of biologically active glycosphingolipids from the sea cucumber *Cucumaria echinata*. *Eur. J. Org. Chem.* **1998**, *1998*, 371–378. [CrossRef]
158. Miyamoto, T.; Yamamoto, A.; Wakabayashi, M.; Nagaregawa, Y.; Inagaki, M.; Higuchi, R.; Iha, M.; Teruya, K. Biologically active glycosides from Asteroidea, 40 two new gangliosides, acanthagangliosides I and J from the starfish *Acanthaster planci*. *Eur. J. Org. Chem.* **2000**, *2000*, 2295–2301. [CrossRef]
159. Sisu, E.; Flangea, C.; Serb, A.; Rizzi, A.; Zamfir, A.D. High-performance separation techniques hyphenated to mass spectrometry for ganglioside analysis. *Electrophoresis* **2011**, *32*, 1591–1609. [CrossRef] [PubMed]

160. Sugawara, T.; Aida, K.; Duan, J.; Hirata, T. Analysis of glucosylceramides from various sources by liquid chromatography-ion trap mass spectrometry. *J. Oleo Sci.* **2010**, *59*, 387–394. [CrossRef] [PubMed]
161. Abdelhameed, R.F.A.; Eltamany, E.E.; Hal, D.M.; Ibrahim, A.K.; AboulMagd, A.M.; Al-Warhi, T.; Youssif, K.A.; Abd El-Kader, A.M.; Hassanean, H.A.; Fayez, S.; et al. New cytotoxic cerebrosides from the red sea cucumber *Holothuria spinifera* supported by in-silico studies. *Mar. Drugs* **2020**, *18*, 405. [CrossRef]
162. Darya, M.; Sajjadi, M.M.; Yousefzadi, M.; Sourinejad, I.; Zarei, M. Antifouling and antibacterial activities of bioactive extracts from different organs of the sea cucumber *Holothuria leucospilota*. *Helgol. Mar. Res.* **2020**, *74*, 4. [CrossRef]
163. Drazen, J.C.; Phleger, C.F.; Guest, M.A.; Nichols, P.D. Lipid, sterols and fatty acid composition of abyssal holothurians and ophiuroids from the North-East Pacific Ocean: Food web implications. *Comp. Biochem. Physiol. B Biochem. Mol. Biol.* **2008**, *151*, 79–87. [CrossRef]
164. Guenther, J.; Wright, A.D.; Burns, K.; De Nys, R. Chemical antifouling defences of sea stars: Effects of the natural products hexadecanoic acid, cholesterol, lathosterol and sitosterol. *Mar. Ecol. Prog. Ser.* **2009**, *385*, 137–149. [CrossRef]
165. Pereira, D.M.; Vinholes, J.; De Pinho, P.G.; Valentão, P.; Mouga, T.; Teixeira, N.; Andrade, P.B. A gas chromatography-mass spectrometry multi-target method for the simultaneous analysis of three classes of metabolites in marine organisms. *Talanta* **2012**, *100*, 391–400. [CrossRef]
166. Ruiz-Torres, V.; Rodríguez-Pérez, C.; Herranz-López, M.; Martín-García, B.; Gómez-Caravaca, A.M.; Arráez-Román, D.; Segura-Carretero, A.; Barrajón-Catalán, E.; Micol, V. Marine invertebrate extracts induce colon cancer cell death via ros-mediated dna oxidative damage and mitochondrial impairment. *Biomolecules* **2019**, *9*, 771. [CrossRef]
167. Telahigue, K.; Ghali, R.; Nouiri, E.; Labidi, A.; Hajji, T. Antibacterial activities and bioactive compounds of the ethyl acetate extract of the sea cucumber *Holothuria forskali* from Tunisian coasts. *J. Mar. Biol. Assoc. U. K.* **2020**, *100*, 229–237. [CrossRef]
168. Zakharenko, A.; Romanchenko, D.; Thinh, P.D.; Pikula, K.; Thuy Hang, C.T.; Yuan, W.; Xia, X.; Chaika, V.; Chernyshev, V.; Zakharenko, S.; et al. Features and advantages of supercritical CO2 extraction of sea cucumber *Cucumaria frondosa japonica* Semper, 1868. *Molecules* **2020**, *25*, 4088. [CrossRef] [PubMed]
169. Zhang, X.M.; Han, L.W.; Zhang, S.S.; Li, X.B.; He, Q.X.; Han, J.; Wang, X.M.; Liu, K.C. Targeted discovery and identification of novel nucleoside biomarkers in *Apostichopus japonicus* viscera using metabonomics. *Nucleosides Nucleotides Nucleic Acids* **2019**, *38*, 203–217. [CrossRef] [PubMed]
170. Zhang, H.; Geng, Y.F.; Qin, L.; Dong, X.P.; Xu, X.B.; Du, M.; Wang, Z.Y.; Thornton, M.; Yang, J.F.; Dong, L. Characterization of volatile compounds in different dried sea cucumber cultivars. *J. Food Meas. Charact.* **2018**, *12*, 1439–1448. [CrossRef]
171. Huo, D.; Sun, L.; Zhang, L.; Ru, X.; Liu, S.; Yang, H. Metabolome responses of the sea cucumber *Apostichopus japonicus* to multiple environmental stresses: Heat and hypoxia. *Mar. Pollut. Bull.* **2019**, *138*, 407–420. [CrossRef]
172. Li, L.; Chen, M.; Storey, K.B. Metabolic response of longitudinal muscles to acute hypoxia in sea cucumber *Apostichopus japonicus* (Selenka): A metabolome integrated analysis. *Comp. Biochem. Physiol. Part D Genom. Proteom.* **2019**, *29*, 235–244. [CrossRef]
173. Liu, S.; Sun, J.; Ru, X.; Cao, X.; Liu, J.; Zhang, T.; Zhou, Y.; Yang, H. Differences in feeding, intestinal mass and metabolites between a thermotolerant strain and common *Apostichopus japonicus* under high summer temperature. *Aquac. Res.* **2018**, *49*, 1957–1966. [CrossRef]
174. Yang, Q.; Zhang, X.; Lu, Z.; Huang, R.; Tran, N.T.; Wu, J.; Yang, F.; Ge, H.; Zhong, C.; Sun, Q.; et al. Transcriptome and metabolome analyses of sea cucumbers *Apostichopus japonicus* in Southern China during the summer aestivation period. *J. Ocean Univ. China* **2021**, *20*, 198–212. [CrossRef]
175. Zhang, Y.; Wang, Y.; Liu, X.; Ding, B.; Sun, Y.; Chang, Y.; Ding, J. Metabolomics analysis for skin ulceration syndrome of *Apostichopus japonicus* based on UPLC/Q-TOF MS. *J. Oceanol. Limnol.* **2021**, *39*, 1559–1569. [CrossRef]
176. Guo, C.; Wang, Y.; Wu, Y.; Han, L.; Gao, C.; Chang, Y.; Ding, J. UPLC-Q-TOF/MS-based metabonomics study on *Apostichopus japonicus* in various aquaculture models. *Aquac. Res.* **2021**, *53*, 2004–2014. [CrossRef]
177. Jiang, J.; Zhao, Z.; Gao, S.; Chen, Z.; Dong, Y.; He, P.; Wang, B.; Pan, Y.; Wang, X.; Guan, X.; et al. Divergent metabolic responses to sex and reproduction in the sea cucumber *Apostichopus Japonicus*. *Comp. Biochem. Physiol. Part D Genom. Proteom.* **2021**, *39*, 100845. [CrossRef] [PubMed]
178. Ru, X.; Zhang, L.; Liu, S.; Yang, H. Reproduction affects locomotor behaviour and muscle physiology in the sea cucumber, *Apostichopus japonicus*. *Anim. Behav.* **2017**, *133*, 223–228. [CrossRef]
179. Xing, L.; Sun, L.; Liu, S.; Zhang, L.; Yang, H. Comparative metabolomic analysis of the body wall from four varieties of the sea cucumber *Apostichopus Japonicus*. *Food Chem.* **2021**, *352*, 129339. [CrossRef] [PubMed]
180. Xing, L.; Sun, L.; Liu, S.; Zhang, L.; Sun, J.; Yang, H. Metabolomic analysis of white, green and purple morphs of sea cucumber *Apostichopus japonicus* during body color pigmentation process. *Comp. Biochem. Physiol. Part D Genom. Proteom.* **2021**, *39*, 100827. [CrossRef] [PubMed]
181. Zhao, G.; Zhao, W.; Han, L.; Ding, J.; Chang, Y. Metabolomics analysis of sea cucumber (*Apostichopus japonicus*) in different geographical origins using UPLC–Q-TOF/MS. *Food Chem.* **2020**, *333*, 127453. [CrossRef]
182. Ding, K.; Zhang, L.; Zhang, T.; Yang, H.; Brinkman, R. The effect of melatonin on locomotor behavior and muscle physiology in the sea cucumber *Apostichopus japonicus*. *Front. Physiol.* **2019**, *10*, 221. [CrossRef]
183. Ding, K.; Zhang, L.; Fan, X.; Guo, X.; Liu, X.; Yang, H. The effect of pedal peptide-type neuropeptide on locomotor behavior and muscle physiology in the sea cucumber *Apostichopus japonicus*. *Front. Physiol.* **2020**, *11*, 559348. [CrossRef]

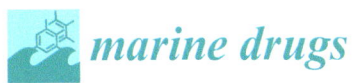

Review

Sphingolipids of Asteroidea and Holothuroidea: Structures and Biological Activities

Timofey V. Malyarenko [1,2,*], Alla A. Kicha [1], Valentin A. Stonik [1,2] and Natalia V. Ivanchina [1,*]

[1] G.B. Elyakov Pacific Institute of Bioorganic Chemistry, Far Eastern Branch of the Russian Academy of Sciences, Pr. 100-let Vladivostoku 159, 690022 Vladivostok, Russia; kicha@piboc.dvo.ru (A.A.K.); stonik@piboc.dvo.ru (V.A.S.)
[2] Department of Bioorganic Chemistry and Biotechnology, School of Natural Sciences, Far Eastern Federal University, Sukhanova Str. 8, 690000 Vladivostok, Russia
* Correspondence: malyarenko-tv@mail.ru (T.V.M.); ivanchina@piboc.dvo.ru (N.V.I.); Tel.: +7-423-2312-460 (T.V.M.); Fax: +7-423-2314-050 (T.V.M.)

Abstract: Sphingolipids are complex lipids widespread in nature as structural components of biomembranes. Commonly, the sphingolipids of marine organisms differ from those of terrestrial animals and plants. The gangliosides are the most complex sphingolipids characteristic of vertebrates that have been found in only the Echinodermata (echinoderms) phylum of invertebrates. Sphingolipids of the representatives of the Asteroidea and Holothuroidea classes are the most studied among all echinoderms. In this review, we have summarized the data on sphingolipids of these two classes of marine invertebrates over the past two decades. Recently established structures, properties, and peculiarities of biogenesis of ceramides, cerebrosides, and gangliosides from starfishes and holothurians are discussed. The purpose of this review is to provide the most complete information on the chemical structures, structural features, and biological activities of sphingolipids of the Asteroidea and Holothuroidea classes.

Keywords: sphingolipids; ceramides; cerebrosides; gangliosides; sialic acid; Asteroidea; Holothuroidea; biological activity; neuritogenic activity

Citation: Malyarenko, T.V.; Kicha, A.A.; Stonik, V.A.; Ivanchina, N.V. Sphingolipids of Asteroidea and Holothuroidea: Structures and Biological Activities. *Mar. Drugs* **2021**, *19*, 330. https://doi.org/10.3390/md19060330

Academic Editor: Vassilios Roussis

Received: 14 May 2021
Accepted: 2 June 2021
Published: 8 June 2021

Publisher's Note: MDPI stays neutral with regard to jurisdictional claims in published maps and institutional affiliations.

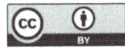

Copyright: © 2021 by the authors. Licensee MDPI, Basel, Switzerland. This article is an open access article distributed under the terms and conditions of the Creative Commons Attribution (CC BY) license (https://creativecommons.org/licenses/by/4.0/).

1. Introduction

Being the second-largest clade in a superphylum Deuterostomia after chordates, Echinodermata (echinoderms) is a phylum of exclusively marine invertebrates, inhabiting all the oceans in all the depths. These animals are characterized by radial symmetry, a particular water vascular system, and calcareous particles (ossicles) embedded in the dermis of their body walls. In some habitats, echinoderms are the dominant species in marine communities. There are five living classes of Echinodermata: Holothuroidea (sea cucumbers), Asteroidea (starfish), Ophiuroidea (brittle stars), Echinoidea (sea urchins), and Crinoidea (sea lilies and feather stars). These invertebrates present a rich source of diverse low molecular biologically active metabolites, including triterpene glycosides, polar steroids, and their glycosides, peptides, fatty acids, carotenoids, quinoid pigments, and different lipids, including sphingolipids. Our group is carrying out long-term studies on natural products from echinoderms [1–6], but sphingolipids from these invertebrates [7] so far were not in our main spotlight. However, our recent metabolomic studies on secondary metabolites from echinoderms, showing their extremal diversity [8–13], and successful attempts of application of some compounds as chemotaxonomic markers required the examination of perspectives of similar use of sphingolipids.

Sphingolipids, a group of heterogeneous lipids known as constituents of the plant, fungal, and animal cellular membranes, play a fundamental role in important phenomena such as cell-cell recognition and antigenic specificity [14,15]. Sphingolipids include ceramides, the hydrophobic molecules, involving a long-chain base (LCB) and an amide-linked fatty acid residue (FAR) and their glycoconjugated derivatives. Glycosylated ceramides are named cerebrosides, except for the corresponding oligoglycosides with carbohydrate chains, comprising one, two, three, or more sialic acid residues, which are known as gangliosides [16]. Sphingolipids were isolated from a number of biological sources, including marine invertebrates such as sea anemones [17], sponges [18–20], octocorals [21], ascidians [22], and representatives of other taxa. Various biological activities of ceramides, cerebrosides, and gangliosides, including plant growth stimulatory action [23], anti-inflammatory effects [24], the improving of the barrier function of the skin [25], cancer-protective action [26], proangiogenic action [27] have been reported.

In their majority, reviews about sphingolipids from marine organisms [28], including those concerning the corresponding natural products from echinoderms, were published from 12 to 20 years ago [29–31]. The present review includes data concerning chemical structures of sphingolipids from two classes of the phylum Echinodermata and their biological activities and covers the literature from 2000 to March 2021. We have focused our attention on the structures of these compounds, modern methods of analyses of complicated fractions of these lipids, and their bioactivities. Current problems of these studies are also discussed.

2. Ceramides

Ceramides are biosynthesized at the reaction of S-acyl-coenzyme A (usually C_{16}-CoA) with serine, catalyzed by serine palmitoyl transcriptase or related enzymes, followed by reduction of carbonyl group by ketosphinganine reductase and the N-acylation by ceramide synthase. Surprisingly, hydroxylation of long-chain bases (LCBs) that leads to so-called phytosphinganine derivatives, takes a place in plants and in many echinoderms. When hydroxylases act on fatty acid residues (FARs) in these invertebrates, an additional hydroxyl is introduced also into α–position of FARs [32]. As result, four main types of ceramides are known from different organisms including echinoderms, namely, A—containing sphinganine bases and nonhydroxylated fatty acid residues, B—consisting of sphinganine bases and α–hydroxylated fatty acids, C—containing phytosphinganine bases and nonhydroxylated fatty acids, and D—consisting of phytosphinganine bases and α–hydroxylated fatty acids (Figure 1). Both bases and fatty acids moieties in this type of natural products may contain normal chains, as well as those with *iso-* and/or *anteiso-*branching. Therefore, ceramides have great structural variety.

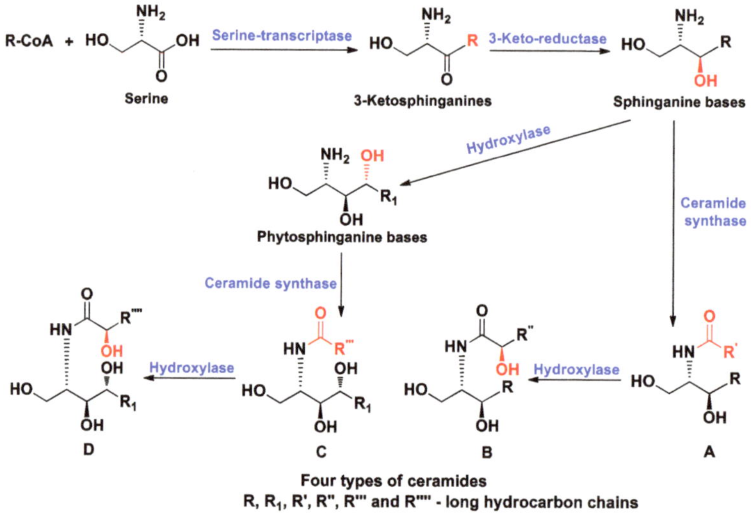

Figure 1. Scheme of biosynthesis and structures of main types of ceramides in echinoderms.

Class Asteroidea

Three ceramides **1**–**3** were isolated from the starfish *Distolasterias nipon* collected off the coast of the East Sea, Republic of Korea [33]. Structures of **1**–**3** were established by spectroscopic techniques and chemical transformations as (2*S*,3*R*,4*E*,8*E*,10*E*)-2-[(2*R*)-2-hydroxyhexadecanoylamino]-9-methyl-4,8,10-octadecatriene-1,3-diol (**1**), (2*S*,3*S*,4*R*,7*Z*)-2-[(2*R*)-2-hydroxyhexadecanoylamino]-7-docosene-1,3,4-triol (**2**), and (2*S*,3*R*,4*E*,7*E*)-2-[(2*R*)-2-hydroxyhexadecanoylamino]-7-docosene-1,3,4-triol (**4**) (Figure 2). Later ceramides **2** and **3** (iteratively) and **4**–**11** (additionally) were extracted from the same species of starfish and purified by silica gel column chromatography and reversed-phase high-performance liquid chromatography [34]. The high-energy collision-induced dissociation (CID) spectra of ceramides with various structures, differing from each other in the number and positions of double bonds on both the *N*-acyl and sphingoid chains as well as in the presence of hydroxy groups or a double bond at the C-4 position of the sphingoid chains as well as an additional α-hydroxy group in *N*-acyl chains, were established. The CID mass spectrum of the monosodiated ion [M + Na]$^+$ of each ceramide molecular species provided structural data concerning fatty acyl chains and sphingoid long-chain bases. This technique allowed determining complete structures of ceramides and cerebrosides in a mixture of sphingoid lipids and showed great potential for analysis of other sphingolipids isolated from various biological sources [34].

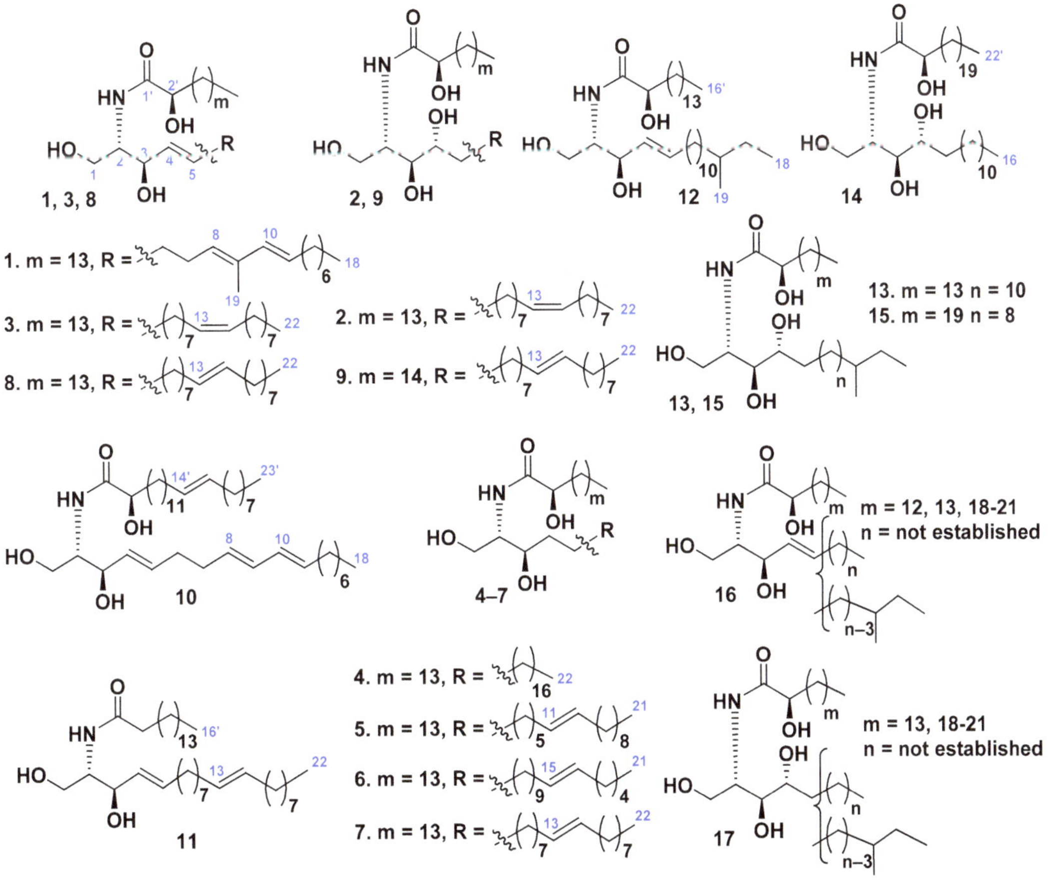

Figure 2. Ceramides from the starfish *Distolasterias nipon* and *Luidia maculata*.

A sphingosine-type ceramide LMCer-1-1 (**12**) and three phytosphingosine-type ceramides, LMCer-2-1 (**13**), LMCer-2-6 (**14**), and LMCer-2-7 (**15**), were isolated from the ceramide molecular species LMCer-1 (**16**) and LMCer-2 (**17**), obtained from the chloroform–methanol extract of the whole bodies of *Luidia maculata* [35]. The structures of ceramides **12**–**15** were determined on the basis of spectroscopic and chemical evidence as ($2S,3R,4E$)-2-[($2R$)-2-hydroxyhexadecanoylamino]-16-methyl-4-octadecene-1,3-diol (**12**), ($2S,3S,4R$)-2-[($2R$)-2-hydroxyhexadecanoylamino]-16-methyl-octadecane-1,3,4-triol (**13**), ($2S,3S,4R$)-2-[($2R$)-2-hydroxydocosanoylamino]-hexadecane-1,3,4-triol (**14**), and ($2S,3S,4R$)-2-[($2R$)-2-hydroxydocosanoylamino]-14-methyl-hexadecane-1,3,4-triol (**15**) (Figure 2).

The phytosphingosine-type ceramide asteriaceramide A was isolated from the whole bodies of the Northern Pacific starfish *Asterias amurensis* [23]. The structure of this compound was determined as identical to compound **2**. Asteriaceramide A (**2**) showed a stimulatory activity toward root growth of *Brassica campestris*. The plant growth activity of the ceramide was reported for the first time.

Since 2000, there were no data on the isolation, structure elucidation, and determination of biological activities of sea cucumber ceramides.

Thus, representatives of all the above-mentioned structural groups of ceramides (Figure 1A–D) were found from starfish. The structural diversity of these metabolites is connected with the presence of many variants of both sphingoid and fatty acid moieties. It should be noted that generally ceramides from starfish were studied worse than other groups of sphingolipids. Perhaps this is due to the difficulty of isolation of individual ceramides or their molecular species.

3. Cerebrosides

Cerebrosides are glycosylceramides that contain glucose, galactose, or other monosaccharide residues in their carbohydrate moieties. These compounds are synthesized by enzymes: UDP-glucose:ceramide β-D-glucosyl-transferase, UDP-galactose:ceramide β-D-galactose-transferase, and other glycosyl-transferases [32]. Cerebrosides can be divided into three classes: monoglycosides, biglycosides (mainly lactosides), and oligoglycosides. This class of complex lipids can contain an aminosugar residue (globosides) in their carbohydrate moieties or be sulfated at a terminal monosaccharide residue [30]. Cerebrosides, such as ceramides, are part of the plasmatic membranes of cells and perform a number of important biological functions: they take part in the formation of new membranes, such as phospholipids, sterols, and cellular membrane proteins, and also participate in the transmission of cellular signals [14]. Moreover, the cerebrosides in cellular membranes act as cell surface antigens and receptors. Interest in sphingolipids and their derivatives mainly is associated with their high biological significance. Some studies have shown that sphingolipids can inhibit the growth of microalgae, fungi, and bacteria. The presumptive mechanism of this action is associated with the ability of this type of compound to perforate cell membrane, in addition, in the presence of sphingolipids, the ability of bacterial cells to adhere is reduced [36–38]. The ability of sphingolipids to stimulate plant growth [23], demonstrate an anti-inflammatory effect [24], and improve the barrier function of the skin [25] has also been shown.

An even larger variety of cerebrosides containing one or more monosaccharide residues, in comparison with ceramides, was isolated from starfish and sea cucumbers.

3.1. Class Asteroidea

From the chloroform–methanol–water extract of gonads and body walls of the Patagonian starfish *Allostichaster inaequalis*, glucosylceramides were isolated [39], along with the previously known phalluside-1 and two glucosylceramides earlier isolated from the starfish *Cosmasterias lurida* [40]. Compounds were described as ($2S,3R,4E,8E,10E$)-1-O-(β-D-glucopyranosyl)-2-[($2R$)-2-hydroxy-15-tetracosenoylamino]-4,8,10-octadecatrien-3-ol (**18**) and ($2S,3R,4E,15Z$)-1-O-(β-D-glucopyranosyl)-2-[($2R$)-2-hydroxyhexadecanoylamino]-4,15-docosadien-3-ol (**19**) using spectroscopic and chemical methods (Figure 3).

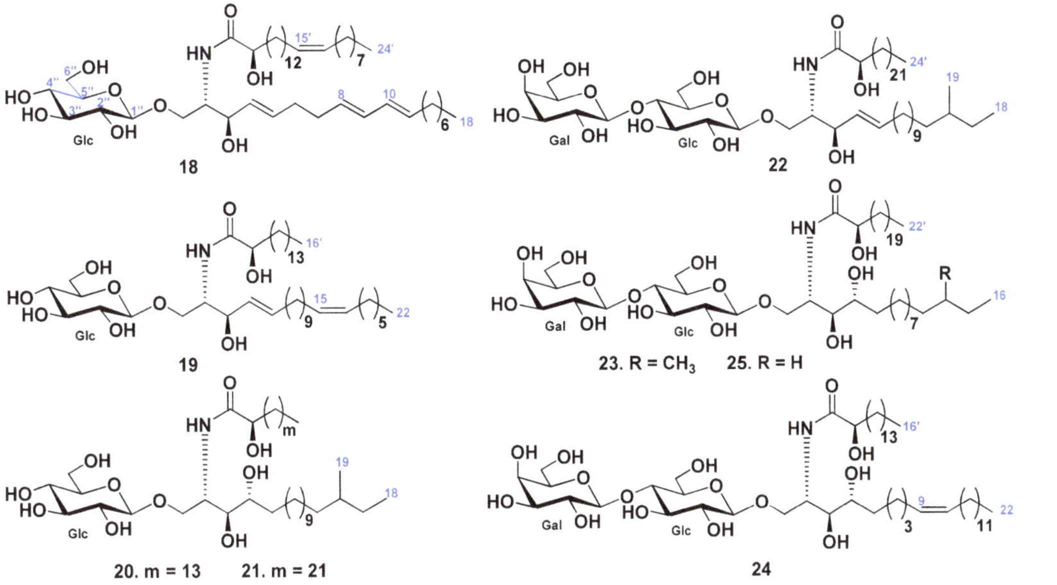

Figure 3. Cerebrosides from the starfish *Allostichaster inaequalis* and *Luidia maculata*.

Glucosylcerebrosides, luidiacerebrosides A (**20**) and B (**21**), were isolated from the cerebroside fraction obtained from the extract of the starfish *Luidia maculata* using HPLC [41]. The structures of cerebrosides were determined as 1-O-β-D-glucopyranoside of (2S,3S,4R)-2-[(2R)-2-hydroxyhexadecanoylamino]-16-methyl-octadecane-1,3,4-triol (**20**) and (2S,3S,4R)-2-[(2R)-2-hydroxytetracosanoylamino]-16-methyl-octadecane-1,3,4-triol (**21**), respectively [41]. In continuation of the studies on sphingolipids from the same starfish four cerebrosides, luidialactosides A–D (**22–25**), were isolated from its the water-insoluble lipid fraction [42]. They were proved to contain lactosyl carbohydrate chains attached to C-1 of 2-[(2R)-2-hydroxytetracosanoylamino]-16-methyl-4-octadecene-1,3-diol (**22**), 2-[(2R)-2-hydroxydocosanoylamino]-14-methyl-1,3,4-hexadecanetriol (**23**), 2-[(2R)-2-hydroxyhexadecanoylamino]-9-docosene-1,3,4-triol (**24**), and 2-[(2R)-2-hydroxydocosanoylamino]-1,3,4-hexadecanetriol (**25**) (Figure 3).

Eight glucosylceramides were found in the Patagonian starfish *Anasterias minuta* [43]. One of these constituents, anasterocerebroside A (**26**), was identified as a new glucosylceramide, while the earlier known glucosylceramide (**27**) was isolated and characterized for the first time as a pure compound. It was earlier isolated in a mixture with related glucosylceramides from the Patagonian starfish *Cosmasterias lurida* [40]. The structures of these sphingolipids were established by different spectroscopic and chemical methods as (2S,3R,4E,8E,10E)-1-O-(β-D-glucopyranosyl)-2-[(2R)-2-hydroxy-14-tricosenoylamino]-4,8,10-octadecatrien-3-ol (**26**) and (2S,3R,4E,8E,10E)-1-O-(β-D-glucopyranosyl)-2-[(2R)-2-hydroxy-15-tetracosenoylamino]-9-methyl-4,8,10-octadecatrien-3-ol (**27**) (Figure 4).

The glucocerebroside, linckiacerebroside A (**28**), and known glucocerebroside S-2a-3 were isolated from the chloroform–methanol extract of the starfish *Linckia laevigata*, together with three pseudo homogeneous glucocerebrosides [44]. The structures of this cerebroside were determined as (2S,3S,4R)-1-O-(β-D-glucopyranosyl)-2-[(2R)-2-hydroxyhexadecanoylamino]-16-methyl-heptadecane-1,3,4-triol (**28**) (Figure 4).

A galactocerebroside molecular species CNC-2 (**29**) were isolated from the extract of the tropical starfish *Culcita novaeguineae* [45] as a phytosphingosine type galactocerebroside with nonhydroxylated and hydroxylated fatty acyl moieties (Figure 4).

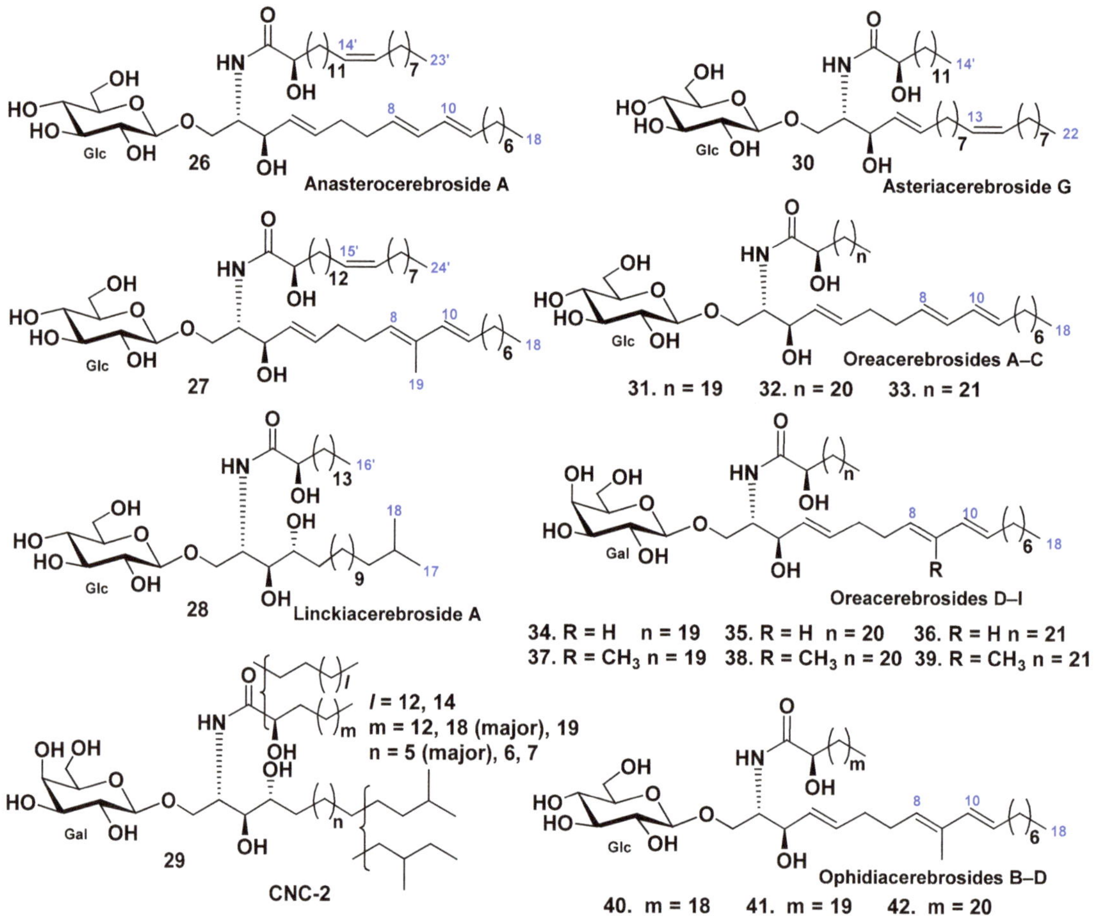

Figure 4. Structures of cerebrosides from the starfish *Anasterias minuta*, *Cosmasterias lurida*, *Linckia laevigata*, *Culcita novaeguineae*, *Oreaster reticulatus*, and *Narcissia canariensis*.

The glucocerebroside, asteriacerebroside G (**30**), and two known cerebrosides, asteriacerebrosides A and B, were isolated from the chloroform–methanol extract of the whole bodies of the Northern Pacific starfish *Asterias amurensis* [23]. The structure of **30** was determined on the basis of chemical and spectroscopic evidence as (2S,3R,4E,13Z)-1-O-(β-D-glucopyranosyl)-2-[(2R)-2-hydroxytetradecanoylamino]-4,13-docosadiene-1,3-diol (Figure 4). Asteriacerebrosides A, B, and G exhibited growth-promoting activity for the whole body of *Brassica campestris*.

The starfish *Oreaster reticulatus* contains nine glycosphingolipids named oreacerebrosides A–I (**31–39**) (along with earlier known ophidiacerebrosides C–E [46], Figure 4). All these compounds have a 4,8,10-triunsaturated sphingoid base. Oreacerebrosides A–C (**31–33**) are β-glucosylceramides in contrast with oreacerebrosides D–I (**34–39**), all these compounds were the first examples of β-galactosylceramides containing this unusual sphingoid base. Four representative glycosphingolipids were tested for cytotoxic activity on rat glioma C6 cells and shown to be mildly cytotoxic. Previously, it was established that the glucosylceramides were more active than the galactosylceramides. In addition, oreacerebroside I (**39**) was shown to exert proangiogenic activity and was able to increase VEGF-induced human endothelial cell proliferation.

Mixtures of three known glucocerebrosides (F13-3), ophidiacerebrosides B–D (**40–42**), were isolated from the starfish *Narcissia canariensis* collected off the coasts of Dakar, Senegal [47]. This fraction included three homologous cerebrosides identified as peracetylated derivatives on the basis of spectroscopic and chemical data (Figure 4). These compounds contain a β-glucopyranose as a sugar unit, 9-methyl-branched 4,8,10-triunsaturated long-chain aminoalcohols as sphingoid bases, and amide-linked 2-hydroxy fatty acid chains. The major component (63%) has an amide-linked 2-hydroxydocosanoic acid chain and was identified as ophidiacerebroside C (**41**), isolated from the starfish *Ophidiaster ophidianus* for the first time [48]. The minor components of F13-3 had one more or one less methylene group and were identified as ophidiacerebrosides B (**40**) and D (**42**). The cytotoxic activity of F13-3 was detected using KB cells. It was shown that three human cancerous cell lines, KMS-11 (adherent plasma cells obtained from patients with multiple myeloma) were inhibited by these cerebrosides with $IC_{50} = 15.2 \pm 4$ µM, GBM (astrocytoma cells obtained after tumor resection of patients with glioblastoma multiforme-primary culture) with $IC_{50} = 34.6 \pm 5.1$ µM, and HCT-116 (colorectal adenocarcinoma cells derived from a patient with Lynch's syndrome) with $IC_{50} = 18 \pm 3.9$ µM.

In total, 21 galactocerebrosides, including 16 new compounds (**43–58**) (Figure 5), were identified as cerebroside molecular species obtained from the chloroform–methanol extract of pyloric caeca cut out from the starfish *Protoreaster nodosus* [49]. These compounds were phytosphingosine-type galactocerebrosides with hydroxylated fatty acyl moieties. It is important, that GC–MS analysis, followed by methanolysis and periodate oxidation of these metabolites, gave reliable structural information of ceramide moiety rapidly in minute amounts. The structures of earlier known compounds were the same as those of galactosylcerebrosides previously found from other starfish and even mammalians.

Six glucocerebrosides (**59–64**) were isolated from the eggs of the starfish *Asterias amurensis* by extraction and different type of column chromatography, including HPLC [50]. It was shown that the structures of cerebrosides could be completely characterized, based on their sodium-adducted molecules, using FAB tandem mass spectrometry. The lipid part of the glucocerebrosides **59–64** consisted of saturated and monounsaturated α-hydroxy fatty acids and sphinganine type of the long-chain base (Figure 5).

Glucosyl ceramides (GlcCers) were later isolated from the viscera of the starfish *Asterias amurensis* [51]. Degraded GlcCers generated *A. amurensis* sphingoid bases (ASBs) that mainly consisted of the triene-type bases d18:3 and 9-methyl-d18:3. Actions of these bases on ceramide synthesis and content were analyzed using normal human epidermal keratinocytes (NHEKs). The bases significantly raised the de novo ceramide synthesis in NHEKs and expression of genes, encoding enzymes such as serinepalmitoyltransferase and ceramide synthase. Total ceramide (GlcCers) and sphingomyelin contents increased highly upon ASB treatment. In particular, GlcCers bearing fatty acids with large carbon atoms ($\geq$ C28) exhibited a significant content increasing. These ASB-induced enhancements on de novo ceramide synthesis were only observed in undifferentiated NHEKs. This stimulation of de novo sphingolipid synthesis may improve skin barrier functions.

Four cerebrosides (**65–68**) were isolated from the starfish *Distolasterias nipon* by extraction and different type of column chromatography, including reverse-phase HPLC [34]. Structural elucidation was conducted using tandem mass spectrometry of monosodiated ions desorbed by fast atom bombardment. Fatty acids in glucocerebrosides **65–68** were identified as saturated and monounsaturated α-hydroxylated derivatives. The glucocerebroside long-chain bases were found to be of di- and triunsaturated sphingenine types (Figure 5).

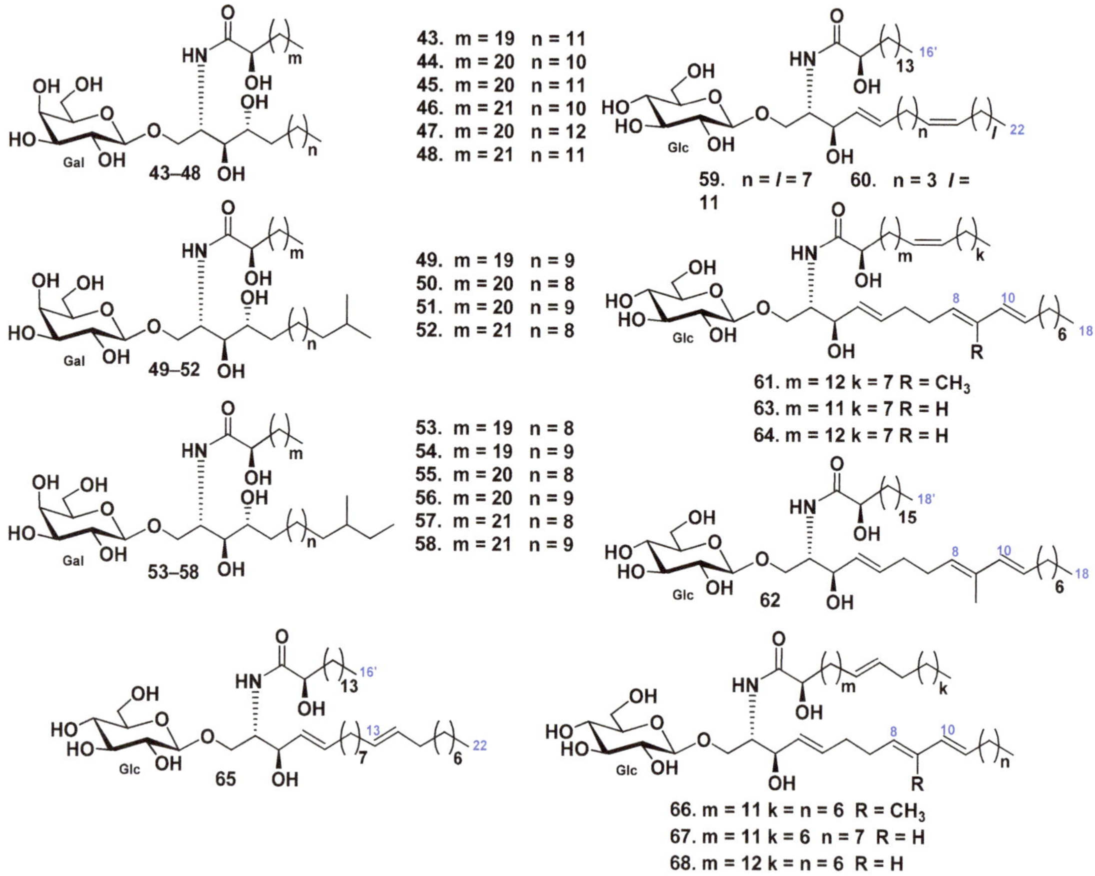

Figure 5. Cerebrosides from the starfish *Protoreaster nodosus*, *Asterias amurensis*, and *Distolasterias nipon*.

3.2. Class Holothuroidea

Overall, 18 glucocerebrosides (**69–86**) were detected in admixture from the sea cucumber *Holothuria coronopertusa* [52]. Their structures were established on the basis of liquid-secondary ion mass spectrometry (LSIMS) experiments. The CID mass spectrum of the lithiated molecules ([M + Li]$^+$) led to diagnostic fragment ions, which were further identified by tandem mass spectrometry (MS/MS). Fatty acids in glucocerebrosides **69–86** were indicated as saturated and monounsaturated α-hydroxyl fatty acids. The glucocerebroside long-chain bases were of sphingosine type (Figure 6).

Moreover, 10 glucocerebrosides, HPC-3-A–HPC-3-J (**87–96**), were isolated from the extract of the sea cucumber *Holothuria pervicax* [53]. All these compounds were mixtures of regio-isomers for terminal methyl groups in the LCB moiety, namely, mixtures of *iso*- and *anteiso*-isomers (Figure 6).

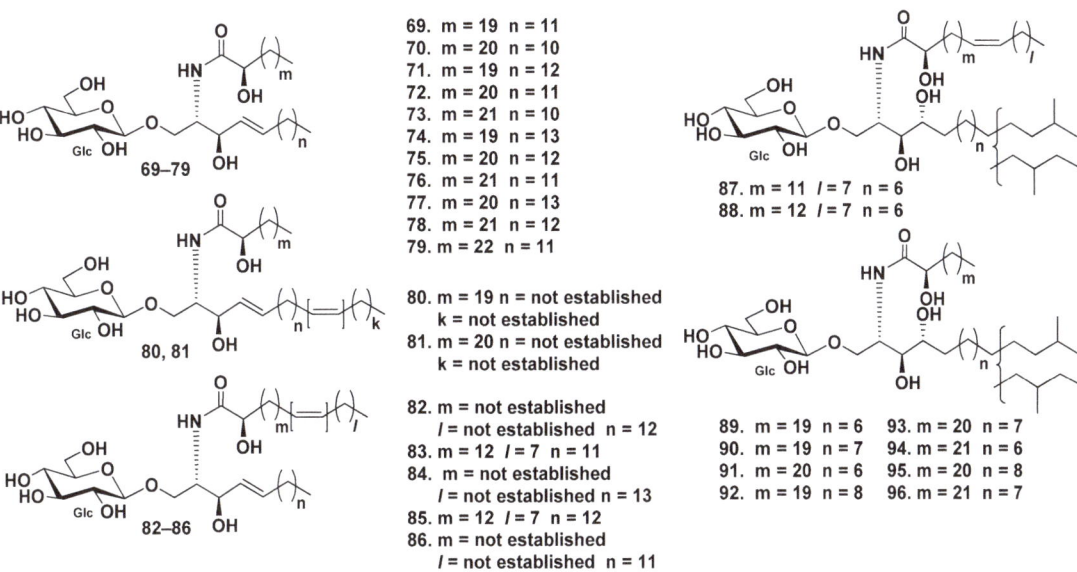

Figure 6. Cerebrosides from the sea cucumbers *Holothuria coronopertusa* and *Holothuria pervicax*.

Five glucocerebroside molecular species (SJC-1-SJC-5, **97–101**) were isolated from the extract of the sea cucumber *Stichopus japonicus* [54]. Cerebrosides **97–99** were sphingosine- and phytosphingosine type derivatives with nonhydroxylated and hydroxylated fatty acyl moieties. At the same time, cerebroside molecular species **100** and **101** were also sphingosine-type glucocerebroside molecular species with hydroxylated fatty acid moieties, although they were new compounds with unique sphingosine bases containing additional two hydroxy groups (Figure 7).

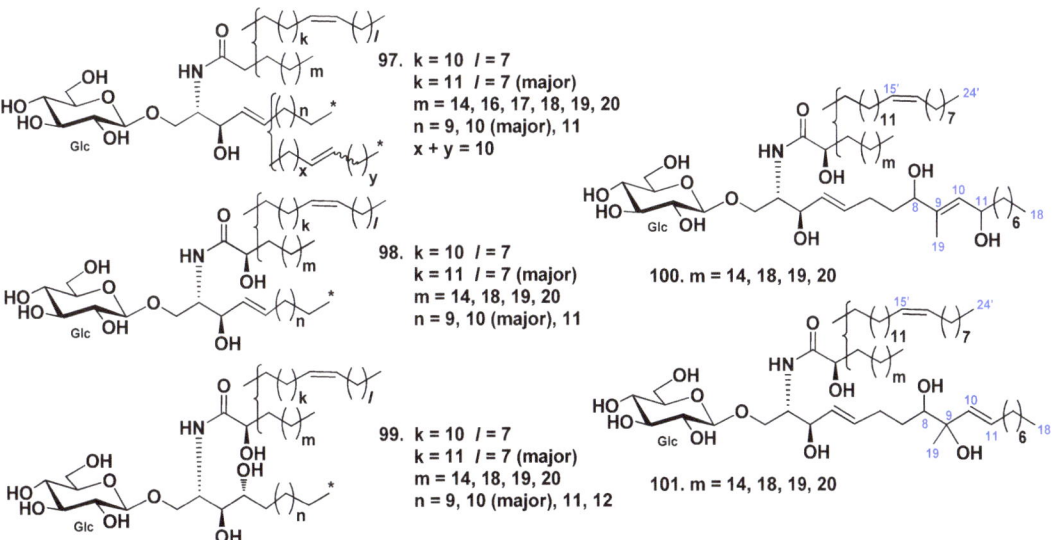

* terminal moieties of LCB parts contain *iso-* and *anteiso-* forms

Figure 7. Cerebrosides molecular species from the sea cucumber *Stichopus japonicus*.

Later, the content and components of cerebrosides from the sea cucumber *Stichopus japonicus* were analyzed by Duan et al. [55]. The absorption of cerebrosides from *S. japonicus* was studied with an in vivo lipid absorption assay. The result revealed that *S. japonicus* was a rich source of cerebrosides that contained considerable amounts of odd carbon chain sphingoid bases. The cumulative recoveries of d17:1 and d19:2 consisting cerebrosides were $0.31 \pm 0.16\%$ and $0.32 \pm 0.10\%$, respectively, for 24 h after administration. In addition, dietary supplementation with sea cucumber cerebrosides to hairless mouse improved the skin barrier function and increased the short-chain fatty acid content in caecal fraction, which demonstrated its effects on host.

An *anteiso*-type regio-isomer on the LCB moiety HLC-2-A (**102**) from the extract of the sea cucumber *Holothuria leucospilota* were isolated from its glucocerebroside molecular species HLC-2 (**104**), composed of *iso*- and *anteiso*-isomers [56]. Other glucocerebroside molecular species HLC-1(**103**) and HLC-3 (**105**) were indicated together with HLC-2 (Figure 8).

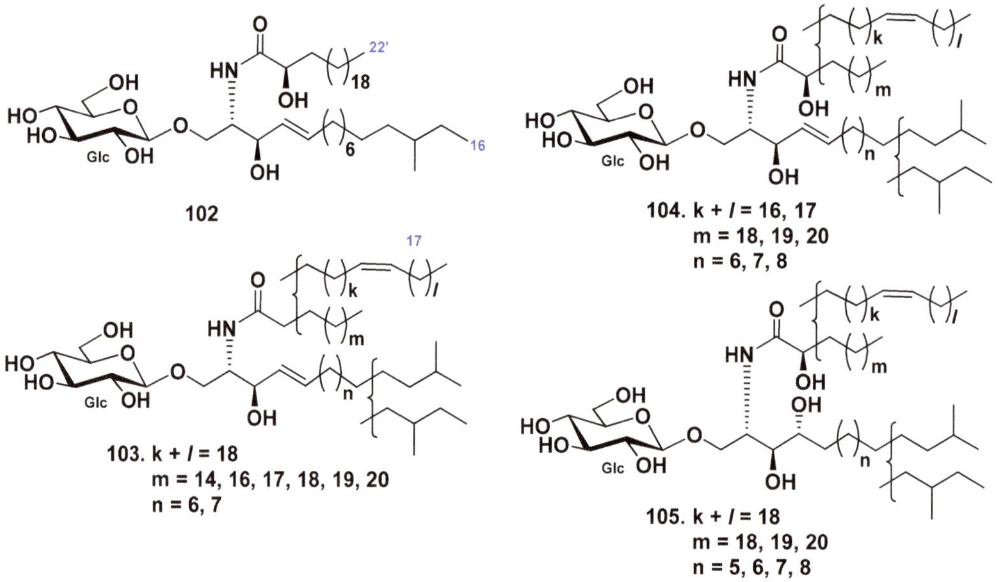

Figure 8. Cerebrosides from the sea cucumber *Holothuria leucospilota*.

Sugavara et al. reported the sphingoid base composition of cerebrosides from sea cucumber (species was not identified) and their cytotoxicity against human colon cancer cell lines [57]. The composition of sphingoid bases obtained from a sea cucumber was different from that of mammals, and the major constituents were supposed from mass spectra as containing branched C-17–C-19 alkyl chains with 1–3 double bounds. The viability of DLD-1, WiDr, and Caco-2 cells treated with sea cucumber sphingoid bases was reduced in a dose-dependent manner and was similar to that of cells treated with sphingosine. The sphingoid bases induced such a morphological change as condensed chromatin fragments and increased caspase-3 activity, indicating that these sphingoid bases reduced the cell viability by causing apoptosis in the above-mentioned cells.

The galactocerebroside BAC-4-4a (**106**) was isolated from its parent galactocerebroside molecular species BAC-4 (**107**), which was obtained from the extract of the sea cucumber *Bohadschia argus* [58]. BAC-4 was obtained together with earlier known glucocerebroside molecular species [53,54,56]. The structure of **106** was determined as (2*S*,3*R*,4*E*)-1-*O*-(β-D-galactopyranosyl)-2[(2R,15Z)-2-hydroxytetracosenoylamino]-4-heptadecene-1,3-diol (Figure 9). Before this study, galactocerebrosides were not found in sea cucumbers.

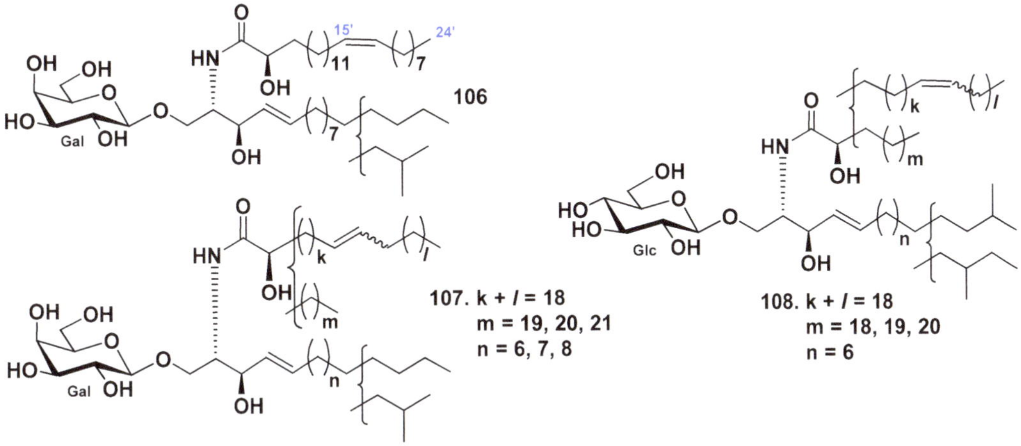

Figure 9. Cerebrosides from the sea cucumbers *Bohadschia argus* and *Acaudina molpadioides*.

The cerebroside molecular species AMC-2 (**108**) was isolated from the extract of the sea cucumber *Acaudina molpadioides* [59]. The amide-linked fatty acid units were established to contain four saturated and monounsaturated α-hydroxy fatty acids, the long-chain dihydroxy sphingoid base, having one double bond, and the glucose residue (Figure 9). It was shown the anti-fatty liver activity of **108** in rats with fatty liver, induced by orotic acid. AMC-2 (**108**) significantly reduced hepatic triglyceride and total cholesterol levels at a diet supplement of 0.03% and 0.006%. The indexes of stearoyl–CoA desaturase activity and mRNA expression were significantly decreased by **108**. This indicated that AMC-2 (**108**) ameliorated nonalcoholic fatty liver disease through suppression of stearoyl–CoA desaturase activity and impaired the biosynthesis of monounsaturated fatty acids in the livers of the rats.

Glucocerebrosides from three specimens of sea cucumbers, specifically, *Acaudina molpadioides*, *Cucumaria frondosa*, and *Apostichopus japonicus*, were rapidly identified by liquid chromatography–ion trap–time-of-flight mass spectrometry [60]. Various long-chain bases of glucosylcerebrosides were detected in these sea cucumbers. Two of the most common LCBs were identified as 2-amino-1,3-dihydroxy-4-heptadecene (d17:1) and 4,8-sphingadienine (d18:2), which were acylated to form saturated and monounsaturated nonhydroxylated and monohydroxylated fatty acids with 18–25 carbon atoms. The glucocerebroside fractions were the most complicated in the sea cucumber *C. frondosa* and were the simplest in the sea cucumber *A. molpadioides*.

It was found that a continuous oral administration of cerebrosides obtained from the sea cucumber *Acaudina molpadioides* at the dose of 50 mg/kg body mass per day suppressed body weight loss through alleviating adipose atrophy in cancer-associated cachexia mice [61]. The long-chain base, hydrolyzed from the cerebroside, contains 2-amino-1,3-dihydroxy-4-heptadecene (d17:1), which is a typical predominant sphingoid base in sea cucumbers. The possible mechanism by which dietary cerebrosides prevent adipose atrophy in cancer-associated cachexia mice was related to reducing serum inflammatory cytokine levels, regulating over lipolysis, enhancing the function of lipogenesis, and decreasing the lipid over-utilization. To elucidate the structure–activity relationships of cerebrosides and their long-chain base, the antitumor activities were compared between them. The results indicated that LCBs exhibited a more prominent antitumor effect both in vivo and in vitro.

In addition, sea cucumber cerebrosides and their main structural units, long-chain bases, were obtained from *Acaudina molpadioides* and then administered to high fat diet-induced obese C57BL/6J mice at a diet supplement dosage of 0.025% for 5 weeks to evaluate their effects on obesity-related metabolic disorders [62]. Cerebrosides and long-chain bases significantly decreased epididymal adipose tissue weights, lowered hepatic triacylglycerol levels, and reduced serum glucose, insulin levels, and insulin resistance HOMA-IR index in mice. The activities of hepatic lipogenetic proteins including FAS, ME, and the mRNA levels encoding proteins SREBP-1c and FAS were reduced by cerebrosides and long-chain bases treatment. However, cerebrosides and LCBs showed no effect on the hepatic lipolysis pathway. Moreover, cerebrosides and LCBs efficiently upregulated the gene expression of SREBP-1c, FAS, ACC, ATGL, and HSL, and downregulated the gene expression of LPL and VLDL-r in the adipose tissue. These results demonstrated that cerebrosides and LCBs were effective in suppressing hepatic SREBP-1c mediated lipogenesis, inhibiting lipid uptake, and increasing TG catabolism in the adipose tissue. The ameliorative degree and regulatory mechanisms of these two groups of natural products were basically the same, suggesting that long-chain bases are the key active structural units of cerebrosides [62].

Three glucocerebrosides, CF-3-1, CF-3-2, and CF-3-3 (**109–111**), were isolated from the cerebroside fraction, which was obtained from the chloroform–methanol extract of the sea cucumber *Cucumaria frondosa* by La et al. [63]. The structures of these cerebrosides were determined as 1-O-β-D-glucopyranosides of (2S,3S,4R)-2-[(2R,15Z)-2-hydroxy-15-tetracosenoylamino]-14-methylhexadecane-1,3,4-triol (**109**), (2S,3R,4E)-2-[(2R,15Z)-2-hydroxy-15-tetracosenoylamino]-15-methyl-4-hexadecene-1,3-diol (**110**), and (**111**) (2S,3R,4E,8Z)-2-[(2R,15Z)-2-hydroxy-15-tetracosenoylamino]-4,8-octadecadiene-1,3-diol (Figure 10). Compounds **110** and **111** were obtained as pure compounds for the first time.

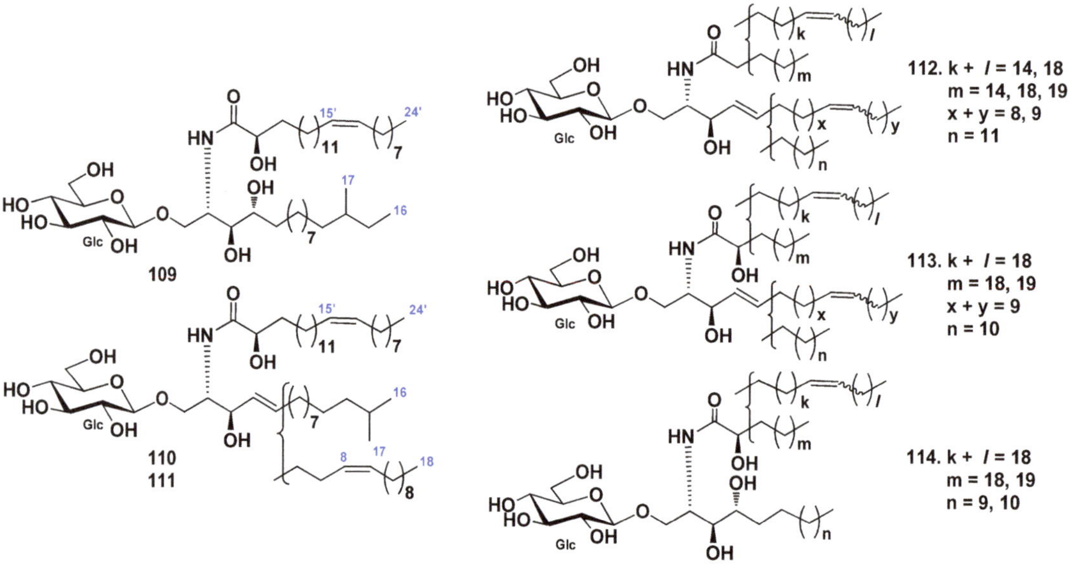

Figure 10. Cerebrosides from the sea cucumber *Cucumaria frondosa*.

Three glucocerebroside molecular species (CFC-1, CFC-2, and CFC-3, **112–114**) were isolated from total cerebrosides from the sea cucumber *Cucumaria frondosa* by Xu et al. (Figure 10) [64]. The structures of these substances were elucidated on the basis of spectroscopic and chemical evidence: fatty acids were identified mainly as saturated (C22:0 and C18:0), monounsaturated (C24:1 and C20:1), and α-hydroxylated derivatives (C24:1h, C23:0h, C23:1h, and C22:0h), the LCB were identified as dihydroxy (d17:1, d18:2, and d18:1) and trihydroxy (t17:0 and t16:0) compounds. The composition analysis of long-chain bases showed that the ratio of d18:2 and d17:1 was approximately 2:1. Four glucocerebrosides and long-chain bases from sea cucumber *Cucumaria frondosa* were evaluated for their cytotoxic activities against Caco-2 colon cancer cells in in vitro assays. The obtained results indicated that both glucocerebrosides and LCB demonstrated an inhibitory effect on cell proliferation. Moreover, **114** was the most effective substance from these four glucocerebrosides in the Caco-2 cell viability test. The inhibitory effects of long-chain bases were much stronger than glucocerebrosides.

Glucocerebrosides, isolated from the sea cucumber *Cucumaria frondosa* (CFC), were investigated on their antiadipogenic activity in vitro [65]. These glucocerebrosides inhibited the lipid accumulation of 3T3-L1 cells and suppressed PPARγ and C/EBPα expressions, which confirmed their antiadipogenic effect. Furthermore, CFCs suppressed lipogenesis in mature adipocytes. Glucocerebrosides enhanced β-catenin expression, promoted its nuclear translocation, and upregulated the expression of CCND1 and c-myc, two target genes of β-catenin. Moreover, after cells were treated with the β-catenin inhibitor 21H7, β-catenin nuclear translocation and transcription activity can be recovered by CFC. These findings suggested that glucocerebrosides from *Cucumaria frondosa* promoted the activation of the WNT/β-catenin pathway. Additionally, CFCs enhanced the expressions of Wnt-receptor frizzled-like protein variant 1(FZ1), low-density lipoprotein receptor-related proteins LRP5, and LRP6, while they had no effect on the expressions of Wnt10b and GSK3β proteins. These findings also confirmed that glucocerebrosides exhibit their antiadipogenic activity through enhancing the activation of the WNT/β-catenin pathway, which was mediated by FZs and LRPs.

Over the past two decades, about a hundred individual cerebrosides and their molecular species were isolated from starfish and sea cucumbers. The isolated compounds contain both sphingosine and phytosphingosine bases of *normal-*, *iso-* and *anteiso-*types. In most cases, long-chain bases include from 16 to 19 carbon atoms, but there were also longer ones, up to C-22. In addition, many LCBs were unsaturated and contained one or two double bonds. In particular, (4*E*,8*E*,10*E*)-sphinga-4,8,10-trienine; (4*E*,8*E*,10*E*)-9-methyl-sphinga-4,8,10-trienine; (4*E*,13*Z*)-sphinga-4,13-dienine; (4*E*,15*Z*)-sphinga-4,15-dienine; and (9*Z*)-4-hydroxy-9-sphingenine long-chain bases were often found. At the same time, unique oxidized LCB (4*E*,9*E*)-9-methyl-8,11-dihydroxy-sphinga-4,9-dienine, and (4*E*,10*E*)-9-methyl-8,9-dihydroxy-sphinga-4,10-dienine were found in the sea cucumber *Stichopus japonicus*.

In most cases, the fatty acids in the cerebrosides were long-chain C-22–C-24 (2*R*)-2-hydroxy acids of *normal-*, *iso-*, and *anteiso-*types. However, shorter FAs such as C-18, C-16, and even C-14 were also found. Some fatty acids in the isolated cerebrosides were unsaturated and most of them had the (15*Z*)-double bond. In contrast to cerebrosides from starfish, cerebrosides from sea cucumbers contained non-α-hydroxylated FA with different long polymethylene chains.

The carbohydrates in cerebrosides of starfish and sea cucumbers were represented by the β-D-glucopyranose and, more rarely, the β-D-galactopyranose. Thus far, no other types of monosaccharide residues have been found in cerebrosides of starfish and sea cucumbers. In addition, cerebrosides lactosides (with Gal-(1→4)-Glc-(1→1)-Cer moieties) were isolated from the starfish *Luidia maculata*. Other variants of cerebroside biglycosides or oligoglycosides in starfish and sea cucumbers have not been found.

The following types of biological activity of cerebrosides from starfish and sea cucumbers were established: *i*. growth-promoting activity on *Brassica campestris*, *ii*. cytotoxic activity against epidermal carcinoma of the mouth KB cells and rat glioma C6 cells; and *iii*.proangiogenic activity. More detailed data are given in Table 1. The conducted studies showed the promising prospects of the practical use of cerebrosides of starfish and sea cucumbers. Accordingly, further expansion of the studies on the biological activity of this class of glycolipids is required, as well as additional data concerning the molecular mechanisms of their action.

Table 1. Composition and biological activity of starfish and sea cucumber sphingolipids mentioned in this review.

Order	Family	Scientific Name	Compounds			Type of Biological Activity	Ref.
			Ceramides	Cerebrosides	Gangliosides		
		Class Asteroidea					
Forcipulatida	Asteriidae	Allostichaster inaequalis		18, 19			[39]
		Anasterias minuta		26, 27			[43]
		Asterias amurensis	2	30, 59–64		Stimulating root growth *Brassica campestris* (**2**, **30**);	[23,50]
		Distolasterias nipon	1–11	65–68			[33,34]
		Evasterias echinosoma			117, 118		[66]
		Evasterias retifera			125, 126		[67]
		Cosmasterias lurida		27			[40]
Paxillosida	Luidiidae	Luidia maculata	12–17	20–25	122–124	Neuritogenic activity toward the rat pheochromocytoma PC12 cells in the presence of NGF (**124**)	[35,41,42,68,69]
Valvatida	Acanthasteridae	Acanthaster planci			115, 116	Binding epitope of AG2 pentasaccharide to human Siglec-2	[70–73]
	Asterinidae	Patiria (=Asterina) pectinifera			127	Neuritogenic activity toward the rat pheochromocytoma PC12 cells in the presence of NGF	[74]
	Ophidiasteridae	Linckia laevigata		28	119–121	Neuritogenic activity toward the rat pheochromocytoma PC12 cells in the presence of NGF (**120**)	[44,75–77]
	Oreasteridae	Culcita novaeguineae		29			[45]
		Protoreaster nodosus		43–58	128–130		[49,78]
		Oreaster reticulatus		31–39		(1) Mildly cytotoxic activity on the rat glioma C6 cells (**31–39**); (2) exertion of proangiogenic activity and increase of VEGF-induced human endothelial cell proliferation (**39**).	[46]

Table 1. Cont.

Order	Family	Scientific Name	Compounds			Type of Biological Activity	Ref.
			Ceramides	Cerebrosides	Gangliosides		
		Narcissia canariensis		40–42		Cytotoxic activity against KB cells (40)	[47]
			Class Holothuroidea				
Holothuriida	Holothuriidae	Holothuria coronopertusa		69–86			[52]
		Holothuria pervicax		87–96	131	Neuritogenic activity toward the rat pheochromocytoma PC12 cell line (131)	[53,79,80]
		Holothuria leucospilota		102–105	132–134	Neuritogenic activity toward the rat pheochromocytoma PC12 cell line (132–134)	[56,81]
		Bohadschia argus		106, 107			[58]
Synallactida	Stichopodidae	Stichopus japonicus		97–101	135	(1) Absorption of cerebrosides in vivo and improving skin barrier functions (97–101); (2) neuritogenic activity toward the rat pheochromocytoma PC12 cells in the presence of NGF (135).	[54,55,82,83]
		Stichopus chloronotus			136–138	Neuritogenic activity toward the rat pheochromocytoma PC12 cells in the presence of NGF	[84]
Molpadida	Caudinidae	Acaudina molpadioides		108		(1) Anti-fatty liver activity of 108 in the rats with fatty liver induced by orotic acid; (2) alleviating adipose atrophy in the cancer-associated cachexia mice; (3) effects of cerebrosides on the obesity-related metabolic disorders in mice.	[59,61,62]
Dendrochirotida	Cucumariidae	Cucumaria frondosa		109–114		(1) In vitro cytotoxic activity against Caco-2 colon cancer cells (112–114); (2) in vitro antiadipogenic activity of cerebrosides.	[63–65]
		Cucumaria echinata			139–141, 144–146, 142, 143	Neuritogenic activity toward the rat pheochromocytoma PC12 cells in the presence of NGF	[85,86]

4. Gangliosides

Gangliosides are known as additionally hydroxylated derivatives of cerebrosides with one or more sialic acid residues in their carbohydrate chains. Sialic acids are a group of higher carbohydrates with nine carbon atoms, which includes several dozens of derivatives of neuraminic acid (NeuAc) [87]. Gangliosides were so named for the first time because they were isolated from brain ganglion cells. It is considered that gangliosides are metabolites of vertebrates; however, they were also found in all classes of Echinoderms and may indicate a high organization of their nervous system. To designate gangliosides, they most often use abbreviated names according to Svennerholm's nomenclature, in which gangliosides are divided into so-called series, indicated by the number of sialic acid units and their position in the carbohydrate chain. Gangliosides are biosynthesized from the corresponding cerebrosides by sialyltransferases on the inner plasma membrane or in the Golgi apparatus, and then they are incorporated into the plasmatic membrane, where these glycosphingolipids perform their biological functions [88]. Gangliosides play an important role in binding to some lectins and affect the activity of receptor protein kinases, taking part in the transmission of cellular signals. In addition, gangliosides, similar to other sphingolipids and cholesterol, play an important role in stabilizing plasma membranes with positive curvature and also affect the surface charge of the membrane. Finally, gangliosides can act as receptors for viruses, bacteria, and toxins, thus being part of the immune system [88].

It is known that gangliosides play an extremely important role in the development of various neurodegenerative diseases, as well as in the regulation of proliferation and energy metabolism of tumor cells [89–91].

Thus, the search for new structural types of gangliosides in echinoderms, as well as a comprehensive study of their biological activity, is an actual scientific task.

4.1. Class Asteroidea

The ganglioside molecular species, AG-1, were obtained from the whole body of the starfish *Acanthaster planci* [70]. Enzymatic hydrolysis by endoglycoceramidase gave an oligosaccharide and ceramides, quantitatively. The oligosaccharide moiety was determined mainly by 2D-NMR experiments as β-Fuc$_f$-(1→4)-α-Gal$_p$-(1→4)-α-NeuAc-(2→3)-β-Gal$_p$-(1→4)-Glc$_p$. The sphingoid moiety was elucidated as the mixture of (2*S*,2′*S*,3*S*,4*R*)-2-((2*R*)-2-hydroxydocosanoylamino)-1,3,4-trihydroxyhexadecane and (2*S*,2′*S*,3*S*,4*R*)-2-((2*R*)-2-hydroxytetracosanoylamino)-1,3,4-trihydroxyhexadecane. Reversed-phase HPLC of AG-1 gave two kinds of gangliosides named acanthagangliosides I (**115**) and J (**116**). It is clear that the oligosaccharide moiety of AG-1 is different in its terminal monosaccharide when compared with AG-2 and AG-3, which were isolated from *A. planci* earlier [71,72]. The terminal β-Gal$_f$ of AG-2 and AG-3 is linked to C-3 of α-Gal$_p$, while the terminal β-Fuc$_f$ of AG-1 is linked to C-4 of α-Gal$_p$. This interesting difference in terminal sugar linkages seems to be derived from the coexistence of different glycosyltransferases, namely, β-1,3-galactofuranosyl transferase and β-1,4-fucofuranosyl transferase. The gangliosides of *A. planci* characteristically have a terminal furanose-type sugar unit (Figure 11).

It was found by performing ^{1}H NMR and saturation transfer difference (STD) NMR experiments that AG2 pentasaccharide (structure not shown) binds to human Siglec-2 (a mammalian sialic acid-binding protein expressed on B-cell surfaces, which involved in the modulation of B-cell mediated immune response [73]. STD NMR experiments indicated that the C-7–C-9 carbohydrate-chain and the acetamide moiety of the central sialic acid residue were located in the binding face of human Siglec-2. The binding epitope of AG2 pentasaccharide to human Siglec-2 was determined as the α-Gal$_p$(1→4)-α-NeuAc-(2→3)-Gal$_p$ unit. The information concerning the binding epitope of AG2 pentasaccharide is of value toward the development of potent Siglec-2 inhibitors.

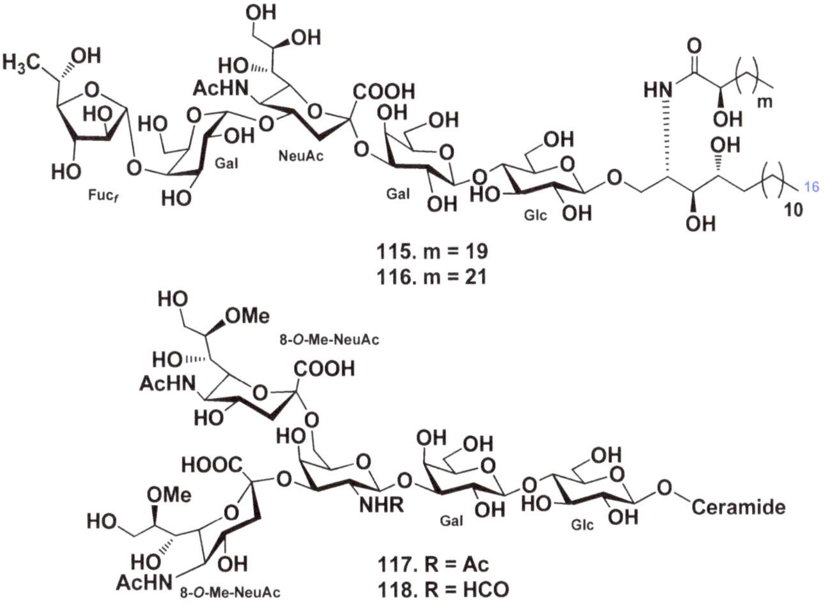

Figure 11. Gangliosides from the starfish *Acanthaster planci* and *Evasterias echinosoma*.

Gangliosides molecular species were isolated from the starfish *Evasterias echinosoma*, and their structures were elucidated [66]. Two major sphingolipids (**117, 118**) were found to be disialogangliosides, whose carbohydrate chain is based on the trisaccharide β-*N*-acylgalactopyranosaminyl-(1→3)-β-galactopyranosyl-(1→4)-β-glucopyranose (acyl is formyl or acetyl). Both residues of 8-*O*-methyl-*N*-acetylneuraminic acid are attached to the *N*-acylgalactosamine residue at positions C-3 and C-6. Compound **118** is the first example of when an *N*-formyl derivative of an amino sugar was found in gangliosides. The lipid part of the gangliosides molecular species consists of monounsaturated sphingoid base and nonhydroxylated fatty acids (mainly, palmitic and stearic acids) (Figure 11).

The ganglioside (**119**) was isolated from the starfish *Linckia laevigata*, and its structure was determined by spectroscopic and chemical methods [75]. The carbohydrate part was proved to be 8-*O*-Me-(*N*-glycolyl-α-D-neuraminosyl)-(2→3)-β-D-galactopyranosyl-(1→4)-β-D-glucopyranoside. The lipid moiety of this ganglioside consists of nonhydroxylated fatty acids (the major component is palmitic acid) and *iso*-C18:1-sphingenine. Based on the structure of the carbohydrate moiety, ganglioside **119** belongs to the hematoside type, characteristic of erythrocytes of vertebrates. It differs from the other known hematosides in the nature of the sialic acid. A hematoside with 8-*O*-methyl-*N*-glycolylneuraminic acid unit was found for the first time (Figure 12).

Continuing research on gangliosides of the starfish *Linckia laevigata*, ganglioside molecular species LLG-5 (**120**) were obtained from the water-soluble portion of its lipid fraction [76]. On the basis of spectroscopic and chemical data, the structure of **120** was elucidated as 8-*O*-methyl-(*N*-glycolyl-α-D-neuraminosyl)-(2→11)-(*N*-glycolyl-α-D-neuraminosyl)-(2→11)-(*N*-glycolyl-α-D-neuraminosyl)-(2→3)-β-D-galactopyranosyl-(1→4)-β-D-glucopyranoside of a ceramide composed of phytosphingosines and 2-hydroxy *n*-fatty acids. The major components of the fatty acids and long-chain bases moieties of **120** were identified as (2*R*)-2-hydroxy *n*-docosanoic acid and (2*S*,3*S*,4*R*)-2-amino-1,3,4-octadecanetriol, respectively. This was the first isolation and characterization of a trisialo-ganglioside from Asteroidea (Figure 12). Furthermore, **120** is a new ganglioside molecular species containing a 2→11 linked trisialosyl moiety. The ganglioside molecular species LLG-5 (**120**) exhibited neuritogenic activity in rat pheochromocytoma PC12 cells in the presence of nerve growth factor (NGF). The proportion of cells with neurites longer than the diameter of the cell body at a concentration of 10 μM or 120 was 59.3% when compared with the control (NGF, 5 ng/mL: 20.6%). Furthermore, their effect was greater than that of the mammalian ganglioside GM1 (47.0%).

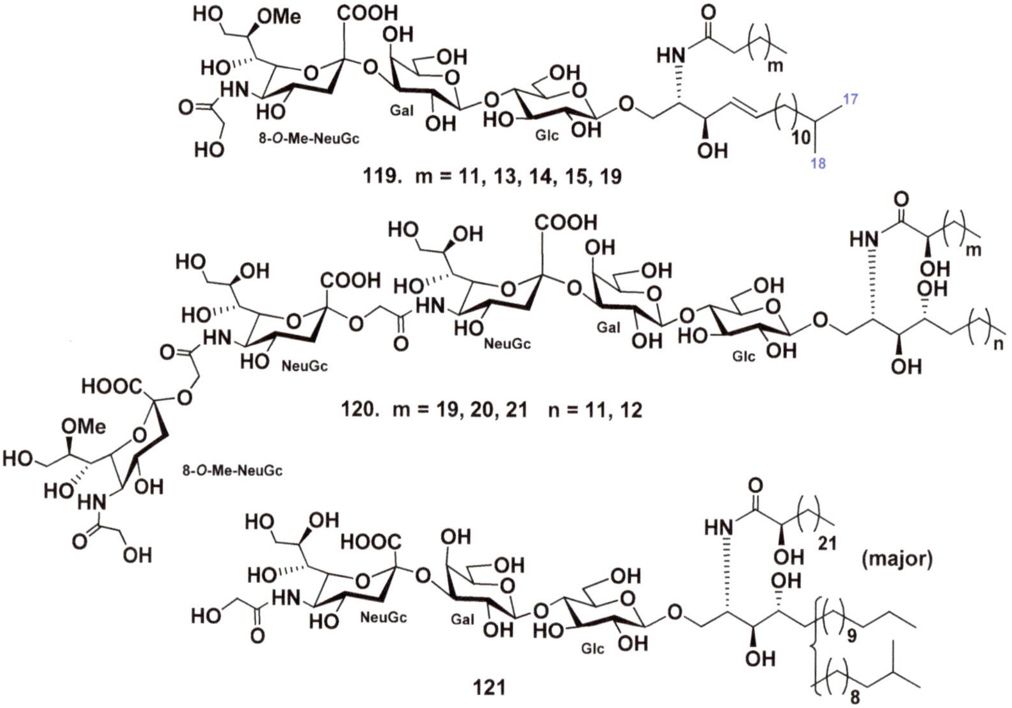

Figure 12. Gangliosides from the starfish *Linckia laevigata*.

In addition, the hematoside-type ganglioside LLG-1 (**121**) was obtained from the polar lipid fraction of the starfish *Linckia laevigata* [77]. The structure of LLG was elucidated on the basis of spectroscopic and chemical evidence as 1-*O*-[(*N*-glycolyl-α-D-neuraminosyl)-(2→3)-β-D-galactopyranosyl-(1→4)-β-D-glucopyranosyl]-ceramide. The ceramide moiety was composed of 2-hydroxy fatty acids and phytosphingosine units (*normal*- and *iso*-type long-chain bases). This was the first report on the isolation and structure elucidation of naked hematoside-type ganglioside from echinoderms (Figure 12).

Two monomethylated GM3-type ganglioside molecular species (**122** and **123**) were isolated from the extract of the starfish *Luidia maculata* [68]. The structures of these gangliosides were determined as 1-*O*-[8-*O*-methyl-(*N*-acetyl-α-D-neuraminosyl)-(2→3)-β-D-galactopyranosyl-(1→4)-β-D-glucopyranosyl]-ceramide (**122**) and 1-*O*-[8-*O*-methyl-(*N*-glycolyl-α-D-neuraminosyl)-(2→3)-β-D-galactopyranosyl-(1→4)-β-D-glucopyranosyl]-ceramide (**123**). The ceramide moieties were composed of heterogeneous nonhydroxylated fatty acid, 2-hydroxy fatty acid, sphingosine, and phytosphingosine units. Compound **122**, designated as LMG-3, represented new ganglioside molecular species. Compound **123** was identified as a known ganglioside molecular species (Figure 13).

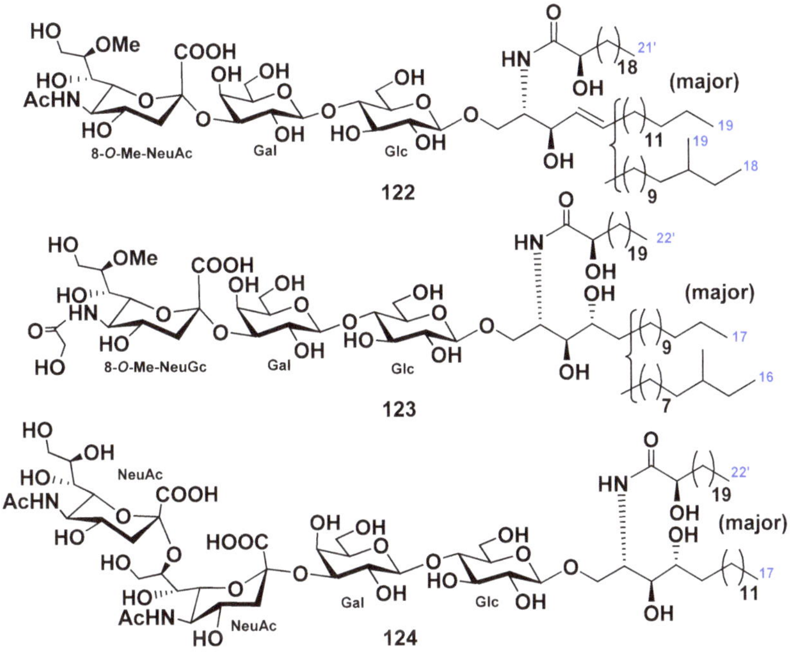

Figure 13. Ganglioside molecular species from the starfish *Luidia maculata*.

In addition, the GD3-type ganglioside molecular species LMG-4 (**124**) was obtained from the extract of the starfish *L. maculata* [69]. The structure of this compound was determined on the basis of spectroscopic and chemical evidence to be 1-*O*-[(*N*-acetyl-α-D-neuraminosyl)-(2→8)-(*N*-acetyl-α-D-neuraminosyl)-(2→3)-β-D-galactopyranosyl-(1→4)-β-D-glucopyranosyl]-ceramide. The ceramide moiety was composed of 2-hydroxy fatty acid and phytosphingosine moieties. GD3-type ganglioside was isolated and its particular structure elucidated for the first time from echinoderms (Figure 13). LMG-4 (**124**) exhibited neuritogenic activity toward the rat pheochromocytoma PC12 cells in the presence of NGF. The proportion of the neurite-bearing cells of **124** at a concentration of 10 µM was 47.7%, in comparison with the control (NGF, 5 ng/mL: 20.6%). The effect of **124** was the same as that of the mammalian ganglioside GM1 (47.0%).

Mono- and disialogangliosides (**125**, **126**) were isolated from gonads of the starfish *Evasterias retifera* [67]. Their structures were elucidated by spectroscopic and chemical evidence, including enzymatic hydrolysis with neuraminidase. The monosialoganglioside has the structure α-8-*O*-Me-NeuGc-(2→3)-β-GalNAc-(1→3)-β-Gal-(1→4)-β-Glc-(1→1)-Cer, while the disialoganglioside contains an additional NeuAc residue, which glycosylates GalNAc in position C-6. The lipid moieties of both gangliosides contain phytosphingosine bases (mainly C18:0) and two types of fatty acids, nonhydroxylated (mainly C16:0 and C18:0) and α-hydroxylated (mainly α-hydroxy-C16:0) (Figure 14).

The molecular species GP-3 (**127**) was obtained from the starfish *Patiria* (=*Asterina*) *pectinifera* [74]. The structure of the ganglioside was determined as 1-*O*-α-L-arabinofuranosyl-(1→3)-α-D-galactopyranosyl-(1→4)-(*N*-acetyl-α-D-neuraminosyl)-(2→6)-β-D-galactofuranosyl-(1→3)-[α-L-arabinofuranosyl-(1→4)]-α-D-galactopyranosyl-(1→4)-(*N*-acetyl-α-D-neuraminosyl)-(2→3)-β-D-galactopyranosyl-(1→4)-β-D-glucopyranoside of ceramide composed of heterogeneous (2*S*,3*S*,4*R*)-phytosphingosine (*iso*-C-17-phytosphingosine as the major component) and (2*R*)-2-hydroxy fatty acid units (docosanoic acid as the major component) (Figure 14). Compound **127** represents new ganglioside molecular species possessing two residues of sialic acids at the inner part of the sugar moiety. A ganglioside molecular species GP-3

(**127**) exhibits neuritogenic activity toward the rat pheochromocytoma cell line PC12, in the presence of NGF. The proportion of the cells with neurite longer than the diameter of the cell body at the use of **127** at a concentration of 10 µM was 38.2% when compared with the control (NGF, 5 ng/mL: 20.6%). The effect of **127** was lower than that of the mammalian ganglioside GM1 (47.0%).

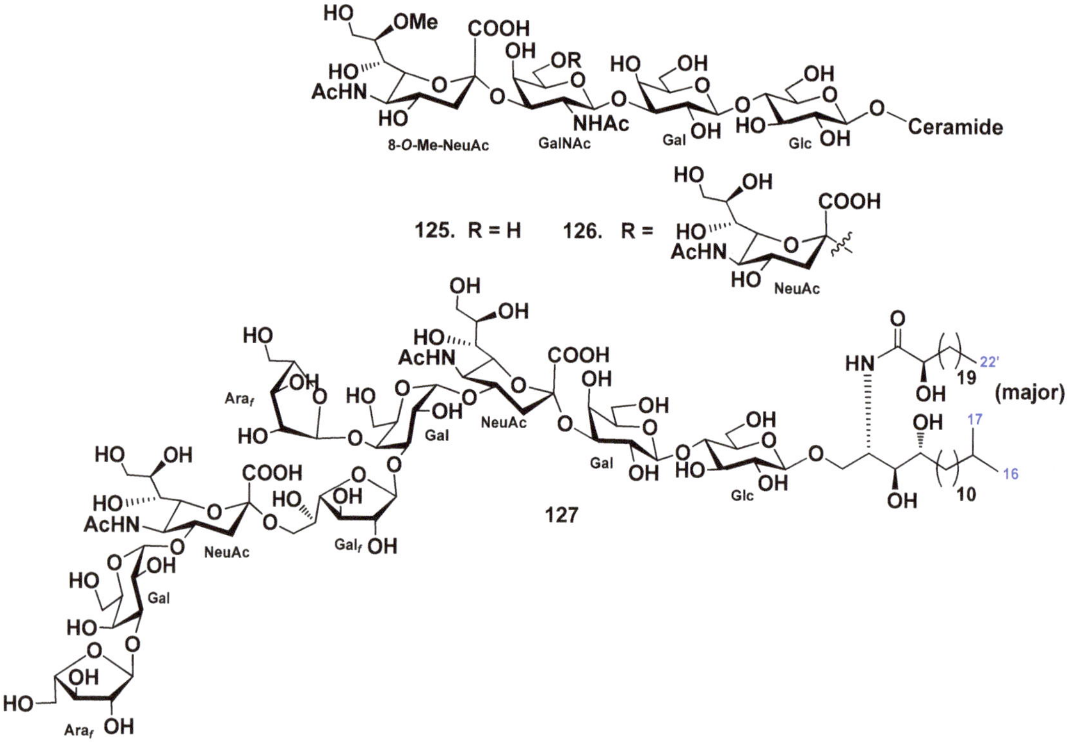

Figure 14. Gangliosides from the starfish *Evasterias retifera* and *Patiria* (=*Asterina*) *pectinifera*.

Three ganglioside molecular species PNG-1 (**128**), PNG-2A (**129**), and PNG-2B (**130**) were isolated from pyloric caeca of the starfish *Protoreaster nodosus* [78]. Their structures as 1-*O*-[8-*O*-methyl-(*N*-acetyl-α-neuraminosyl)-(2→3)-β-galactopyranosyl]-ceramide (**128**), 1-*O*-[β-galactofuranosyl-(1→3)-α-galactopyranosyl-(1→4)-8-*O*-methyl-(*N*-acetyl-α-neuraminosyl)-(2→3)-β-galactopyranosyl]-ceramide (**129**), and 1-*O*-[β-galactofuranosyl-(1→3)-α-galactopyranosyl-(1→9)-(*N*-acetyl-α-neuraminosyl)-(2→3)-β-galactopyranosyl]-ceramide (**130**) were elucidated by a combination of spectroscopic and chemical methods. The ceramide moieties of ganglioside molecular species consisted of (2S,3S,4R)-phytosphingosines (*iso*-C-18-phytosphingosine as the major component) and (2R)-2-hydroxy fatty acid units (docosanoic acid as the major component). PNG-2A (**129**) and PNG-2B (**130**) represent the first GM4 elongation products in nature (Figure 15).

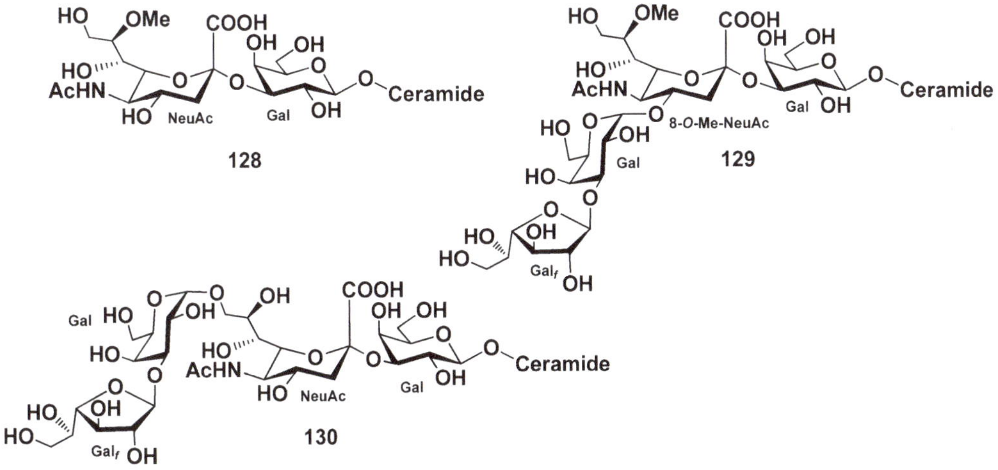

Figure 15. Gangliosides molecular species from the starfish *Protoreaster nodosus*.

4.2. Class Holothuroidea

The ganglioside molecular species HPG-7 (**131**) was isolated from the chloroform–methanol extract of the sea cucumber *Holothuria pervicax* [79]. On the basis of the spectroscopic and chemical evidence, the structure of the major component of **131** was determined as 1-O-[α-L-fucopyranosyl-(1→4)-(N-acetyl-α-D-neuraminosyl)-(2→11)-(N-glycolyl-α-D-neuraminosyl)-(2→4)-(N-acetyl-α-D-neuraminosyl)-(2→6)-β-D-glucopyranosyl]-(2S,3S,4R)-[(2R)-2-hydroxytetracosanoylamino]-14-methyl-hexadecane-1,3,4-triol (Figure 16). The trisialo-ganglioside was isolated for the first time from sea cucumbers. HPG-7 (**131**) was studied for neuritogenic action toward the PC12 rat pheochromocytoma cell line. It was shown that **131** does not have neuritogenic activity, in comparison with control, at a concentration of above 10 μg/mL, similar to three other ganglioside molecular species (HPG-1, HPG-3, and HPG-8) [80].

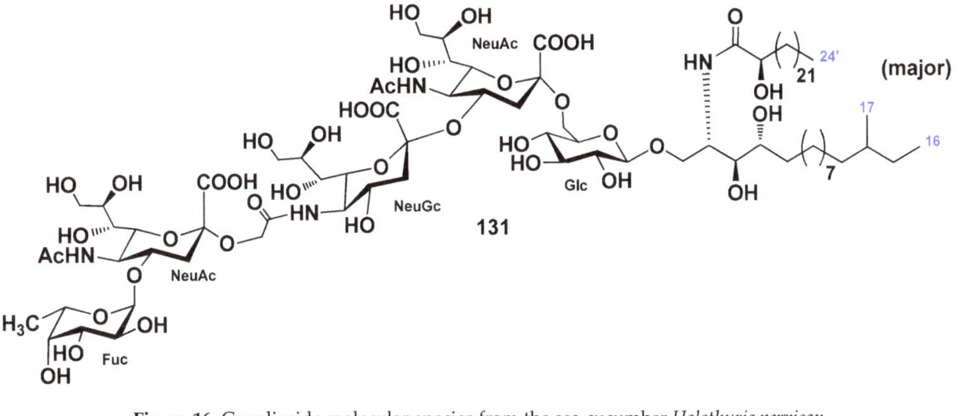

Figure 16. Ganglioside molecular species from the sea cucumber *Holothuria pervicax*.

Three ganglioside molecular species, HLG-1 (**132**), HLG-2 (**133**), and HLG-3 (**134**), were isolated from the extract of the sea cucumber *Holothuria leucospilota* [81]. Structures of these gangliosides were determined as 1-O-[(N-glycolyl-α-D-neuraminosyl)-(2→6)-β-D-glucopyranosyl]-ceramide (**132**), 1-O-[(N-glycolyl-α-D-neuraminosyl)-(2→4)-(N-acetyl-α-

D-neuraminosyl)-(2→6)-β-D-glucopyranosyl]-ceramide (**133**), and 1-*O*-[α-L-fucopyranosyl-(1→11)-(*N*-glycolyl-α-D-neuraminosyl)-(2→4)-(*N*-acetyl-α-D-neuraminosyl)-(2→6)-β-D-glucopyranosyl]-ceramide (**134**), respectively. The ceramide moieties were composed of phytosphingosines or sphingosines and 2-hydroxy fatty acids (Figure 17). Compounds **133** and **134** represent new ganglioside molecular species. These three substances showed slight neuritogenic activity toward the rat pheochromocytoma cell line PC12 cell in the presence of NGF.

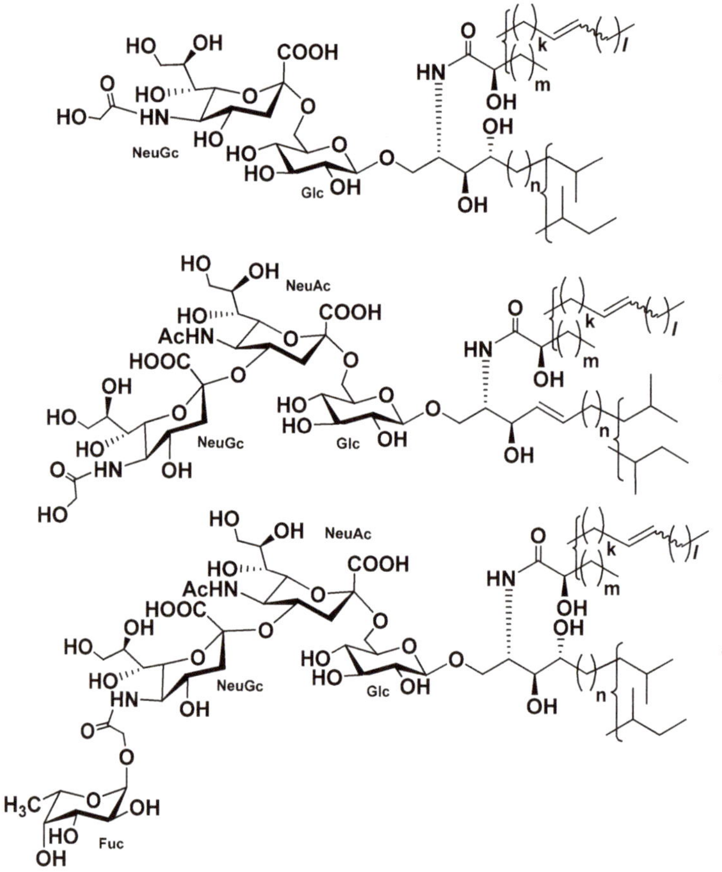

132. k + *l* = 19
m = 19, 20, 21
n = 9, 10, 11

133. k + *l* = 19
m = 19, 20, 21
n = 8

134. k + *l* = 19
m = 19, 20, 21
n = 9, 10, 11

Figure 17. Ganglioside molecular species from the sea cucumber *Holothuria leucospilota*.

The ganglioside molecular species SJG-2 (**135**) was obtained from the extract of the sea cucumber *Stichopus japonicus* [82]. On the basis of spectroscopic and chemical studies, the structure of SJG-2 (**135**) was determined as α-NeuAc-(2→4)-α-NeuAc-(2→3)-β-Gal-(1→8)-α-NeuAc-(2→3)-β-GalNAc-(1→3)-β-Gal-(1→4)-β-Glc-(1→1)-Cer. The ganglioside **135**, possessing a unique carbohydrate moiety, is the first corresponding substance with a branched sugar chain moiety and *N*-acetylgalactosamine residue isolated from sea cucumbers (Figure 18). Ganglioside SJG-2 (**135**) exhibited neuritogenic activity toward the rat pheochromocytoma cell line PC12 cells in the presence of NGF. The proportion of neurite-bearing cells at the use of SJG-2 (64.8 ± 7.6%) was larger than that induced by the previously isolated SJG-1 [83], (35.4 ± 4.0%) when compared with the control (NGF, 5 ng/mL: 20.6 ± 2.2%). Furthermore, the effect of SJG-2 (**135**) was more considerable than that of the mammalian ganglioside GM1 (47.0 ± 2.5%).

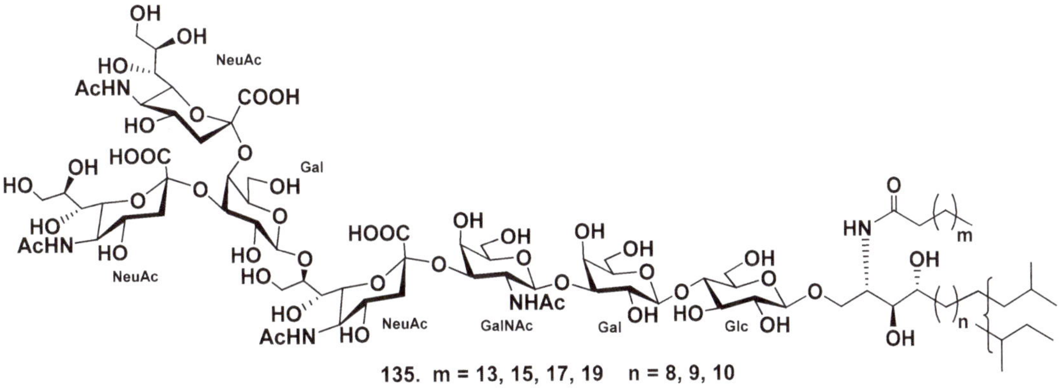

Figure 18. Ganglioside molecular species from the sea cucumber *Stichopus japonicus*.

Three ganglioside molecular species, SCG-1 (**136**), SCG-2 (**137**), and SCG-3 (**138**), were isolated from the extract of the sea cucumber *Stichopus chloronotus* [84]. On the basis of spectroscopic and chemical evidence, the structures of these gangliosides were determined to be 1-O-[(N-glycolyl-α-D-neuraminosyl)-(2→6)-β-D-glucopyranosyl]-ceramide (**136**), 1-O-[8-O-sulfo-(N-acetyl-α-D-neuraminosyl)-(2→6)-β-D-glucopyranosyl]-ceramide (**137**), and 1-O-[α-L-fucopyranosyl-(1→11)-(N-glycolyl-α-D-neuraminosyl)-(2→6)-β-D-glucopyranosyl]-ceramide (**138**). The ceramide moieties were composed of isomeric long-chain bases and fatty acid units. The molecular species **138** is the first representative of gangliosides containing fucopyranose in the sialosyl trisaccharide moiety (Figure 19). Gangliosides **136**–**138** exhibited neuritogenic activity toward the rat pheochromocytoma PC12 cells in the presence of NGF. The proportions of the neurite-bearing cells at a concentration of **136**–**138** of 3.3 µg/mL were 34.1%, 24.4%, and 24.5%, respectively. These effects were compared with that of the mammalian ganglioside GM1 (22.1% at a concentration of 3.3 mg/mL).

Three monosialo-gangliosides, CEG-3 (**139**), CEG-4 (**140**), and CEG-5 (**141**), were obtained, together with two previously known gangliosides, SJG-1 (**142**, structure not shown, [83]) and CG-1 (**143**, structure not shown, [92]), from the extract of the sea cucumber *Cucumaria echinata* [85]. In addition, three disialo- or trisialo-gangliosides, CEG-6 (**144**), CEG-8 (**145**), and CEG-9 (**146**), were also obtained along with the known ganglioside, HLG-3 (**134**, [81]) from this species of sea cucumbers [86]. Structures of these gangliosides were determined as 1-O-[(4-O-acetyl-α-L-fucopyranosyl)-(1→11)-(N-glycolyl-α-D-neuraminosyl)-(2→6)-β-D-glucopyranosyl]-ceramide (**139**), 1-O-[α-L-fucopyranosyl-(1→11)-(N-glycolyl-α-D-neuraminosyl)-(2→6)-β-D-glucopyranosyl]-ceramides (**140**, **141**), 1-O-[α-L-fucopyranosyl-(1→11)-(N-glycolyl-α-D-neuraminosyl)-(2→4)-(N-acetyl-α-D-neuraminosyl)-(2→6)-β-D-glucopyranosyl]-ceramide (**144**), and homologous to each other 1-O-[(N-glycolyl-D-neuraminosyl)-(2→11)-(N-glycolyl-D-neuraminosyl)-(2→4)-(N-acetyl-D-neuraminosyl)-(2→6)-D-glucopyranosyl]-ceramides (**145**, **146**). The ceramide moieties of each compound were composed of sphingosine or phytosphingosine bases and 2-hydroxy- or nonhydroxylated fatty acid units (Figure 20). Gangliosides **134**, **139**–**146** demonstrated neuritogenic activity toward the rat pheochromocytoma cell line PC12 in the presence of NGF. The proportions of cells with neurites longer than the diameter of the cell body after the treatment with compounds **134**, **139**–**146** at concentration of 10 µM were of 40.2%, 50.8%, 34.0%, 35.7%, 39.1%, 43.0%, 43.0%, 40.2%, and 35.1%, respectively, in comparison with the control experiments (NGF, 5 ng/mL: 7.5%). The effects of **134**, **139**, and **142**–**145** were stronger than that of the mammalian ganglioside GM1 (35.6%). Compound **139** with an acetyl group at the terminal fucopyranosyl unit showed the most potent activity.

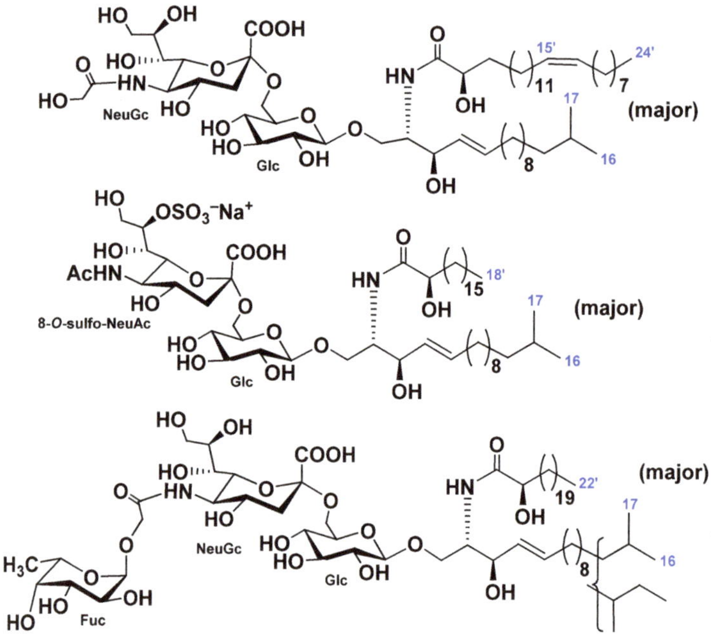

Figure 19. Ganglioside molecular species from the sea cucumber *Stichopus chloronotus*.

Enantiomeric pairs of sialic acids (D- and L-NeuAc) were converted to D- and L-arabinose, respectively, by chemical degradation [93]. Using this approach, the absolute configurations of the sialic acid residues NeuAc and NeuGc as D-forms were determined in the gangliosides from the sea cucumber *Cucumaria echinata*. Although naturally occurring sialic acids have been believed to have D-configurations on the basis of biosynthetic evidence, this is the first report describing the determination of the absolute configuration of the sialic acid residues in gangliosides using chemical methods.

Starfish and sea cucumbers gangliosides remain to be less studied, in comparison with cerebrosides. At the same time, about 30 new compounds and/or molecular species have been isolated since 2000. The carbohydrate chains of the starfish and sea cucumber gangliosides differ markedly from the carbohydrate chains of mammals as well as from each other. Generally, besides sialic acid residues, these compounds contain lactoside fragment (Gal-(1→4)-Glc-(1→1)-Cer) and analogous fragment additionally glycosylated with galactosamine (GalNAc-(1→3)-Gal-(1→4)-Glc-(1→1)-Cer). Part of them are derivatives of galactosylceramides having (Gal-(1→1)-Cer) moiety.

In the sea cucumbers gangliosides, containing fragments of only two cerebrosides were found: lactosides glycosylated with galactosamine (GalNAc-(1→3)-Gal-(1→4)-Glc-(1→1)-Cer), and glucosylceramides (Glc-(1→1)-Cer).

Both starfish and sea cucumber gangliosides contain unusual sialic acid residues, including sialic acids within carbohydrate chains as well as additional monosaccharide residues and unusual types of glycosidic bonds between them. For example, terminal β-D-Fuc$_f$ was found in the gangliosides from the starfish *Acanthaster planci*, 8-O-Me-NeuAc and 8-O-Me-NeuGc were found in the gangliosides from the starfish *Linckia laevigata* as well as the glycosidic bond 2→11 between sialic acid residues. The ganglioside from the starfish *Evasterias echinosoma* contains an unusual β-D-N-formyl-galactosamine residue, while the carbohydrate chains from gangliosides of the starfish *Patiria* (=*Asterina*) *pectinifera* bears the terminal α-L-arabinofuranose residue and has three forms of galactose (β-D-Gal$_p$, β-D-Gal$_f$, and α-D-Gal$_p$). These gangliosides contain the maximum number of monosaccharide residues (up to nine), in comparison with other echinoderm gangliosides.

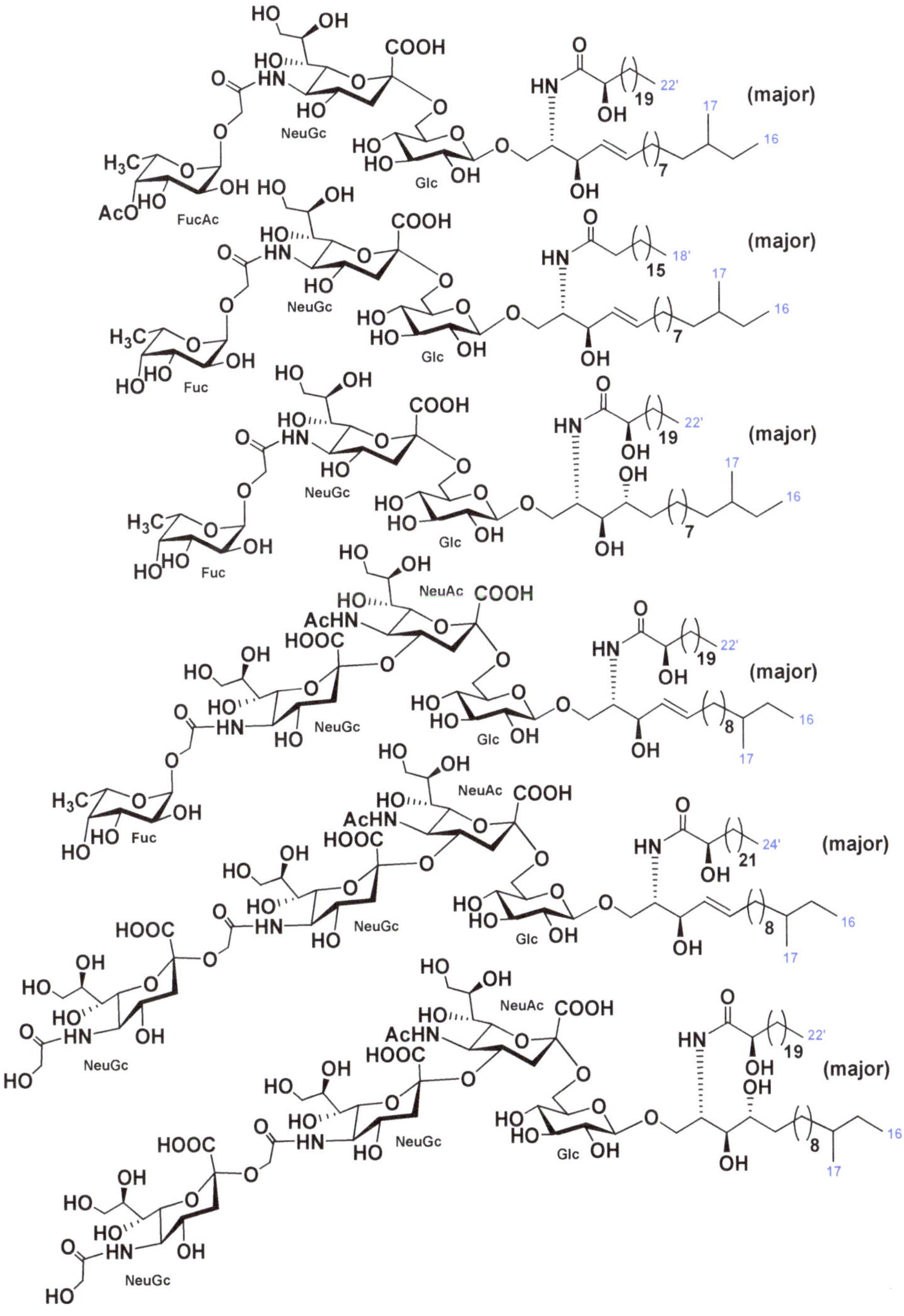

139

140

141

144

145

146

Figure 20. Gangliosides from the sea cucumber *Cucumaria echinata*.

Gangliosides with the terminal α-L-Fuc$_p$ were identified in several species of sea cucumbers along with NeuAc and NeuGc residues within carbohydrate chains. A unique 8-O-sulfo-NeuAc residue was found in the corresponding substances from the sea cucumber *Stichopus chloronotus*. The maximum length of the carbohydrate chain in the sea cucumbers gangliosides was found in the ganglioside from *Stichopus japonicus*, which contained seven monosaccharide residues.

Lipid parts of gangliosides from both starfish and sea cucumbers were similar and contained both sphingosine and phytosphingosine bases of *normal-*, *iso-* and *anteiso-*types. Predominantly (2R)-2-hydroxy fatty acids of the normal type were found in these substances. For gangliosides of starfish and sea cucumbers, only one type of biological activity was studied, neuritogenic activity toward the rat pheochromocytoma cell line PC12 in the presence of NGF. In a number of cases, starfish and sea cucumbers gangliosides showed a higher neuritogenic effect at concentration 10 μM than the mammalian ganglioside GM1, while some gangliosides exhibited slighter action at the same concentration.

5. Conclusions

To the best of our knowledge, sphingolipids of 15 starfish and 9 sea cucumbers, mainly common Pacific Ocean inhabitants, have been studied (Table 1). In total, these 24 echinoderm species were used for the isolation and identification of about 150 sphingolipids. This indicates that echinoderms and, in particular, starfish and sea cucumbers are a rich source of sphingolipids, structures of which may differ markedly from the corresponding metabolites of plants and terrestrial animals.

Ceramides are the least studied group of echinoderms sphingolipids. Moreover, since 2000, only studies on starfish ceramides have been carried out. Nevertheless, a big variety of structural types of the isolated ceramides was detected, for instance, sphingosine and phytosphingosine LCBs of various lengths, *normal-*, *iso-*, and *anteiso-*types, often having one or two additional double bonds, were found in starfish ceramides. Fatty acid residues in starfish ceramides were most often identified as (2R)-2-hydroxy derivatives of various lengths (usually from C-18 to C-22) with normal hydrocarbon chains, which can also contain one additional double bonds. The "gray spot" in the study of starfish ceramides is the lack of data on biological activity, with the exception of the stimulating root growth of *Brassica campestris* activity by ceramides from *Asterias amurensis*.

Cerebrosides are the most studied class of starfish and sea cucumbers sphingolipids. Generally, about one hundred individual cerebrosides and their molecular species have been isolated from these animals. As in ceramides, sphingosine and phytosphingosine LCBs of various lengths with *normal-*, *iso-*, and *anteiso-*structures were found in starfish and sea cucumber cerebrosides. Unique oxidized sphingosine LCBs with additional hydroxy groups at either C-8 and C-9 or C-8 and C-11 were indicated in the sea cucumber *Stichopus japonicus*. Mainly saturated and monounsaturated (2R)-2-hydroxy fatty acids with normal hydrocarbon chains having various lengths were identified as constituents of these cerebrosides, but nonhydroxylated FAs were sometimes also detected. Almost all the isolated cerebrosides were monoglycosides and contained glucose or galactose residues. Cerebroside lactosides were isolated from the starfish *Luidia maculata*.

The following types of biological activities of starfish and sea cucumbers cerebrosides were studied: growth-promoting activity of *Brassica campestris*, anti-fatty liver activity in rats treated by orotic acid, alleviating adipose atrophy action in cancer-associated cachexia mice, effects on obesity-related metabolic disorders in mice, cytotoxic activities against KB, rat glioma C6 cells, and colon cancer Caco-2cells, and proangiogenic action. As result, it was shown that starfish and sea cucumbers cerebrosides possess various types of biological activities that are important for their practical application in the human diet and in the composition of food supplements (Table 1).

Starfish and sea cucumber gangliosides were also studied for some species, and their structural diversity was proved to be great. Carbohydrate chains of starfish and sea cucumbers gangliosides have interesting structural features and differ from gangliosides of terrestrial animals. Really, the residues of β-D-Fuc$_f$, 8-O-Me-NeuAc, and 8-O-Me-NeuGc, β-D-N-formyl-galactosamine, as well as terminal α-L-Ara$_f$ were recently found in the starfish gangliosides. In gangliosides from holothurians (sea cucumbers), the terminal α-L-Fuc$_p$, α-L-FucAc$_p$, and 8-O-sulfo-NeuAc were detected.

For starfish and sea cucumbers gangliosides, only one type of biological activity was studied, namely, neuritogenic activity toward the rat pheochromocytoma cell line PC12 in the presence of NGF. Therefore, further research of other types of biological activities including antitumor and anti-inflammatory properties might be of interest. It is noteworthy that the starfish and sea cucumber gangliosides, as a rule, are species specific. Therefore, they could be taxonomic markers, such as some unusual starfish polar steroidal compounds [94,95] and sea cucumber triterpene glycosides [96]. However, the structures of gangliosides were less studied than those of other secondary metabolites of starfish and sea cucumbers and require further research.

Previously, we studied the metabolic profile of polar steroid compounds of three species of starfish and their changes under stress conditions, as well as the metabolic profile of triterpene glycosides from the sea cucumber *Eupentacta fraudatrix* [8–13]. The study of the metabolomic profiles of sphingolipids and their changes under various environmental conditions can also be one of the directions of metabolomics research. However, first of all, it is necessary to systematize the literature data on the structures of all types of sphingolipids, including ceramides, cerebrosides, and gangliosides, in these animals. We believe this review can help meet this challenge.

Author Contributions: Writing—original draft preparation and writing—review and editing, T.V.M., A.A.K. and N.V.I.; conceptualization and validation, V.A.S. All authors have read and agreed to the published version of the manuscript.

Funding: This work was carried out with the support of the Russian Science Foundation (RSF) Grant Number 20-14-00040.

Conflicts of Interest: The authors declare no conflict of interest.

References

1. Stonik, V.A.; Kalinin, V.I.; Avilov, S.A. Toxins from sea cucumbers (holothuroids): Chemical structures, properties, taxonomic distribution, biosynthesis and evolution. *J. Nat. Toxins* **1999**, *8*, 235–248. [PubMed]
2. Stonik, V.A. Marine polar steroids. *Russ. Chem. Rev.* **2001**, *70*, 673–715. [CrossRef]
3. Stonik, V.A.; Ivanchina, N.V.; Kicha, A.A. New polar steroids from starfish. *Nat. Prod. Commun.* **2008**, *3*, 1587–1610. [CrossRef]
4. Ivanchina, N.V.; Kicha, A.A.; Stonik, V.A. Steroid glycosides from marine organisms. *Steroids* **2011**, *76*, 425–454. [CrossRef]
5. Ivanchina, N.V.; Kicha, A.A.; Malyarenko, T.V.; Stonik, V.A. *Advances in Natural Products Discovery*; Gomes, A.R., Rocha-Santos, T., Duarte, A., Eds.; Nova Science Publishers: New York, NY, USA, 2017; Volume 6, pp. 191–224.
6. Stonik, V.A.; Kicha, A.A.; Malyarenko, T.V.; Ivanchina, N.V. Asterosaponins: Structures, taxonomic distribution, biogenesis and biological activities. *Mar. Drugs* **2020**, *18*, 584. [CrossRef] [PubMed]
7. Fattorusso, E.; Mangoni, A. Marine glycolipids. *Prog. Chem. Org. Nat. Prod.* **1997**, *72*, 215–301.
8. Popov, R.S.; Ivanchina, N.V.; Kicha, A.A.; Malyarenko, T.V.; Dmitrenok, P.S.; Stonik, V.A. Metabolite profiling of polar steroid constituents in the Far Eastern starfish *Aphelasterias japonica* using LC–ESI MS/MS. *Metabolomics* **2014**, *10*, 1152–1168. [CrossRef]
9. Popov, R.S.; Ivanchina, N.V.; Kicha, A.A.; Malyarenko, T.V.; Dmitrenok, P.S.; Stonik, V.A. LC-ESI MS/MS profiling of polar steroid metabolites of the Far Eastern starfish *Patiria (=Asterina) pectinifera*. *Metabolomics* **2016**, *12*, 21. [CrossRef]
10. Popov, R.S.; Ivanchina, N.V.; Kicha, A.A.; Malyarenko, T.V.; Grebnev, B.B.; Dmitrenok, P.S.; Stonik, V.A. LC-MS-based metabolome analysis on steroid metabolites from the starfish *Patiria (=Asterina) pectinifera* in conditions of active feeding and stresses. *Metabolomics* **2016**, *12*, 106. [CrossRef]
11. Popov, R.S.; Ivanchina, N.V.; Kicha, A.A.; Malyarenko, T.V.; Dmitrenok, P.S. Structural characterization of polar steroid compounds of the Far Eastern starfish *Lethasterias fusca* by nanoflow liquid chromatography coupled to quadrupole time-of-flight tandem mass spectrometry. *J. Am. Soc. Mass Spectrom.* **2019**, *30*, 743–764. [CrossRef]
12. Popov, R.S.; Ivanchina, N.V.; Kicha, A.A.; Malyarenko, T.V.; Grebnev, B.B.; Stonik, V.A.; Dmitrenok, P.S. The distribution of asterosaponins, polyhydroxysteroids and related glycosides in different body components of the Far Eastern starfish *Lethasterias fusca*. *Mar. Drugs* **2019**, *17*, 523. [CrossRef]
13. Popov, R.S.; Ivanchina, N.V.; Silchenko, A.S.; Avilov, S.A.; Kalinin, V.I.; Dolmatov, I.Y.; Stonik, V.A.; Dmitrenok, P.S. Metabolite profiling of triterpene glycosides of the Far Eastern sea cucumber *Eupentacta fraudatrix* and their distribution in various body components using LC-ESI QTOF-MS. *Mar. Drugs* **2017**, *15*, 302. [CrossRef]

14. Degroote, S.; Wolthoorn, J.; van Meer, G. The cell biology of glycosphingolipids. *Semin. Cell Dev. Biol.* **2004**, *15*, 375–387. [CrossRef]
15. Hakomori, S.; Igarashi, Y. Functional role of glycosphingolipids in cell recognition and signaling. *J. Biochem.* **1995**, *118*, 1091–1103. [CrossRef] [PubMed]
16. Fahy, E.; Subramaniam, S.; Brown, H.A.; Glass, C.K.; Merrill, A.H., Jr.; Murphy, R.C.; Raetz, C.R.H.; Russell, D.W.; Seyama, Y.; Shaw, W.; et al. A comprehensive classification system for lipids. *J. Lipid Res.* **2005**, *46*, 839–861. [CrossRef]
17. Chebane, K.; Guyot, M. Occurrence of *erythro*-docosasphinga-4,8-dienine, as an ester, in *Anemonia sulcata*. *Tetrahedron Lett.* **1986**, *27*, 1495–1496. [CrossRef]
18. Costantino, V.; Fattorusso, E.; Imperatore, C.; Mangoni, A. Glycolipids from sponges. 13.1 Clarhamnoside, the first rhamnosylated α-galactosylceramide from *Agelas clathrodes*. Improving spectral strategies for glycoconjugate structure determination. *J. Org. Chem.* **2004**, *69*, 1174–1179. [CrossRef] [PubMed]
19. Mansoor, T.A.; Shinde, P.B.; Luo, X.; Hong, J.; Lee, C.O.; Sim, X.; Son, B.W.; Jung, J.H. Renierosides, cerebrosides from a marine sponge *Haliclona* (*Reniera*) sp. *J. Nat. Prod.* **2007**, *70*, 1481–1486. [CrossRef] [PubMed]
20. Costantino, V.; Fattorusso, E.; Imperatore, C.; Mangoni, A.; Freigang, S.; Teyton, L. Corruguside: A new immunostimulatory α-galactoglycosphingolipid from the marine sponge *Axinella corrugata*. *Bioorg. Med. Chem.* **2008**, *16*, 2077–2085. [CrossRef] [PubMed]
21. Cheng, S.Y.; Wen, Z.H.; Chiou, S.F.; Tsai, C.W.; Wang, S.K.; Hsu, C.H.; Dai, C.F.; Chiang, M.Y.; Wang, W.H.; Duh, C.Y. Ceramide and cerebrosides from the octocoral *Sarcophyton ehrenbergi*. *J. Nat. Prod.* **2009**, *72*, 465–468. [CrossRef]
22. Durán, R.; Zubia, E.; Ortega, M.J.; Naranjo, S.; Salvá, J. Phallusides, new glucosphingolipids from the ascidian *Phallusia fumigata*. *Tetrahedron* **1998**, *54*, 14597–14602. [CrossRef]
23. Ishii, T.; Okino, T.; Mino, Y. A ceramide and cerebroside from the starfish *Asterias amurensis* Lütken and their plant-growth promotion activities. *J. Nat. Prod.* **2006**, *69*, 1080–1082. [CrossRef]
24. Duan, J.; Sugawara, T.; Sakai, S.; Aida, K.; Hirata, T. Oral glucosylceramide reduces 2,4-dinitrofluorobenzene induced inflammatory response in mice by reducing TNF-alpha levels and leukocyte infiltration. *Lipids* **2011**, *46*, 505–512. [CrossRef] [PubMed]
25. Duan, J.; Sugawara, T.; Hirose, M.; Aida, K.; Sakai, S.; Fujii, A.; Hirata, T. Dietary sphingolipids improve skin barrier functions via the upregulation of ceramide synthases in the epidermis. *Exp. Dermatol.* **2012**, *21*, 448–452. [CrossRef]
26. Dillehay, D.L.; Webb, S.K.; Schmelz, E.M.; Merrill, A.H., Jr. Dietary sphingomyelin inhibits 1,2-dimethylhydrazine-induced colon cancer in CF1 mice. *J. Nutr.* **1994**, *124*, 615–620. [CrossRef] [PubMed]
27. Carmeliet, P. Angiogenesis in health and disease. *Nat. Med.* **2003**, *9*, 653–660. [CrossRef] [PubMed]
28. Muralidhar, P.; Radhika, P.; Krishna, N.; Venkata Rao, D. Bheemasankara Rao, Ch. Sphingolipids from marine organisms: A review. *Nat. Prod. Sci.* **2003**, *9*, 117–142.
29. Higuchi, R.; Inagaki, M.; Yamada, K.; Miyamoto, T. Biologically active gangliosides from echinoderms. *J. Nat. Med.* **2007**, *61*, 367–370. [CrossRef]
30. Yamada, K. Chemo-pharmaceutical studies on the glycosphingolipid constituents from Echinoderm, sea cucumbers, as the medicinal materials. *Yakugaku Zasshi* **2002**, *122*, 1133–1143. [CrossRef]
31. Inagaki, M. Structure and biological activity of glycosphingolipids from starfish and feather star. *Yakugaku Zasshi* **2008**, *128*, 1187–1194. [CrossRef]
32. Sperling, P.; Heinz, E. Plant sphingolipids: Structural diversity, biosynthesis, first genes and functions. *Biochim. Biophys. Acta* **2003**, *1632*, 1–15. [CrossRef]
33. Rho, J.-R.; Kim, Y.H. Isolation and structure determination of three new ceramides from the starfish *Distolasterias nipon*. *Bull. Korean Chem. Soc.* **2005**, *26*, 1457–1460. [CrossRef]
34. Yoo, J.S.; Park, T.; Bang, G.; Lee, C.; Rho, J.R.; Kim, Y.H. High-energy collision-induced dissociation of [M+Na]$^+$ ions desorbed by fast atom bombardment of ceramides isolated from the starfish *Distolasterias nipon*. *J. Mass Spectrom.* **2013**, *48*, 164–171. [CrossRef]
35. Inagaki, M.; Ikeda, Y.; Kawatake, S.; Nakamura, K.; Tanaka, M.; Misawa, E.; Yamada, M.; Higuchi, R. Isolation and structure of four new ceramides from the starfish *Luidia maculata*. *Chem. Pharm. Bull.* **2006**, *54*, 1647–1649. [CrossRef]
36. Bibel, D.J.; Aly, R.; Shinefield, H.R. Antimicrobial activity of sphingosines. *J. Investig. Dermatol.* **1992**, *98*, 269–273. [CrossRef]
37. Fischer, C.L.; Drake, D.R.; Dawson, D.V.; Blanchette, D.R.; Brogden, K.A.; Wertz, P.W. Antibacterial activity of sphingoid bases and fatty acids against gram-positive and gram-negative bacteria. *Antimicrob. Agents Chemother.* **2012**, *56*, 1157–1161. [CrossRef] [PubMed]
38. Murshid, S.S.A.; Badr, J.M.; Youssef, D.T.A. Penicillosides A and B: New cerebrosides from the marine-derived fungus *Penicillum* species. *Rev. Bras. Farmacognosia.* **2016**, *26*, 29–33. [CrossRef]
39. De Vivar, M.E.D.; Seldes, A.M.; Maier, M.S. Two novel glucosylceramides from gonads and body walls of the Patagonian starfish *Allostichaster inaequalis*. *Lipids* **2002**, *37*, 597–603. [CrossRef]
40. Maier, M.S.; Kuriss, A.; Seldes, A.M. Isolation and structure of glucosylceramides from the starfish *Cosmasterias lurida*. *Lipids* **1998**, *33*, 825–827. [CrossRef]
41. Kawatake, S.; Nakamura, K.; Inagaki, M.; Higuchi, R. Isolation and structure determination of six glucocerebrosides from the starfish *Luidia maculata*. *Chem. Pharm. Bull.* **2002**, *50*, 1091–1096. [CrossRef]
42. Inagaki, M.; Nakamura, K.; Kawatake, S.; Higuchi, R. Isolation and structural determination of four new ceramide lactosides from the Starfish *Luidia maculata*. *Eur. J. Org. Chem.* **2003**, 325–331. [CrossRef]

43. Chludil, H.D.; Seldes, A.M.; Maier, M.S. Anasterocerebroside A, a new glucosylceramide from the Patagonian starfish *Anasterias minuta*. *Z. Naturforsch. C* **2003**, *58*, 433–440. [CrossRef]
44. Maruta, T.; Saito, T.; Inagaki, M.; Shibata, O.; Higuchi, R. Biologically active glycosides from Asteroidea, 41. Isolation and structure determination of glucocerebrosides from the starfish *Linckia laevigata*. *Chem. Pharm. Bull.* **2005**, *53*, 1255–1258. [CrossRef] [PubMed]
45. Inagaki, M.; Nakata, T.; Higuchi, R. Isolation and structure of a galactocerebroside molecular species from the starfish *Culcita novaeguineae*. *Chem. Pharm. Bull.* **2006**, *54*, 260–261. [CrossRef] [PubMed]
46. Costantino, V.; de Rosa, C.; Fattorusso, E.; Imperatore, C.; Mangoni, A.; Irace, C.; Maffettone, C.; Capasso, D.; Malorni, L.; Palumbo, R.; et al. Oreacerebrosides: Bioactive cerebrosides with a triunsaturated sphingoid base from the sea star *Oreaster reticulatus*. *Eur. J. Org. Chem.* **2007**, 5277–5283. [CrossRef]
47. Farokhi, F.; Wielgosz-Collin, G.; Clement, M.; Kornprobst, J.-M.; Barnathan, G. Cytotoxicity on human cancer cells of ophidiacerebrosides isolated from the African starfish *Narcissia canariensis*. *Mar. Drugs* **2010**, *8*, 2988–2998. [CrossRef]
48. Jin, W.; Rinehart, K.L.; Jares-Erijman, E.A. Ophidiacerebrosides: Cytotoxic glycosphingolipids containing a novel sphingosine from a sea star. *J. Org. Chem.* **1994**, *59*, 144–147. [CrossRef]
49. Pan, K.; Inagaki, M.; Ohno, N.; Tanaka, C.; Higuchi, R.; Miyamoto, T. Identification of sixteen new galactocerebrosides from the starfish *Protoreaster nodosus*. *Chem. Pharm. Bull.* **2010**, *58*, 470–474. [CrossRef]
50. Park, T.; Park, Y.S.; Rho, J.-R.; Kim, Y.H. Structural determination of cerebrosides isolated from *Asterias amurensis* starfish eggs using high-energy collision-induced dissociation of sodium-adducted molecules. *Rapid Commun. Mass Spectrom.* **2011**, *25*, 572–578. [CrossRef]
51. Mikami, D.; Sakai, S.; Sasaki, S.; Igarashi, Y. Effects of *Asterias amurensis*-derived sphingoid bases on the de novo ceramide synthesis in cultured normal human epidermal keratinocytes. *J. Oleo Sci.* **2016**, *65*, 671–680. [CrossRef]
52. Hue, N.; Montagnac, A.; Païs, M.; Serani, L.; Laprèvote, O. Structural elucidation of eighteen cerebrosides from *Holothuria coronopertusa* in a complex mixture by high-energy collision-induced dissociation of $[M + Li]^+$ ions. *Eur. J. Mass Spectrom.* **2001**, *7*, 409–417. [CrossRef]
53. Yamada, K.; Sasaki, K.; Harada, Y.; Isobe, R.; Higuchi, R. Constituents of Holothuroidea. 12. Isolation and structure of glucocerebrosides from the sea cucumber *Holothuria pervicax*. *Chem. Pharm. Bull.* **2002**, *50*, 1467–1470. [CrossRef]
54. Kisa, F.; Yamada, K.; Kaneko, M.; Inagaki, M.; Higuchi, R. Constituents of Holothuroidea, 14. Isolation and structure of new glucocerebroside molecular species from the sea cucumber *Stichopus japonicus*. *Chem. Pharm. Bull.* **2005**, *53*, 382–386. [CrossRef] [PubMed]
55. Duan, J.; Ishida, M.; Aida, K.; Tsuduki, T.; Zhang, J.; Manabe, Y.; Hirata, T.; Sugawara, T. Dietary cerebroside from sea cucumber (*Stichopus japonicus*): Absorption and effects on skin barrier and caecal short-chain fatty acids. *J. Agric. Food Chem.* **2016**, *64*, 7014–7021. [CrossRef]
56. Yamada, K.; Wada, N.; Onaka, H.; Matsubara, R.; Isobe, R.; Inagaki, M.; Higuchi, R. Constituents of Holothuroidea. 15. Isolation of ante-iso type regioisomer on long chain base moiety of glucocerebroside from the sea cucumber *Holothuria leucospilota*. *Chem. Pharm. Bull.* **2005**, *53*, 788–791. [CrossRef]
57. Sugawara, T.; Zaima, N.; Yamamoto, A.; Sakai, S.; Noguchi, R.; Hirata, T. Isolation of sphingoid bases of sea cucumber cerebrosides and their cytotoxicity against human colon cancer cells. *Biosci. Biotechnol. Biochem.* **2006**, *70*, 2906–2912. [CrossRef] [PubMed]
58. Ikeda, Y.; Inagaki, M.; Yamada, K.; Zhang, X.W.; Zhang, B.; Miyamoto, T.; Higuchi, R. Isolation and structure of a galactocerebroside from the sea cucumber *Bohadschia argus*. *Chem. Pharm. Bull.* **2009**, *57*, 315–317. [CrossRef]
59. Xu, J.; Wang, Y.M.; Feng, T.Y.; Zhang, B.; Sugawara, T.; Xue, C.H. Isolation and anti-fatty liver activity of a novel cerebroside from the sea cucumber Acaudina molpadioides. *Biosci. Biotechnol. Biochem.* **2011**, *75*, 1466–1471. [CrossRef]
60. Xu, J.; Duan, J.; Xue, C.; Feng, T.; Dong, P.; Sugawara, T.; Hirata, T. Analysis and comparison of glucocerebroside species from three edible sea cucumbers using liquid chromatography–ion trap–time-of-flight mass spectrometry. *J. Agric. Food Chem.* **2011**, *59*, 12246–12253. [CrossRef]
61. Du, L.; Xu, J.; Xue, Y.; Takahashi, K.; Xue, C.H.; Wang, J.F.; Wang, Y.M. Cerebrosides from sea cucumber ameliorates cancer-associated cachexia in mice by attenuating adipose atrophy. *J. Funct. Foods* **2015**, *17*, 352–363. [CrossRef]
62. Liu, X.; Xu, J.; Xue, Y.; Gao, Z.; Li, Z.; Leng, K.; Wang, J.; Xue, C.; Wang, Y. Sea cucumber cerebrosides and long-chain bases from *Acaudina molpadioides* protect against high fat diet-induced metabolic disorders in mice. *Food Funct.* **2015**, *6*, 3428–3536. [CrossRef]
63. La, M.-P.; Shao, J.-J.; Jiao, J.; Yi, Y.-H. Three cerebrosides from the sea cucumber *Cucumaria frondosa*. *Chin. J. Nat. Med.* **2012**, *10*, 105–109. [CrossRef]
64. Xu, J.; Guo, S.; Du, L.; Wang, Y.M.; Sugawara, T.; Hirata, T.; Xue, C.H. Isolation of cytotoxic glucocerebrosides and long-chain bases from sea cucumber *Cucumaria frondosa* using high speed counter-current chromatography. *J. Oleo Sci.* **2013**, *62*, 133–142. [CrossRef]
65. Xu, H.; Wang, F.; Wang, J.; Xu, J.; Wang, Y.; Xue, C. The WNT/β-catenin pathway is involved in the anti-adipogenic activity of cerebrosides from the sea cucumber *Cucumaria frondosa*. *Food Funct.* **2015**, *6*, 2396–2404. [CrossRef]
66. Smirnova, G.P. Gangliosides from the starfish *Evasterias echinosoma*: Identification of a disialoganglioside containing 8-O-methyl-N-acetylneuraminic acid and N-formylgalactosamine. *Russ. Chem. Bull.* **2000**, *49*, 159–164. [CrossRef]
67. Smirnova, G.P. Structure of gangliosides from gonads of the starfish *Evasterias retifera*. *Russ. Chem. Bull.* **2003**, *52*, 2270–2275. [CrossRef]

68. Kawatake, S.; Inagaki, M.; Isobe, R.; Miyamoto, T.; Higuchi, R. Isolation and structure of monomethylated GM$_3$-type ganglioside molecular species from the starfish *Luidia maculata*. *Chem. Pharm. Bull.* **2002**, *50*, 1386–1389. [CrossRef]
69. Kawatake, S.; Inagaki, M.; Isobe, R.; Miyamoto, T.; Higuchi, R. Isolation and structure of a GD$_3$-type ganglioside molecular species possessing neuritogenic activity from the starfish *Luidia maculata*. *Chem. Pharm. Bull.* **2004**, *52*, 1002–1004. [CrossRef]
70. Miyamoto, T.; Yamamoto, A.; Wakabayashi, K.; Nagaregawa, Y.; Inagaki, M.; Higuchi, R.; Iha, M.; Teruya, K. Biologically active glycosides from Asteroidea. 40. Two new gangliosides, acanthagangliosides I and J from the starfish *Acanthaster planci*. *Eur. J. Org. Chem.* **2000**, 2295–2301. [CrossRef]
71. Kawano, Y.; Higuchi, R.; Komori, T. Biologically active glycosides from Asteroidea. XIX. Glycosphingolipids from the starfish *Acanthaster planci*. 4. Isolation and structure of five new gangliosides. *Liebigs Ann. Chem.* **1990**, 43–50. [CrossRef]
72. Miyamoto, T.; Inagaki, M.; Isobe, R.; Tanaka, Y.; Higuchi, R.; Iha, M.; Teruya, K. Biologically active glycosides from Asteroidea. 36. Re-examination of the structure of acanthaganglioside C, and the identification of three minor acanthagangliosides F, G and H. *Liebigs Ann. Chem.* **1997**, 931–936. [CrossRef]
73. Hanashima, S.; Sato, K.I.; Naito, Y.; Takematsu, H.; Kozutsumi, Y.; Ito, Y.; Yamaguchi, Y. Synthesis and binding analysis of unique AG2 pentasaccharide to human Siglec-2 using NMR techniques. *Bioorg. Med. Chem.* **2010**, *18*, 3720–3725. [CrossRef]
74. Higuchi, R.; Inoue, S.; Inagaki, K.; Sakai, M.; Miyamoto, T.; Komori, T.; Inagaki, M.; Isobe, R. Biologically active glycosides from Asteroidea. 42. Isolation and structure of a new biologically active ganglioside molecular species from the starfish Asterina pectinifera. *Chem. Pharm. Bull.* **2006**, *54*, 287–291. [CrossRef]
75. Smirnova, G.P. Hematoside with 8-*O*-methyl-*N*-glycolylneuraminic acid from the starfish *Linckia laevigata*. *Russ. Chem. Bull.* **2000**, *49*, 165–168. [CrossRef]
76. Inagaki, M.; Miyamoto, T.; Isobe, R.; Higuchi, R. Biologically active glycosides from Asteroidea. 43. Isolation and structure of a new neuritogenic-active ganglioside molecular species from the starfish Linckia laevigata. *Chem. Pharm. Bull.* **2005**, *53*, 1551–1554. [CrossRef] [PubMed]
77. Inagaki, M.; Saito, T.; Miyamoto, T.; Higuchi, R. Isolation and structure of hematoside-type ganglioside from the starfish *Linckia laevigata*. *Chem. Pharm. Bull.* **2009**, *57*, 204–206. [CrossRef]
78. Pan, K.; Tanaka, C.; Inagaki, M.; Higuchi, R.; Miyamoto, T. Isolation and structure elucidation of GM4-type gangliosides from the Okinawan starfish *Protoreaster nodosus*. *Mar. Drugs* **2012**, *10*, 2467–2480. [CrossRef] [PubMed]
79. Yamada, K.; Harada, Y.; Miyamoto, T.; Isobe, R.; Higuchi, R. Constituents of Holothuroidea. 9. Isolation and structure of a new ganglioside molecular species from the sea cucumber *Holothuria pervicax*. *Chem. Pharm. Bull.* **2000**, *48*, 157–159. [CrossRef]
80. Yamada, K.; Harada, Y.; Nagaregawa, Y.; Miyamoto, T.; Isobe, R.; Higuchi, R. Constituents of Holothuroidea. 7. Isolation and structure of biologically active gangliosides from the sea cucumber *Holothuria pervicax*. *Eur. J. Org. Chem.* **1998**, 2519–2525. [CrossRef]
81. Yamada, K.; Matsubara, R.; Kaneko, M.; Miyamoto, T.; Higuchi, R. Constituents of Holothuroidea. 10. Isolation and structure of a biologically active ganglioside molecular species from the sea cucumber *Holothuria leucospilota*. *Chem. Pharm. Bull.* **2001**, *49*, 447–452. [CrossRef]
82. Kaneko, M.; Kisa, F.; Yamada, K.; Miyamoto, T.; Higuchi, R. Structure of a new neuritogenic-active ganglioside from the sea cucumber *Stichopus japonicus*. *Eur. J. Org. Chem.* **2003**, 1004–1008. [CrossRef]
83. Kaneko, M.; Kisa, F.; Yamada, K.; Miyamoto, T.; Higuchi, R. Constituents of Holothuroidea. 8-Structure of neuritogenic active ganglioside from the sea cucumber *Stichopus japonicus*. *Eur. J. Org. Chem.* **1999**, 3171–3174. [CrossRef]
84. Yamada, K.; Hamada, A.; Kisa, F.; Miyamoto, T.; Higuchi, R. Constituents of Holothuroidea. 13. Structure of neuritogenic active ganglioside molecular species from the sea cucumber *Stichopus chloronotus*. *Chem. Pharm. Bull.* **2003**, *51*, 46–52. [CrossRef] [PubMed]
85. Kisa, F.; Yamada, K.; Miyamoto, T.; Inagaki, M.; Higuchi, R. Constituents of Holothuroidea. 17. Isolation and structure of biologically active monosialo-gangliosides from the sea cucumber *Cucumaria echinata*. *Chem. Pharm. Bull.* **2006**, *54*, 982–987. [CrossRef]
86. Kisa, F.; Yamada, K.; Miyamoto, T.; Inagaki, M.; Higuchi, R. Constituents of Holothuroidea. 18. Isolation and structure of biologically active disialo- and trisialo-gangliosides from the sea cucumber *Cucumaria echinata*. *Chem. Pharm. Bull.* **2006**, *54*, 1293–1298. [CrossRef] [PubMed]
87. Traving, C.; Schauer, R. Structure, function and metabolism of sialic acids. *Cell. Mol. Life Sci.* **1998**, *54*, 1330–1349. [CrossRef]
88. Kolter, T. Ganglioside biochemistry. *ISRN Biochem.* **2012**, *2012*, 506160. [CrossRef]
89. Sipione, S.; Monyror, J.; Galleguillos, D.; Steinberg, N.; Kadam, V. Gangliosides in the brain: Physiology, pathophysiology and therapeutic applications. *Front. Neurosci.* **2020**, *14*, 572965. [CrossRef]
90. Schengrund, C.-L. Gangliosides and neuroblastomas. *Int. J. Mol. Sci.* **2020**, *21*, 5313. [CrossRef] [PubMed]
91. Schömel, N.; Geisslingera, G.; Wegnera, M.-S. Influence of glycosphingolipids on cancer cell energy metabolism. *Prog. Lipid Res.* **2020**, *79*, 101050. [CrossRef]
92. Yamada, K.; Hara, E.; Miyamoto, T.; Higuchi, R.; Isobe, R.; Honda, S. Constituents of Holothuroidea, 6-Isolation and structure of biologically active glycosphingolipids from the sea cucumber *Cucumaria echinata*. *Eur. J. Org. Chem.* **1998**, 371–378. [CrossRef]
93. Kisa, F.; Yamada, K.; Miyamoto, T.; Inagaki, M.; Higuchi, R. Determination of the absolute configuration of sialic acids in gangliosides from the sea cucumber *Cucumaria echinata*. *Chem. Pharm. Bull.* **2007**, *55*, 1051–1052. [CrossRef] [PubMed]

94. Kicha, A.A.; Kalinovsky, A.I.; Malyarenko, T.V.; Ivanchina, N.V.; Dmitrenok, P.S.; Menchinskaya, E.S.; Yurchenko, E.A.; Pislyagin, E.A.; Aminin, D.L.; Huong, T.T.; et al. Cyclic steroid glycosides from the starfish *Echinaster luzonicus*: Structures and immunomodulatory activities. *J. Nat. Prod.* **2015**, *78*, 1397–1405. [CrossRef]
95. Malyarenko, T.V.; Kharchenko, S.D.; Kicha, A.A.; Ivanchina, N.V.; Dmitrenok, P.S.; Chingizova, E.A.; Pislyagin, E.A.; Evtushenko, E.V.; Antokhina, T.I.; Minh, C.V.; et al. Anthenosides L-U, steroidal glycosides with unusual structural features from the starfish *Anthenea aspera*. *J. Nat. Prod.* **2016**, *79*, 3047–3056. [CrossRef]
96. Mondol, M.A.M.; Shin, H.J.; Rahman, M.A.; Islam, M.T. Sea cucumber glycosides: Chemical structures, producing species and important biological properties. *Mar. Drugs* **2017**, *15*, 317. [CrossRef]

MDPI
St. Alban-Anlage 66
4052 Basel
Switzerland
Tel. +41 61 683 77 34
Fax +41 61 302 89 18
www.mdpi.com

Marine Drugs Editorial Office
E-mail: marinedrugs@mdpi.com
www.mdpi.com/journal/marinedrugs

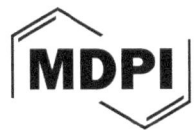

www.ingramcontent.com/pod-product-compliance
Lightning Source LLC
LaVergne TN
LVHW072348090526
838202LV00019B/2502